T0324985

METHODS IN PHARMACOLOGY AND TOXICOLOGY

Series Editor
Y. James Kang
University of Louisville
School of Medicine
Prospect, Kentucky, USA

For further volumes:
http://www.springer.com/series/7653

Immunotherapy and Biomarkers in Neurodegenerative Disorders

Edited by

Martin Ingelsson and Lars Lannfelt

Department of Public Health and Caring Sciences/Geriatrics, Uppsala University, Uppsala, Sweden

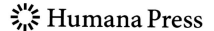 Humana Press

Editors
Martin Ingelsson
Department of Public Health
  and Caring Sciences/Geriatrics
Uppsala University
Uppsala, Sweden

Lars Lannfelt
Department of Public Health
  and Caring Sciences/Geriatrics
Uppsala University
Uppsala, Sweden

ISSN 1557-2153   ISSN 1940-6053   (electronic)
Methods in Pharmacology and Toxicology
ISBN 978-1-4939-3558-1   ISBN 978-1-4939-3560-4   (eBook)
DOI 10.1007/978-1-4939-3560-4

Library of Congress Control Number: 2016934446

Cover illustration: Light microscopy image of amyloid plaques in the brain from an Alzheimer patient, 400 × magnification. This image was taken by Paul O'Callaghan

Printed on acid-free paper

This Humana Press imprint is published by Springer Nature
The registered company is Springer Science+Business Media LLC New York

Preface

Neurodegenerative disorders represent significant unmet medical needs and major costs to the health care system. In the search for more efficient treatments, immunotherapy targeting abnormal protein aggregates or inflammatory molecules has emerged as one of the most promising therapeutic strategies.

Today immunomodulatory therapies are used to treat multiple sclerosis, and similar concepts are currently being tested for the treatment of Alzheimer's disease. In the latter disorder, pathological forms of the amyloid-β peptide and the tau protein accumulate as plaques and tangles between and inside the brain neurons, respectively. In a pioneering study, immunization against amyloid-β was proven to prevent and reverse pathology in transgenic mice with Alzheimer-like brain pathology. These promising preclinical findings spurred a clinical trial on Alzheimer patients, in which advantageous effects could be observed on both neuropathological and biochemical markers, along with some clinical benefits. Unfortunately, the trial had to be halted due to the development of meningoencephalitis in 6 % of the immunized patients.

In the last decade, there has been a focus on passive immunization with monoclonal antibodies against amyloid-β, which may represent a safer and more reliable approach. Overall, therapeutic antibodies represent one of the fastest growing areas in the pharmaceutical industry for the treatment of cancer, autoimmune disorders, and now also for neurodegenerative disorders. Monoclonal antibodies have appealing drug characteristics such as high target specificity, long half-life, and an ability to reach chemically non-tractable targets.

As for the antibody-based clinical trials for Alzheimer's disease that have been conducted so far, potential treatment effects have been reported in some of the studies whereas other trials have failed to find any obvious beneficial effects. The relative lack of success may be explained by several factors. For example, a certain percentage of the patients included may not have been accurately diagnosed and instead have had a different brain pathology. Moreover, the patients might have been recruited at a too late stage of the disease, when a high degree of brain atrophy and neuronal loss have already been present. Yet another possibility is that the targets have not been optimally chosen. Neither the monomeric, presumably functional, form of the protein nor the ready-formed aggregates seem to possess particularly toxic properties. Instead, the prefibrillar soluble aggregates—oligomers and protofibrils—seem to exert a more toxic effect on cells, and some investigators therefore now regard them as more suitable immunotherapeutic targets.

The successful example of antibody-based treatment for multiple sclerosis and the ongoing efforts to design immunotherapy protocols for Alzheimer's disease are now being followed by a similar development for several other neurodegenerative disorders. Researchers have also begun to explore the possibility of targeting the other pathological proteins that form brain aggregates believed to be central in their respective disease processes. For Parkinson's disease, the α-synuclein protein deposits as intracellular Lewy bodies and Lewy neurites. After administrating vaccine or antibodies against α-synuclein on transgenic Parkinson mouse models, several research groups have shown that the formation of such aggregates and their associated toxicity can be prevented. Such preclinical observations have also encouraged the development of therapeutics for human use, and the first α-synuclein-based clinical trials are currently underway. Also for Huntington's disease, amyotrophic lateral sclerosis, and prion disorders, such as Creutzfeldt–Jakob disease, initial experiments on cell culture systems and animal models have been successful in reducing the protein pathology that occurs in the respective disorders.

To efficiently battle these diseases, the treatment most likely has to be initiated at an early stage. Thus, along with the development of efficacious drugs, there will be an increasing need for novel ways to diagnose these disorders at a time point when there still has been no or only limited damage to the central nervous system. Thus, there is currently also a focus on designing new diagnostic tests based on more sensitive and specific biomarkers. In general, such biomarkers reflect either the brain deposition of the disease-specific proteins or their presence in cerebrospinal fluid (CSF) and plasma. One example is the ELISA-based assays that can measure decreased levels of amyloid-β 42 along with increased levels of tau and hyperphosphorylated tau in CSF from subjects with Alzheimer's disease. As for imaging, novel magnetic resonance imaging (MRI) and positron emission tomography (PET)-based techniques have emerged that in a better way can visualize the pathological alterations that are known to occur in the degenerating brain. One of the most successful examples is the development of PET ligands that can selectively bind to aggregating amyloid-β and enable imaging of ongoing amyloid deposition in the living brain from an Alzheimer patient. This technique enables not only early diagnosis and a possibility to monitor therapeutic efficacy but also a more accurate recruitment of patients for the clinical trials. In addition, major efforts are underway to design ligands that instead can bind to the other disease-related protein aggregates, such as tau and α-synuclein. Once developed and evaluated, such ligands could enable early detection also of disorders such as frontotemporal dementia and Parkinson's disease.

In this book, we have tried to select a number of topics that will give the reader a thorough understanding of the current status of immunotherapy and diagnostic markers for neurodegenerative disorders. There is an emphasis on the development within the field of Alzheimer's disease, but we also cover a number of other disorders in which most of the activities are still on the preclinical level. In the years to come, we will hopefully witness continued progress in the development of novel immune-based drugs and diagnostic tools for several of these devastating brain diseases.

Uppsala, Sweden   *Martin Ingelsson*
                                                                                                                            Lars Lannfelt

Contents

Preface.. *v*

Contributors... *ix*

PART I   IMMUNOTHERAPY AGAINST AMYLOID-B IN ALZHEIMER'S DISEASE

1   Immunotherapy Against Amyloid-β in Alzheimer's Disease: An Overview   3
    Niels D. Prins

2   Active Immunization Against the Amyloid-β Peptide....................   19
    Enchi Liu and J. Michael Ryan

3   Immunotherapy Against N-Truncated Amyloid-β Oligomers..............   37
    Thomas A. Bayer and Oliver Wirths

4   Immunotherapy Against Amyloid-β Protofibrils: Opportunities
    and Challenges   51
    Lars Lannfelt

PART II   IMMUNOTHERAPY IN OTHER NEURODEGENERATIVE DISORDERS

5   Immunotherapy Against α-Synuclein Pathology   63
    Elvira Valera and Eliezer Masliah

6   Extracellular α-Synuclein as a Target for Immunotherapy.............   73
    Jun Sung Lee and Seung-Jae Lee

7   Immunotherapy of Parkinson's Disease   85
    Achim Schneeberger, Suzanne Hendrix, and Markus Mandler

8   Tau Immunotherapy.. 109
    Einar M. Sigurdsson

9   Active and Passive Immunotherapy Against Tau: Effects
    and Potential Mechanisms.. 121
    Kiran Yanamandra, Marc I. Diamond, and David M. Holtzman

10 Immunotherapy on Experimental Models for Huntington's Disease 139
    Anne Messer

PART III   BIOMARKERS FOR NEURODEGENERATIVE DISORDERS

11 Cerebrospinal Fluid Biomarkers in Alzheimer's Disease 153
    Henrik Zetterberg and Jonathan M. Schott

12 Volumetric MRI as a Diagnostic Tool in Alzheimer's Disease.............. 181
    Eric Westman, Lena Cavalin, and Lars-Olof Wahlund

13 PET Imaging as a Diagnostic Tool in Alzheimer's Disease............... 199
    Juha O. Rinne

14 Alpha-Synuclein as a Diagnostic Biomarker for Parkinson's Disease   215
    Joakim Bergström and Martin Ingelsson
15 Imaging as a Diagnostic Tool in Parkinson's Disease   235
    Johan Wikström and Torsten Danfors
16 Mass Spectrometry-Based Proteomics in Biomarker Discovery
    for Neurodegenerative Diseases.   253
    Sravani Musunuri, Ganna Shevchenko, and Jonas Bergquist

Index *283*

Contributors

THOMAS A. BAYER • *Division of Molecular Psychiatry, Department of Psychiatry and Psychotherapy, University Medical Center Göttingen (UMG), Georg-August-University, Göttingen, Germany*

JONAS BERGQUIST • *Analytical Chemistry, Department of Chemistry-BMC, SciLifeLab Uppsala University, Uppsala, Sweden*

JOAKIM BERGSTRÖM • *Department of Public Health & Caring Sciences/Geriatrics, Uppsala University, Uppsala, Sweden*

LENA CAVALIN • *Department of Clinical Science, Intervention and Technology, Karolinska Institutet, Stockholm, Sweden; Department of Radiology, Karolinska University Hospital, Stockholm, Sweden*

TORSTEN DANFORS • *Section for Nuclear Medicine & PET, Department of Surgical Sciences, Uppsala University, Uppsala, Sweden*

MARC I. DIAMOND • *Department of Neurology and Neurotherapeutics, University of Texas, Southwestern Medical Center, Dallas, TX, USA*

SUZANNE HENDRIX • *Pentara Corporation, Salt Lake City, UT, USA*

DAVID M. HOLTZMAN • *Department of Neurology, Hope Center for Neurological Disorders, Knight Alzheimer's Disease Research Center, Washington University School of Medicine, St. Louis, MO, USA*

MARTIN INGELSSON • *Department of Public Health & Caring Sciences/Geriatrics, Uppsala University, Uppsala, Sweden*

LARS LANNFELT • *Department of Public Health & Caring Sciences/Geriatrics, Uppsala University, Uppsala, Sweden*

JUN SUNG LEE • *Department of Medicine, Neuroscience Research Institute, Seoul National University College of Medicine, Seoul, South Korea*

SEUNG-JAE LEE • *Department of Medicine, Neuroscience Research Institute, Seoul National University College of Medicine, Seoul, South Korea*

ENCHI LIU • *Prothena Biosciences, Inc., South San Francisco, CA, USA*

MARKUS MANDLER • *AFFiRiS AG, Vienna, Austria*

ELIEZER MASLIAH • *Department of Neurosciences, University of California, San Diego, La Jolla, CA, USA; Department of Pathology, University of California, San Diego, La Jolla, CA, USA*

ANNE MESSER • *Neural Stem Cell Institute, Rensselaer, NY, USA*

SRAVANI MUSUNURI • *Analytical Chemistry, Department of Chemistry-BMC, SciLifeLab Uppsala University, Uppsala, Sweden*

NIELS D. PRINS • *Alzheimer Center and Department of Neurology, Neuroscience Campus Amsterdam, Vrije Universiteit Medical Center, Amsterdam, The Netherlands; Alzheimer Research Center, Amsterdam, The Netherlands*

JUHA O. RINNE • *Turku PET Centre and Division of Clinical Neurosciences, University of Turku and Turku University Hospital, Turku, Finland*

J. MICHAEL RYAN • *Novartis Pharmaceuticals Corporation, East Hanover, NJ, USA*

ACHIM SCHNEEBERGER • *AFFiRiS AG, Vienna, Austria*

JONATHAN M. SCHOTT • *Dementia Research Centre, UCL Institute of Neurology, Queen Square, London, UK*

GANNA SHEVCHENKO • *Analytical Chemistry, Department of Chemistry-BMC, SciLifeLab Uppsala University, Uppsala, Sweden*

EINAR M. SIGURDSSON • *Department of Neuroscience and Physiology, New York University School of Medicine, New York, NY, USA; Department of Psychiatry, New York University School of Medicine, New York, NY, USA*

ELVIRA VALERA • *Department of Neurosciences, University of California, San Diego, La Jolla, CA, USA*

LARS-OLOF WAHLUND • *Department of Neurobiology, Care Sciences and Society, Karolinska Institutet, Stockholm, Sweden*

ERIC WESTMAN • *Department of Neurobiology, Care Sciences and Society, Karolinska Institutet, Stockholm, Sweden*

JOHAN WIKSTRÖM • *Department of Surgical Sciences, Section of Radiology, Uppsala University, Uppsala, Sweden*

OLIVER WIRTHS • *Division of Molecular Psychiatry, Department of Psychiatry and Psychotherapy, University Medical Center Göttingen (UMG), Georg-August-University, Göttingen, Germany*

KIRAN YANAMANDRA • *Department of Neurology, Hope Center for Neurological Disorders, Knight Alzheimer's Disease Research Center, Washington University School of Medicine, St. Louis, MO, USA*

HENRIK ZETTERBERG • *Clinical Neurochemistry Laboratory, Institute of Neuroscience and Physiology, Department of Psychiatry and Neurochemistry, The Sahlgrenska Academy at the University of Gothenburg, Mölndal, Sweden; Department of Molecular Neuroscience, UCL Institute of Neurology, Queen Square, London, UK*

Part I

Immunotherapy Against Amyloid-β in Alzheimer's Disease

Chapter 1

Immunotherapy Against Amyloid-β in Alzheimer's Disease: An Overview

Niels D. Prins

Abstract

Therapeutic options in Alzheimer's disease (AD) are limited to symptomatic treatments that show only modest clinical effects. Disease-modifying treatments are urgently needed, and the amyloid cascade hypothesis thus far provides the best basis for the development of such therapies. Preclinical studies in mouse models of AD showed that immunization with amyloid-β (Aβ) as well as passive vaccination with monoclonal antibodies against Aβ may be effective in preventing and treating AD. This has led to the development and testing of immunotherapeutic agents in patients with prodromal AD or AD dementia. Passive immunotherapy with monoclonal antibodies against several Aβ species has been tested in phase 3 clinical trials, with thus far disappointing results. Whether the dosage level, target specificity, and/or stage of the disease is to be blamed for these failures is not fully clear. New mAbs specifically aimed at protofibrils of Aβ species that are thought to be most toxic have been developed and are currently being tested in phase 1 and 2 clinical trials. The first active immunotherapy with AN1792 was halted because of severe side effects. New-generation active vaccination programs with compounds avoiding inflammatory T cell activation are in clinical development. Amyloid-related imaging abnormalities (ARIA) consisting of cerebral edema (ARIA-E) or hemorrhage (ARIA-H) are side effects associated with immunotherapy. It has been suggested that immunotherapy may be most effective when administered early in the disease course, and several studies with mAbs in subjects with preclinical AD are now being performed.

Key words Immunotherapy, Monoclonal antibody, Active vaccination, Alzheimer's disease, Mild cognitive impairment, Amyloid-related imaging abnormalities

1 Introduction

As the global population ages, the worldwide prevalence of Alzheimer's disease (AD) is increasing [1]. Despite increased knowledge of the pathogenesis of AD over the past two decades, therapeutic options are still limited. The currently available cholinesterase inhibitors and the N-methyl-d-aspartate receptor agonists have modest clinical effects but do not modify the underlying pathophysiology [2, 3]. Therefore, new drugs that delay the onset, slow the progression, or improve the symptoms of AD are desperately needed.

Martin Ingelsson and Lars Lannfelt (eds.), *Immunotherapy and Biomarkers in Neurodegenerative Disorders*, Methods in Pharmacology and Toxicology, DOI 10.1007/978-1-4939-3560-4_1, © Springer Science+Business Media New York 2016

The amyloid cascade hypothesis is the main theory for the pathology of AD and forms the basis for the development of disease-modifying drugs against AD [4–6]. Excess of amyloid-β (Aβ) causes aggregation and in turn leads to microglial and astrocytic activation with subsequent formation of neurofibrillary tangles and associated neurodegeneration. The soluble oligomeric forms of Aβ ("protofibrils") are thought to be particularly pathogenic [7].

Immunotherapy, both passive and active, may be a way to intervene in the amyloid cascade and to slow down clinical progression or even prevent the disease to become clinically manifest. Treatment with monoclonal antibodies (mAbs) directed at Aβ species or administration of Aβ in order to elicit production of anti-Aβ antibodies is a potential disease-modifying treatment for AD [8–10]. To date, the large clinical trials with mAbs have shown disappointing results, and the central question now is how these failures may be explained. An underlying explanation may be the characteristics of the drugs themselves, such as the specific Aβ species that they target or their side effect profile. Another possibility is that the failures can be related to factors associated with the study designs, such as inappropriate dosages or selection of the wrong patients and outcome measures. If the failures are drug specific, another question will be whether next-generation mAbs will be more successful. The first active vaccination program in humans had a dramatic course with the occurrence of serious side effects in a substantial number of participants and was therefore discontinued. However, a new generation of vaccines are currently being evaluated in phase 2 clinical trials.

We here provide a general overview of immunotherapy in AD, a discussion of general concepts in passive and active immunotherapy, the status of ongoing clinical trials, as well as perspectives for the future.

2   Immunotherapy in Neurodegeneration

2.1   Alzheimer's Disease

Alzheimer's disease (AD) is the most common form of dementia, accounting for 60–80 % of all dementia cases [11]. The estimated worldwide prevalence of AD in 2012 was as high as 24 million. Given that both established and developing nations are rapidly aging, the frequency is expected to double every 20 years until 2040 [1, 12]. Clinically, AD is characterized by memory loss and impairments in other cognitive functions, such as language, visuospatial skills, and executive function, coupled with behavioral changes. Most patients require assistance with activities of daily living (ADL), and many eventually require full-time care and supervision [13]. Terminally, patients may become bedridden, incontinent, and unable to communicate [14]. Alzheimer's disease imposes a high burden on healthcare systems, society, patients, and their families, and is one of the leading contributors to disability among older people. Therapeutic interventions for AD that can slow or perhaps even prevent disease progression are urgently needed.

Alzheimer's disease is a slowly progressive brain disease and there is evidence that biomarkers reflecting the pathophysiological process of AD can be abnormal for as long as 20 years before clinical symptoms emerge [15]. Three stages of AD are acknowledged. In the preclinical stage, subjects show abnormal AD biomarkers but have no objective cognitive impairment. In the prodromal stage, also referred to as mild cognitive impairment (MCI), patients have cognitive impairment that is not severe enough to interfere with the instrumental activities of daily living (iADL). Finally, a dementia stage is characterized by cognitive impairment in two or more domains and iADL interference. In 2011 (revised) criteria were published for preclinical AD, mild cognitive impairment (MCI) due to AD, and dementia due to AD [16–18].

The hallmark pathologies of AD are the progressive interneuronal accumulation of the protein fragment Aβ as plaques and twisted intraneuronal strands (tangles) of the protein tau [19]. The predominant pathophysiological theory of AD is the amyloid cascade hypothesis, which suggests that an increased production or decreased degradation of Aβ leads to aggregation and subsequent synaptic changes and deposition of Aβ as diffuse plaques. The aggregation of Aβ is believed to explain the microglial and astrocytic activation, which in turn leads to changes in neuronal homeostasis and to oxidative stress. Subsequently, neurofibrillary tangles are formed, leading to neurodegeneration and synaptic loss [4–6].

Several mutations in rare genetic forms of AD are responsible for early-onset AD, either by increased Aβ production or by elevating the Aβ 42/40 ratio [20]. Higher Aβ levels accelerate aggregation of the peptide. There is increasing evidence that prefibrillar, soluble oligomeric forms of Aβ, also referred to as protofibrils, are particularly pathogenic, and therefore able to cause synapse loss and neuronal injury [7]. There are many different soluble forms of Aβ, as a result of differential cleavage from the amyloid precursor protein (APP) [5–7]. First, APP is cleaved by a β-secretase (also called β-amyloid-cleaving enzyme-1, BACE-1), at the amino terminus of the Aβ domain. Next, the large ectodomain is released into the luminal and extracellular fluid with the carboxy-terminal stub left in the cell membrane. Thereafter, the 99-amino-acid-long stub is cleaved by γ-secretase, releasing Aβ. Three principal forms of Aβ, comprising 38, 40, or 42 amino acid residues, respectively, are produced depending on the point of cleavage. The Aβ 42 form is more likely to oligomerize and form fibrils than the more frequent Aβ 40. The Aβ oligomers are thought to exert their harmful effects by binding directly to the membranes of neurons, or to specific receptors needed for neuronal signaling, although more research is needed to fully understand the negative effects of the oligomers [6, 7, 21]. The self-association of Aβ results in aggregates with varying morphology and molecular weight. The activated monomeric state is in rapid equilibrium with low-molecular-weight aggregates. A large variation of Aβ aggregates have been described, including dimers, trimers, and smaller oligomers [7]. These species can further associate and form larger, still soluble oligomers and protofibrils that eventually may accumulate as Aβ fibrils into senile plaques. Recently, a rare polymorphism for the APP has been identified that appears to decrease synthesis of Aβ by approximately 40 % and thereby reduce the risk of AD [22]. The late-onset sporadic forms of AD are not clearly associated with Aß overproduction and may be more closely related to decreased Aß clearance [15].

2.2 Pharmacological Treatment of Alzheimer's Disease

Despite a significant increase in our understanding of the pathogenesis of AD over the past decades, the therapeutic options are still modest. Approved drugs for AD consist of symptomatic treatment with either cholinesterase inhibitors (donepezil, rivastigmine, galantamine) in the mild-to-moderate stages of the disease or an N-methyl-d-aspartate receptor antagonist (memantine) in the severe stage [2, 3]. These drugs are able to provide some symptomatic relief in some patients, but most likely do not slow down the underlying disease process. In contrast to symptomatic treatments, disease-modifying treatments aim to halt the pathogenic process by intervening in the amyloid cascade, thereby preventing clinical progression. There are currently three main therapeutic intervention strategies targeting Aβ: facilitating Aβ clearance, reducing Aβ production, and preventing Aβ aggregation. In the following, we focus on the clearance of Aβ with passive and active immunotherapy.

2.3 Immunotherapy in AD: Concept and Preclinical Work

Immunotherapy is the prevention or treatment of a disease with substances that stimulate the immune response. It can be divided into passive immunotherapy, where individuals are treated with ready-made antibodies, and active immunotherapy where individuals are treated with a specific antigen that stimulates an intrinsic immune response. With regard to AD treatment, this translates into treatment with either monoclonal antibodies directed at Aβ species or administration of Aβ or Aβ fractions with the goal of eliciting an immune response that produces anti-Aβ antibodies. The possibility that immunization with Aβ may be effective in preventing and treating AD was raised by a seminal work by Schenk and colleagues. In a study in PDAPP mice, active immunization with Aβ42 of young animals prevented the development of Aβ plaque deposition, whereas treatment of older animals reduced the extent and progression of AD-like neuropathologies [23]. These findings have been corroborated by other active vaccination studies both in transgenic mice and nonhuman primates [24, 25].

Moreover, passive immunization studies in transgenic mice showed that peripherally administered antibodies against Aβ were able to enter the central nervous system, decorate plaques, and induce clearance of preexisting amyloid [26–28]. In preclinical studies, the reduction of amyloid pathology has been associated with the rescue of synaptic electrophysiological functions and neurotransmission, signs of neuroprotection, and restored behavioral functions [29–31].

2.4 Passive Immunotherapy with Monoclonal Antibodies

Monoclonal antibodies are antibodies that are produced by identical immune cells which are all clones of a unique parent cell, and that bind to the same epitope (monovalent affinity) [32]. The mAbs designed to treat AD are either "humanized mAbs" or "fully human mAbs." Murine antibodies are relatively easy to produce, but their use in AD treatment is limited by their immunogenicity: the human immune system will see these antibodies as foreign and target them in an immune response against them. To overcome this problem, some parts of the mouse antibody proteins can be replaced with human components, leading to chimeric antibodies that contain a mixture of mouse and human components, known as chimeric antibodies. In humanized mAbs, even more protein sequences have been modified to increase their similarity to antibody variants produced naturally in humans, which further reduce their immunogenicity. Fully human mAbs are derived either from transgenic mice technologies or phage-display technologies, and these can avoid some of the side effects still associated with humanized antibodies. Thus, they are thought to be safer and also more effective than humanized mAbs [33]. For the disease-modifying treatment of AD, several mAbs have been designed at various species of Aβ. These mAbs can be administered via intravenous infusion or subcutaneous injections.

Table 1 lists different mAbs that have been developed for the treatment of AD and have been tested in various phases of clinical trial development. So far, three large phase 3 trials with mAbs have shown disappointing results (Table 1). Two large phase 3 trials with bapineuzumab, a humanized mAb directed at the amino terminus of amyloid-β, in mild-to-moderate AD patients who were stratified according to ApoE genotype, were negative with regard to the primary cognitive or functional outcome measures [34, 35]. Biomarker results showed that bapineuzumab did lower phospho-tau in the cerebrospinal fluid (CSF). Due to these disappointing results the program was halted. Another two large phase 3 trials with solanezumab, a humanized mAb against the central part of soluble Aβ, also did not meet primary cognitive and functional endpoints. However, a prespecified secondary analysis of pooled subjects from the two trials was performed and showed that solanezumab-treated patients with milder symptoms (Mini-Mental State Examination (MMSE) 20–26 at entry) had less cognitive decline as measured with the ADAS-cog and MMSE [36].

Table 1
Overview of passive immunotherapy for AD

Compound	Company	Epitope	Trial results	References
AAB-003, Fc-engineered bapineuzumab	Janssen/Pfizer	N-terminus	Phase 1 trial completed in August 2014	[54]
Aducanumab, fully human IgG1	Biogen	Conformational epitope found on Aβ	Phase 1 trial showed target engagement and cognitive benefit	[38, 55]
BAN2401, humanized mAb158	Eisai Inc.	Binds large-size amyloid-β protofibrils (>100 kDa)	Phase 1 trial showed compound was safe and well tolerated. Phase 2b study ongoing	[56]
Bapineuzumab, humanized 3D6	Janssen/Pfizer	N-terminus	Phase 3 trials did not meet cognitive and functional endpoints	[34, 35]
Crenezumab, humanized IgG4	Genentech	Conformational epitopes including oligomeric and protofibrillar forms	Phase 2 open-label extension trial in AD and prevention trial in preclinical AD ongoing	[57, 58]
Gammagard, intravenous immunoglobulin, IVIg	Baxter Healthcare	Polyclonal antibodies directed against Aβ	Phase 3 trial did not meet cognitive and functional endpoint	[59]
Gantenerumab, full human	Hoffmann-La Roche	N-terminus and central potions of amyloid-β	Phase 3 in MCI failed futility analysis, phase 3 trial in mild AD ongoing	[60, 61]
GSK 933776, humanized IgG1	GlaxoSmithKline	N-terminus	Phase 1 trial showed that compound was safe and well tolerated	[62]
KHK6640, humanized IgG4	Kyowa Hakko Kirin Pharma	Aβ oligomers and higher molecular species	Phase 1 trial ongoing	[63]
LY3002813	Eli Lilly & Co.	Aβ (p3–42), a pyroglutamate form of Aβ	Phase 1 trial ongoing	[64]
MEDI1814	AstraZeneca	Aβ	Phase 1 trial ongoing	[65]
Ponezumab	Pfizer	C-terminal amino acids 33–40 of Aβ 1-40	Discontinued after phase 1	[66, 67]

(continued)

Table 1
(continued)

Compound	Company	Epitope	Trial results	References
SAR228810, humanized 13C3	Sanofi	Protofibrils, and low-molecular-weight amyloid-β	Phase 1 trial ongoing	[38, 68]
Solanezumab, humanized m266	Eli Lilly	Central (aa 16-24), accessible only on soluble Aβ	Phase 3 trials did not meet functional endpoint, did meet cognitive endpoint in pooled analyses in mild AD. New phase 3 study ongoing	[36, 69]

In another phase 3 trial, the fully human mAb gantenerumab, directed against both the amino terminus and central portions of Aβ, was tested in patients with prodromal AD. The study was halted because a futility analysis showed that the primary endpoint, i.e., less decline on the Clinical Dementia Rating scale Sum of Boxes, could not be met [37]. Possible explanations for these negative results could be that these compounds were administered in a too low dose, that they target the wrong Aβ species, or, in the case of bapineuzumab and solanezumab, that they were given too late in the disease course. Finally, for both of these phase 3 trials, there was no biomarker confirmation for AD pathology, which may have let to inclusion of patients who did not have AD. Several new generation of mAbs targeting various different Aβ epitopes are now being tested in ongoing phase 1, 2, and 3 clinical trials.

A key question relates to which epitope an efficacious mAb should be targeted. The selection of different Aβ species for treatment with mAbs is complicated by the fact that the identification and characterization of these species depend upon the definitions, protocols, and methods used for their preparation and characterization [38]. The lack of a common experimental description of the toxic Aβ oligomer makes interpretation and direct comparison of data between different research groups difficult [21].

The mechanism of action of mAbs comprises firstly the capture of a target and secondly an effector function linked to the Fc domain of the mAb. Several hypotheses have been proposed regarding the mechanism of action of mAbs in clearing amyloid in AD. Antibody binding to amyloid may lead to macrophage phagocytosis and complement activation [26], which assumes that sufficient antibody enters the brain and binds to Aβ to stimulate phagocytosis of resident microglia or infiltrating monocytes/macrophages. An alternative mechanism is the "peripheral sink" hypothesis. Antibodies in the peripheral circulation may contribute to the equilibrium between Aβ in the blood and CNS compartments. If antibody levels are raised, passive diffusion down a concentration gradient can help to clear monomeric Aβ from the brain [8]. Antibodies may also alter Aß clearance by interacting with the transport system that moves Aß into and out of the CNS compartment [39]. It is possible that more than one process takes place during passive Aβ immunotherapy.

2.5 Active Immunotherapy with Amyloid-Beta

The preclinical work by Schenk and others provided proof of concept for a beneficial effect by removing Aβ from the brain through active immunization with amyloid-β [23–25]. Table 2 gives an overview of trials with active immunotherapy in AD. In 2000 Elan/Wyeth initiated a randomized, multiple-dose, dose-escalation, double-blind phase 1 clinical trial with AN1792, a vaccine containing pre-aggregated Aβ1–42 and an immune-stimulating adjuvant. The vaccine was designed to induce a strong cell-mediated immune response. There were no adverse responses detected during the trial portion of the phase 1 study. Another finding was that the antibody response was variable, with many patients failing to develop detectable titers against the antigen. Approximately

Table 2
Overview of active immunotherapy for AD

Compound	Company	Antibody response	Trial results	References
ACI-24	AC Immune SA	Aggregated Aβ peptides	Phase 1/2 trial ongoing	[70]
Affitope AD02	AFFiRiS AG	Synthetic peptide of six amino acids that mimics the N-terminus of Aβ	Phase 2 study did not meet primary and secondary endpoint	[71]
AN-1792	Janssen, Pfizer	Synthetic full-length Aβ peptide with QS-21 adjuvant	Phase 2a trial was suspended when four treated patients developed aseptic meningoencephalitis	[43, 44]
CAD-106	Novartis Pharmaceutical Corporation	Aβ1-6 peptide derived from the N-terminal B cell epitope of Aβ, coupled to a Qβ viruslike particle	Phase 2 trials showed prolonged antibody titers in responders and safety after seven injections and follow-up of two and a half years	[72]
Vanutide cridificar	Janssen	Conjugate of multiple short Aβ fragments linked to a carrier made of inactivated diphtheria toxin	Discontinued after being tested in phase 2	[73]

halfway through the trial, there was a change in the adjuvant to QS-21 in an attempt to enhance this response [40]. In the subsequent phase 2a trial, started in 2001, 372 patients were enrolled with 300 receiving AN1792 (AN1792-to-placebo ratio of 4:1). However, the trial had to be prematurely terminated in January 2002 because of the development of a T-cell-mediated meningoencephalitis in approximately 6 % of the vaccinated patients. Although some patients were asymptomatic, most of these patients presented with confusion, lethargy, and/or headache. Brain MRI showed white matter hyperintensities with or without evidence of brain edema, i.e., amyloid-related imaging abnormalities (ARIA). Apart from giving rise to serious side effects, only approximately 20 % of vaccinated patients showed an antibody response above a therapeutic cutoff level [41]. In a *postmortem* examination performed on a limited number of trial patients who had received AN1792, clearance of parenchymal Aβ plaques had occurred, confirming the validity of the method [42]. Furthermore, AN1792-treated patients showed less amyloid angiopathy, and in some cases almost no insoluble amyloid deposits could be demonstrated [43]. When the active group was compared to the placebo group, no clinical benefits were found [41]. Interestingly, approximately 4.6 years after immunization with AN1792, patients who had shown an antibody response in the phase 2a study maintained sustained anti-AN1792 antibody titers and demonstrated reduced functional decline compared with placebo-treated patients [44].

Despite the dramatic course the AN1792 trial had taken, it is still believed that there is a future for active vaccination as treatment for AD. Active immunization has several advantages over passive vaccination. First, with active vaccination it is possible to generate a prolonged antibody response with a small number of administrations. Second, antibodies that are produced have multiple specificities against Aβ (as they are polyclonal) and over time the affinity may improve due to clonal maturation [8]. Potential disadvantages of active vaccination are the variability in the antibody response across patients, and the possibility of persistent adverse events. Although the development of active immunization for AD has proceeded more slowly than that of passive immunization, several second-generation active vaccination trials have been performed.

CAD106 is an active vaccination that aims to elicit an antibody response while avoiding inflammatory T cell activation. CAD106 is a small Aβ fragment (Aβ1–6) serving as a B-cell epitope, coupled to an adjuvant carrier. It has been tested in subcutaneous and intramuscular injections in several multicenter phase 2 trials. Two 66-week extension trials ending in 2010 and 2011 explored antibody response and tolerability of additional doses, i.e., different longer injection/booster-shot regimens. Prolonged antibody titers were found in responders and no cases of meningitis, meningoencephalitis, or vasogenic edema occurred clinically or by MRI [45].

Another vaccination trial is performed by AC Immune. Their ACI-24 is designed to induce a humoral immune response to Aβ in a predominately β-sheet conformation. Their phase 1/2a trial is testing the safety, immunogenicity, and efficacy in patients aged 40 and older with mild-to-moderate AD who had a positive amyloid PET scan and are on stable acetyl cholinesterase inhibitor therapy [46]. The ACC-001 vaccine from Janssen and Pfizer was tested in a phase 2 trial that used an Aβ [1–6] fragment attached to a carrier protein, using the surface-active saponin adjuvant QS-21. In August 2013, Pfizer's company pipeline listed this immunotherapy as having been discontinued from clinical development [47].

Affitope AD02 is a synthetic peptide of six amino acids that mimics the N-terminus of Aβ. This approach is based on the hypothesis that this fragment enables exclusive recognition of Aβ without cross-reacting with APP, and hence may have a favorable safety profile. A multicenter phase 2 trial of AD02 in patients with early AD was conducted in Europe. The limited data that has been shared suggests that AD02 had not reached either primary or secondary outcome measures [48].

2.6 Amyloid-Related Imaging Abnormalities

Amyloid-related imaging abnormalities (ARIAs) form a spectrum and two main categories can be acknowledged: ARIA-E and ARIA-H. Signal hyperintensities on fluid attenuation inversion recovery (FLAIR) MRI are thought to represent "vasogenic edema" and/or sulcal effusion (ARIA-E). The signal hypointensities on GRE/T2* are believed to be caused by hemosiderin deposits (ARIA-H), including microhemorrhage and cortical superficial siderosis [49]. Barkhof et al. have developed a reproducible and easily implemented MRI for the assessment of ARIA-E [50]. With regard to the etiology of ARIA it has been hypothesized that vascular amyloid is the common pathophysiological mechanism leading to increased vascular permeability. Dose-related vasogenic edema (ARIA-E) was observed in the phase 2 bapineuzumab trial [51], whereas the occurrence of ARIAs in mAb treatment for AD has varied from one compound to another. In the phase 3 solanezumab study the incidence of vasogenic edema (ARIA-E) among antibody-treated subjects was approximately 1 %, which was comparable to the placebo-treated group.

2.7 Preventing AD with Immunotherapy

The development of drugs for the treatment of AD has more and more focused on disease stages before the onset of overt dementia. It has been suggested that the benefits of a disease-modifying therapy may only be found in early prodromal AD or in preclinical AD, before too much neurodegeneration has occurred. However, phase 3 studies on prodromal and mild-to-moderate AD have so far yielded disappointing results. Three consortia are currently investigating the efficacy of mAbs administered at the preclinical stage: the Alzheimer's Prevention Initiative (API), the Dominantly Inherited

Alzheimer Network (DIAN), and the Anti-Amyloid Treatment of Asymptomatic Alzheimer's Disease (A4) study [52]. The API study investigates the efficacy of crenezumab in 300 members of Colombian families, including 100 carriers of disease-causing mutations in the PSEN1 gene. In the DIAN trial, 240 members of families with early-onset AD, of whom 60 have a mutation, are treated with solanezumab and gantenerumab. The A4 initiative will study the effect of solanezumab in 1500 healthy older people, some of whom are at risk for AD on the basis of amyloid-positive brain scans. The European Prevention of Alzheimer's dementia (EPAD) Initiative is a collaborative research initiative and part of the Innovative Medicines Initiative, a joint undertaking between the European Union and the European Federation of Pharmaceutical Industries and Associations, EFPIA [53]. The EPAD initiative aims to establish a European-wide register of 24,000 participants, of which 1500 will be invited to participate in a trial to test new treatments, some of which will likely be immunotherapeutic agents, for prevention of Alzheimer's dementia.

3   Conclusion

Alzheimer's disease is a dreadful disorder for which so far no efficacious disease-modifying treatment is available. On the basis of the amyloid cascade hypothesis, removing Aβ through immunotherapy, either passive with mAbs or active with Aβ fragments, may be an effective method to intervene in the pathophysiology of AD and prevent progression of the disease. However, thus far the results of three large phase 3 mAbs programs with bapineuzumab and solanezumab in AD, and gantenerumab in prodromal AD, have shown disappointing results. This lack of effect may be explained by inappropriate target selection, insufficient dosing, or, in the case of bapineuzumab and solanezumab, a too late intervention in the disease process. New-generation mAbs, primarily targeting protofibrils, may turn out to be more successful, and these compounds are at present being tested in phase 1 and 2 clinical trials. Although the first active immunotherapy with AN1792 had to be stopped because of severe side effects, new active vaccination programs with compounds that avoid inflammatory T cell activation may be safe and efficacious. Immunotherapy may give rise to the occurrence of amyloid-related imaging abnormalities (ARIA) that on the one hand may be associated with clinical symptoms, while on the other hand might signal target engagement and a positive immune response. It has been suggested that the earlier the disease process is targeted, the more efficacious the immunotherapy is likely to be. Several preclinical studies with mAbs, both in patients with autosomal genetic forms of AD and sporadic AD, have started and preparations for a large European prevention study are being made.

References

1. World Alzheimer Report (2014) World Alzheimer Report 2014
2. Hansen RA, Gartlehner G, Webb AP, Morgan LC, Moore CG, Jonas DE (2008) Efficacy and safety of donepezil, galantamine, and rivastigmine for the treatment of Alzheimer's disease: a systematic review and meta-analysis. Clin Interv Aging 3(2):211–225
3. Kaduszkiewicz H, Zimmermann T, Beck-Bornholdt HP, van den Bussche H (2005) Cholinesterase inhibitors for patients with Alzheimer's disease: systematic review of randomised clinical trials. BMJ 331(7512):321–327
4. Hardy J (2009) The amyloid hypothesis for Alzheimer's disease: a critical reappraisal. J Neurochem 110(4):1129–1134
5. Hardy J, Bogdanovic N, Winblad B, Portelius E, Andreasen N, Cedazo-Minguez A, Zetterberg H (2014) Pathways to Alzheimer's disease. J Intern Med 275(3):296–303
6. Selkoe DJ (2008) Soluble oligomers of the amyloid β-protein impair synaptic plasticity and behavior. Behav Brain Res 192(1):106–113, Accessed from http://www.sciencedirect.com/science/article/pii/S0166432808000831
7. Walsh DM, Selkoe DJ (2007) Aβ Oligomers ? a decade of discovery. J Neurochem 101(5):1172–1184
8. Lannfelt L, Relkin NR, Siemers ER (2014) Amyloid-ß-directed immunotherapy for Alzheimer's disease. J Intern Med 275(3):284–295
9. Winblad B, Graf A, Riviere ME, Andreasen N, Ryan JM (2014) Active immunotherapy options for Alzheimer's disease. Alzheimers Res Ther 6(1):7
10. Wisniewski T, Goñi F (2014) Immunotherapy for Alzheimer's disease. Biochem Pharmacol 88(4):499–507
11. What is Alzheimer's? Accessed from: http://www.alz.org/alzheimers_disease_what_is_alzheimers.asp
12. Mayeux R, Stern Y (2012) Epidemiology of Alzheimer disease. Cold Spring Harbor Perspect Med 2(8):a006239
13. Cummings JL, Cole G (2002) Alzheimer disease. JAMA 287(18):2335–2338
14. Lopez OL (2011) The growing burden of Alzheimer's disease. Am J Manag Care 17(Suppl 13):S339–45
15. Bateman RJ, Xiong C, Benzinger TL, Fagan AM, Goate A, Fox NC, Marcus DS, Cairns NJ, Xie X, Blazey TM, Holtzman DM, Santacruz A, Buckles V, Oliver A, Moulder K, Aisen PS, Ghetti B, Klunk WE, McDade E, Martins RN, Masters CL, Mayeux R, Ringman JM, Rossor MN, Schofield PR, Sperling RA, Salloway S, Morris JC, Dominantly Inherited Alzheimer Network (2012) Clinical and biomarker changes in dominantly inherited Alzheimer's disease. N Engl J Med 367(9):795–804
16. Sperling RA, Aisen PS, Beckett LA, Bennett DA, Craft S, Fagan AM, Iwatsubo T, Jack CR, Kaye J, Montine TJ, Park DC, Reiman EM, Rowe CC, Siemers E, Stern Y, Yaffe K, Carrillo MC, Thies B, Morrison-Bogorad M, Wagster MV, Phelps CH (2011) Toward defining the preclinical stages of Alzheimer's disease: recommendations from the National Institute on Aging-Alzheimer's Association workgroups on diagnostic guidelines for Alzheimer's disease. Alzheimers Dement 7(3):280–292
17. Albert MS, DeKosky ST, Dickson D, Dubois B, Feldman HH, Fox NC, Gamst A, Holtzman DM, Jagust WJ, Petersen RC, Snyder PJ, Carrillo MC, Thies B, Phelps CH (2011) The diagnosis of mild cognitive impairment due to Alzheimer's disease: recommendations from the National Institute on Aging-Alzheimer's Association workgroups on diagnostic guidelines for Alzheimer's disease. Alzheimers Dement 7(3):270–279
18. McKhann GM, Knopman DS, Chertkow H, Hyman BT, Jack CR, Kawas CH, Klunk WE, Koroshetz WJ, Manly JJ, Mayeux R, Mohs RC, Morris JC, Rossor MN, Scheltens P, Carrillo MC, Thies B, Weintraub S, Phelps CH (2011) The diagnosis of dementia due to Alzheimer's disease: recommendations from the National Institute on Aging-Alzheimer's Association workgroups on diagnostic guidelines for Alzheimer's disease. Alzheimers Dement 7(3):263–269
19. Association A's (2014) 2014 Alzheimer's disease facts and figures. Alzheimers Dement 10(2):e47–e92
20. Loy CT, Schofield PR, Turner AM, Kwok JB (2014) Genetics of dementia. Lancet 383(9919):828–840
21. Benilova I, Karran E, De Strooper B (2012) The toxic Aβ oligomer and Alzheimer's disease: an emperor in need of clothes. Nat Neurosci 15(3):349–357
22. Jonsson T, Atwal JK, Steinberg S, Snaedal J, Jonsson PV, Bjornsson S, Stefansson H, Sulem P, Gudbjartsson D, Maloney J, Hoyte K, Gustafson A, Liu Y, Lu Y, Bhangale T, Graham RR, Huttenlocher J, Bjornsdottir G, Andreassen OA, Jönsson EG, Palotie A, Behrens TW, Magnusson OT, Kong A, Thorsteinsdottir U, Watts RJ, Stefansson K (2012) A mutation in APP protects against Alzheimer's disease and age-related cognitive decline. Nature 488(7409):96–99
23. Schenk D, Barbour R, Dunn W, Gordon G, Grajeda H, Guido T, Hu K, Huang J, Johnson-Wood K, Khan K, Kholodenko D, Lee M, Liao

Z, Lieberburg I, Motter R, Mutter L, Soriano F, Shopp G, Vasquez N, Vandevert C, Walker S, Wogulis M, Yednock T, Games D, Seubert P (1999) Immunization with amyloid-beta attenuates Alzheimer-disease-like pathology in the PDAPP mouse. Nature 400(6740):173–177

24. Janus C, Pearson J, McLaurin J, Mathews PM, Jiang Y, Schmidt SD, Chishti MA, Horne P, Heslin D, French J, Mount HT, Nixon RA, Mercken M, Bergeron C, Fraser PE, St George-Hyslop P, Westaway D (2000) A beta peptide immunization reduces behavioural impairment and plaques in a model of Alzheimer's disease. Nature 408(6815):979–982

25. Lemere CA, Beierschmitt A, Iglesias M, Spooner ET, Bloom JK, Leverone JF, Zheng JB, Seabrook TJ, Louard D, Li D, Selkoe DJ, Palmour RM, Ervin FR (2004) Alzheimer's disease abeta vaccine reduces central nervous system abeta levels in a non-human primate, the Caribbean vervet. Am J Pathol 165(1):283–297

26. Bard F, Cannon C, Barbour R, Burke RL, Games D, Grajeda H, Guido T, Hu K, Huang J, Johnson-Wood K, Khan K, Kholodenko D, Lee M, Lieberburg I, Motter R, Nguyen M, Soriano F, Vasquez N, Weiss K, Welch B, Seubert P, Schenk D, Yednock T (2000) Peripherally administered antibodies against amyloid beta-peptide enter the central nervous system and reduce pathology in a mouse model of Alzheimer disease. Nat Med 6(8):916–919

27. Das P, Howard V, Loosbrock N, Dickson D, Murphy MP, Golde TE (2003) Amyloid-beta immunization effectively reduces amyloid deposition in FcRgamma –/– knock-out mice. J Neurosci 23(24):8532–8538

28. DeMattos RB, Bales KR, Cummins DJ, Dodart JC, Paul SM, Holtzman DM (2001) Peripheral anti-A beta antibody alters CNS and plasma A beta clearance and decreases brain A beta burden in a mouse model of Alzheimer's disease. Proc Natl Acad Sci U S A 98(15):8850–5

29. Morgan D, Diamond DM, Gottschall PE, Ugen KE, Dickey C, Hardy J, Duff K, Jantzen P, DiCarlo G, Wilcock D, Connor K, Hatcher J, Hope C, Gordon M, Arendash GW (2000) A beta peptide vaccination prevents memory loss in an animal model of Alzheimer's disease. Nature 408(6815):982–985

30. Nitsch RM, Hock C (2008) Targeting beta-amyloid pathology in Alzheimer's disease with Abeta immunotherapy. Neurotherapeutics 5(3):415–420

31. Bales KR, Tzavara ET, Wu S, Wade MR, Bymaster FP, Paul SM, Nomikos GG (2006) Cholinergic dysfunction in a mouse model of Alzheimer disease is reversed by an anti-A beta antibody. J Clin Invest 116(3):825–832

32. Morgan D (2011) Immunotherapy for Alzheimer's disease. J Intern Med 269(1):54–63

33. Nelson AL, Dhimolea E, Reichert JM (2010) Development trends for human monoclonal antibody therapeutics. Nat Rev Drug Discov 9(10):767–774

34. Salloway S et al (2012) A randomized, double-blind, placebo-controlled clinical trial of intra-venous bapineuzumab in patients with Alzheimer's disease who are apolipoprotein E e4 non-carriers. Eur J Neurol 19(Suppl 1):70

35. Sperling R et al (2012) A randomized, double-blind, placebo-controlled clinical trial of intra-venous bapineuzumab in patients with Alzheimer's disease who are apolipoprotein E e4 carriers. Eur J Neurol 19(Suppl 1):70

36. Tayeb HO, Murray ED, Price BH, Tarazi FI (2013) Bapineuzumab and solanezumab for Alzheimer's disease: is the 'amyloid cascade hypothesis' still alive? Expert Opin Biol Ther 13(7):1075–1084

37. Delrieu J, Ousset PJ, Vellas B (2012) Gantenerumab for the treatment of Alzheimer's disease. Expert Opin Biol Ther 12(8):1077–1086

38. Moreth J, Mavoungou C, Schindowski K (2013) Passive anti-amyloid immunotherapy in Alzheimer's disease: what are the most promising targets? Immun Ageing 10(1):18

39. Zlokovic BV (2004) Clearing amyloid through the blood-brain barrier. J Neurochem 89(4):807–811

40. Schenk D (2002) Amyloid-beta immunotherapy for Alzheimer's disease: the end of the beginning. Nat Rev Neurosci 3(10):824–828

41. Gilman S, Koller M, Black RS, Jenkins L, Griffith SG, Fox NC, Eisner L, Kirby L, Rovira MB, Forette F, Orgogozo JM, AN1792(QS-21)-201 Study Team (2005) Clinical effects of Abeta immunization (AN1792) in patients with AD in an inter-rupted trial. Neurology 64(9):1553–62

42. Holmes C, Boche D, Wilkinson D, Yadegarfar G, Hopkins V, Bayer A, Jones RW, Bullock R, Love S, Neal JW, Zotova E, Nicoll JA (2008) Long-term effects of Abeta42 immunisation in Alzheimer's disease: follow-up of a randomised, placebo-controlled phase I trial. Lancet 372(9634):216–223

43. Nicoll JA, Wilkinson D, Holmes C, Steart P, Markham H, Weller RO (2003) Neuropathology of human Alzheimer disease after immunization with amyloid-beta peptide: a case report. Nat Med 9(4):448–452

44. Vellas B, Black R, Thal LJ, Fox NC, Daniels M, McLennan G, Tompkins C, Leibman C, Pomfret M, Grundman M, AN1792 (QS-21)-251 Study Team (2009) Long-term follow-up of patients immunized with AN1792: reduced

functional decline in antibody responders. Curr Alzheimer Res 6(2):144–51

45. Farlow MR, Andreasen N, Riviere ME, Vostiar I, Vitaliti A, Sovago J, Caputo A, Winblad B, Graf A (2015) Long-term treatment with active Aβ immunotherapy with CAD106 in mild Alzheimer's disease. Alzheimers Res Ther 7(1):23

46. http://www.alzforum.org/therapeutics/aci-24

47. http://www.alzforum.org/therapeutics/vanutide-cridificar

48. http://www.alzforum.org/therapeutics/affitope-ad02

49. Sperling RA, Jack CR, Black SE, Frosch MP, Greenberg SM, Hyman BT, Scheltens P, Carrillo MC, Thies W, Bednar MM, Black RS, Brashear HR, Grundman M, Siemers ER, Feldman HH, Schindler RJ (2011) Amyloid-related imaging abnormalities in amyloid-modifying therapeutic trials: recommendations from the Alzheimer's Association Research Roundtable Workgroup. Alzheimers Dement 7(4):367–385

50. Barkhof F, Daams M, Scheltens P, Brashear HR, Arrighi HM, Bechten A, Morris K, McGovern M, Wattjes MP (2013) An MRI rating scale for amyloid-related imaging abnormalities with edema or effusion. AJNR Am J Neuroradiol 34:1550–1555

51. Salloway S, Sperling R, Gilman S, Fox NC, Blennow K, Raskind M, Sabbagh M, Honig LS, Doody R, van Dyck CH, Mulnard R, Barakos J, Gregg KM, Liu E, Lieberburg I, Schenk D, Black R, Grundman M, Bapineuzumab 201 Clinical Trial Investigators (2009) A phase 2 multiple ascending dose trial of bapineuzumab in mild to moderate Alzheimer disease. Neurology 73(24):2061–70

52. Miller G (2012) Alzheimer's research. Stopping Alzheimer's before it starts. Science 337(6096):790–2

53. (2015). Accessed from: http://synapse-pi.com/epad/

54. Crespi GA, Ascher DB, Parker MW, Miles LA (2014) Crystallization and preliminary X-ray diffraction analysis of the Fab portion of the Alzheimer's disease immunotherapy candidate bapineuzumab complexed with amyloid-β. Acta Crystallogr F Struct Biol Commun 70(Pt 3):374–7

55. Single ascending dose study of BIIB037 in subjects with Alzheimer's disease [Internet]. Retrieved from: http://www.clinicaltrials.gov/ct2/show/NCT01397539?term=BIIB037&rank=2

56. Lannfelt L, Möller C, Basun H, Osswald G, Sehlin D, Satlin A, Logovinsky V, Gellerfors P (2014) Perspectives on future Alzheimer therapies: amyloid-β protofibrils - a new target for immunotherapy with BAN2401 in Alzheimer's disease. Alzheimers Res Ther 6(2):16

57. Adolfsson O, Pihlgren M, Toni N, Varisco Y, Buccarello AL, Antoniello K, Lohmann S, Piorkowska K, Gafner V, Atwal JK, Maloney J, Chen M, Gogineni A, Weimer RM, Mortensen DL, Friesenhahn M, Ho C, Paul R, Pfeifer A, Muhs A, Watts RJ (2012) An effector-reduced anti-β-amyloid (Aβ) antibody with unique aβ binding properties promotes neuroprotection and glial engulfment of Aβ. J Neurosci 32(28):9677–9689

58. Garber K (2012) Genentech's Alzheimer's antibody trial to study disease prevention. Nat Biotechnol 30(8):731–732

59. Relkin N (2014) Clinical trials of intravenous immunoglobulin for Alzheimer's disease. J Clin Immunol 34(Suppl 1):S74–9

60. Bohrmann B, Baumann K, Benz J, Gerber F, Huber W, Knoflach F, Messer J, Oroszlan K, Rauchenberger R, Richter WF, Rothe C, Urban M, Bardroff M, Winter M, Nordstedt C, Loetscher H (2012) Gantenerumab: a novel human anti-Aβ antibody demonstrates sustained cerebral amyloid-β binding and elicits cell-mediated removal of human amyloid-β. J Alzheimers Dis; 28(1):49–69

61. Ostrowitzki S, Deptula D, Thurfjell L, Barkhof F, Bohrmann B, Brooks DJ, Klunk WE, Ashford E, Yoo K, Xu ZX, Loetscher H, Santarelli L (2012) Mechanism of amyloid removal in patients with Alzheimer disease treated with gantenerumab. Arch Neurol 69(2):198–207

62. Andreasen N, Simeoni M, Ostlund H, Lisjo PI, Fladby T, Loercher AE, Byrne GJ, Murray F, Scott-Stevens PT, Wallin A, Zhang YY, Bronge LH, Zetterberg H, Nordberg AK, Yeo AJ, Khan SA, Hilpert J, Mistry PC (2015) First administration of the Fc-attenuated anti-β amyloid antibody GSK933776 to patients with mild Alzheimer's disease: a randomized, placebo-controlled study. PLoS One 10(3):e0098153

63. A study of single and multiple doses of KHK6640 in subjects with prodromal or mild to moderate Alzheimer's disease [Internet]. [cited 2015]. Retrieved from: https://clinical-trials.gov/ct2/show/NCT02127476

64. Demattos RB, Lu J, Tang Y, Racke MM, Delong CA, Tzaferis JA, Hole JT, Forster BM, McDonnell PC, Liu F, Kinley RD, Jordan WH, Hutton ML (2012) A plaque-specific antibody clears existing β-amyloid plaques in Alzheimer's disease mice. Neuron 76(5):908–920

65. https://www.clinicaltrials.gov/ct2/show/NCT01561053?term=gamunex+AD&rank=1

66. Burstein AH, Zhao Q, Ross J, Styren S, Landen JW, Ma WW, McCush F, Alvey C, Kupiec JW, Bednar MM (2013) Safety and pharmacology of ponezumab (PF-04360365) after a single 10-minute infusion in subjects with mild to moderate Alzheimer disease. Clin Neuropharmacol 36(1):8–13

67. Landen JW, Zhao Q, Cohen S, Borrie M, Woodward M, Billing CB, Bales K, Alvey C, McCush F, Yang J, Kupiec JW, Bednar MM (2013) Safety and pharmacology of a single intravenous dose of ponezumab in subjects with mild-to-moderate Alzheimer disease: a phase I, randomized, placebo-controlled, double-blind, dose-escalation study. Clin Neuropharmacol 36(1):14–23

68. Single and repeated dosing study to assess the safety and the concentration-time profile of SAR228810 in Alzheimer's patients [Internet]. Retrieved from: http://www.clinicaltrials.gov/ct2/show/NCT01485302?term=SAR228810&rank=1

69. Farlow M, Arnold SE, van Dyck CH, Aisen PS, Snider BJ, Porsteinsson AP, Friedrich S, Dean RA, Gonzales C, Sethuraman G, DeMattos RB, Mohs R, Paul SM, Siemers ER (2012) Safety and biomarker effects of solanezumab in patients with Alzheimer's disease. Alzheimers Dement 8(4):261–271

70. Hickman DT, López-Deber MP, Ndao DM, Silva AB, Nand D, Pihlgren M, Giriens V, Madani R, St-Pierre A, Karastaneva H, Nagel-Steger L, Willbold D, Riesner D, Nicolau C, Baldus M, Pfeifer A, Muhs A (2011) Sequence-independent control of peptide conformation in liposomal vaccines for targeting protein misfolding diseases. J Biol Chem 286(16): 13966–13976

71. Schneeberger A, Mandler M, Otawa O, Zauner W, Mattner F, Schmidt W (2009) Development of AFFITOPE vaccines for Alzheimer's disease (AD)--from concept to clinical testing. J Nutr Health Aging 13(3):264–267

72. Kingwell K (2012) Alzheimer disease: amyloid-β immunotherapy CAD106 passes first safety test in patients with Alzheimer disease. Nat Rev Neurol 8(8):414

73. Ryan JM, Grundman M (2009) Anti-amyloid-beta immunotherapy in Alzheimer's disease: ACC-001 clinical trials are ongoing. J Alzheimers Dis. 243

Chapter 2

Active Immunization Against the Amyloid-β Peptide

Enchi Liu and J. Michael Ryan

Abstract

Alzheimer's disease (AD) has a devastating toll not only on the affected individuals but also on their families, caregivers, and society as a whole. Several therapies have been approved to treat AD, all of which provide modest effect on the symptoms of the illness but without slowing or halting the underlying disease processes. Since the last of these therapies was approved, the largest research effort has been devoted to developing therapies targeting amyloid-β, specifically $A\beta_{42}$, as this protein is thought to initiate the cascade of events that lead to the disease. This chapter focuses on active immunotherapy (vaccines) and specifically on therapies that currently are in clinical development.

Key words Alzheimer's disease, Amyloid-β, Active immunotherapy, Therapeutic vaccine

1   Introduction

Alzheimer's disease (AD) is a serious and invariably fatal neurodegenerative disease and the major cause of dementia in the elderly [1–4]. Progressive deterioration in both cognition and function over time leads to serious clinical outcomes including increased dependence and decreased survival. Besides the direct cost for patient care, indirect costs add incrementally to the burden on society. These are represented by care provided by families and other unpaid caregivers of AD patients, by the impact on caregivers in terms of lost time at work, lost wages and depleted finances, as well as increased caregiver emotional stress and medical needs [5, 6]. Even a small delay in the onset, e.g., by 1 year, of AD dementia would result in a significant reduction in the global burden of the disease. A 1-year decrease in both onset and progression of AD dementia would reduce the 2050 global burden by more than nine million cases with the majority of the reduction among the most severe cases [5]. Therefore, any significant effective treatments that delay, halt, or prevent the progression of disease should decrease costs to patients, caregivers, and society as a whole as well as improve patient and caregiver quality of life.

Martin Ingelsson and Lars Lannfelt (eds.), *Immunotherapy and Biomarkers in Neurodegenerative Disorders*, Methods in Pharmacology and Toxicology, DOI 10.1007/978-1-4939-3560-4_2, © Springer Science+Business Media New York 2016

The characteristic progressive loss of memory and other cognitive functions, manifest as progressive dementia in AD, develops in parallel with the hallmark neuropathological changes of extracellular proteinaceous lesions (senile plaques) and intraneuronal neurofibrillary tangles, leading ultimately to neuronal death and neurodegeneration. The predominant component of senile plaques is the amyloid-β (Aβ) peptide, particularly the 42-amino acid isoform (Aβ$_{42}$), which is derived from a larger amyloid precursor protein (APP) [7]. The N-terminus of Aβ is cleaved first by the β-site amyloid precursor protein-cleaving enzyme 1 (BACE-1), and then by γ-secretase at the C-terminus. In the brain, Aβ$_{42}$ can form soluble neurotoxic oligomers, fibrillar parenchymal plaques closely associated with neuritic dystrophy and gliosis, and fibrillar (congophilic) amyloid angiopathy [7, 8].

Research over more than 30 years provides evidence that aberrant Aβ$_{42}$ production or clearance, resulting in a chronic dyshomeostasis of Aβ$_{42}$, is a central part in AD pathogenesis. All known genetically linked forms of AD directly affect either the production or the deposition of Aβ$_{42}$, and Aβ$_{42}$clearance appears to be impaired in AD [7–13]. Mutations in the *APP* and the presenilin genes, *PSEN1* and *PSEN2*, result in rare, early-onset, familial forms of AD and increase the accumulation of Aβ [14]. On the other hand, a recently identified allelic variant of APP (A673T), which is a less efficient substrate for BACE-1, was proposed to be protective against the more common sporadic AD in the wider population [15]. Further, in sporadic AD, the genetic risk factor gene allele ApoE ε4, known to be correlated with greater brain amyloid burden [16, 17], increases the risk for development of AD [14].

Multiple lines of evidence implicate Aβ as having a key precipitating role in the pathogenesis of AD. Mainly, the production and/or deposition of toxic forms of Aβ, along with the slowing of Aβ degradation, are viewed as the central and primary events in AD pathogenesis, while neurofibrillary-tangle formation and neuronal cell death occur downstream in this amyloid cascade [7, 8, 18]. Recent in vitro work has demonstrated that Aβ dimers (the major form of soluble oligomers in the human brain) isolated from patients with AD induce both the abnormal phosphorylation of tau that is characteristic of AD and the degeneration of neurites, providing further confirmation of the pivotal role of Aβ in the pathogenesis of AD [19]. However, the work of Braak and colleagues [20] has suggested a refinement of the amyloid cascade hypothesis, in which tauopathy can occur very early, independent of Aβ pathology, progressing in an age-dependent manner. In this model it is likely that the later development of Aβ pathology exacerbates and drives the further development of tauopathy resulting in clinical AD.

2   Therapeutic Approaches

Currently marketed therapies for the treatment of AD include cholinesterase inhibitors and the NMDA receptor antagonist memantine. These drugs only provide modest transient symptomatic effects, aimed at temporary enhancement of impaired neurotransmitter systems to maximize the remaining activity in neuronal populations not affected by the disease [21–23], but do not alter, slow, or halt progression of the disease. The search for a disease-modifying therapy—that affects the underlying disease pathology and has a measurable and long-lasting effect on the progression of disability—has been intense but so far unsuccessful [24, 25].

The pathologic hallmarks of AD—the accumulation of toxic Aβ with the formation of extracellular plaques, the development of intracellular neurofibrillary tangles, and the degeneration of cerebral neurons—provides potential targets for disease-modifying therapies. However, although the large majority of therapies that have been evaluated in the past 15 years have focused on Aβ, anti-tau therapies are beginning to be tested in the clinic (e.g., Axon Neuroscience SE NCT02031198, NCT01850238; AC Immune SA www.acimmune.com). Moreover, next-generation symptomatic approaches which focus on ameliorating the neuropsychiatric and behavioral symptoms associated with AD are also under evaluation (e.g., Pfizer NCT01712074; Lilly NCT00843518; Elan Pharmaceuticals NCT01735630).

Several therapeutic approaches to reduce cerebral amyloid have been explored. While small-molecule approaches aimed at reducing Aβ production by inhibiting or modulating the enzymatic activities of the BACE-1 and γ secretase continue to be explored, this chapter focuses on large-molecule biologic approaches to reduce/prevent accumulation of Aβ.

2.1   Immunotherapeutic Approaches to Amyloid-β Clearance

The concept of immunotherapy as an approach to treat AD was first introduced by Schenk and colleagues [26], who proposed that the immune system could be harnessed to clear toxic Aβ from the brain [27–29]. These approaches involve immune-mediated interventions either by inducing an oligoclonal response through immunization (active immunotherapy) or by administering monoclonal antibodies directed against Aβ (passive immunotherapy) (Fig. 1).

Passive immunotherapy allows for the precise targeting of Aβ epitopes and obviates the need for patients to mount an antibody response, but requires continuous periodic administration for long-term treatment. Active immunotherapy involves the administration of either full-length Aβ peptides or peptide fragments to activate the patient's immune system in order to produce anti-Aβ antibodies. Moreover, the Aβ peptides or peptide fragments can be conjugated to a carrier protein and may be administered with an adjuvant in order to help stimulate the immune response. Active immunotherapy can induce an oligoclonal (as opposed to monoclonal) response, with antibodies that differ with respect to their binding affinity for a number of toxic Aβ species. Unlike passive immunotherapy, which has to be readministered at frequent intervals, active immunotherapy has the potential to produce persistent levels of anti-Aβ antibody titers with less frequent administration [27–29].

Immunization with aggregated human Aβ$_{42}$ [26] and passive immunotherapy with antibodies directed against the N-terminus of Aβ$_{42}$ [30, 31] have been evaluated in PDAPP mice, an animal model of the ß-amyloidosis and associated cellular changes of AD [32]. These studies have shown a robust reduction or clearance of brain amyloid and have been widely confirmed in other mouse models by many academic and biopharmaceutical research laboratories worldwide [33].

The proof of principle was first demonstrated in the late 1990s [26]. In this study, immunization with intact Aβ$_{1-42}$ resulted in an antibody response that was predominantly directed against an immunodominant epitope located at or near the N-terminus of Aβ$_{1-42}$. In young adult PDAPP mice, immunization generated robust titers of anti-Aβ$_{1-42}$ antibodies and almost entirely prevented the development of AD-like amyloid plaques, neuritic dystrophy,

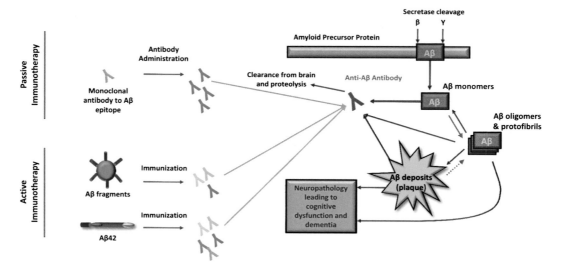

Fig. 1 Passive and active immunotherapeutic approaches to Aβ clearance. Anti-Aβ immunotherapy compounds under development utilize anti-beta-amyloid antibodies, generated through either passive or active immunotherapy approaches (*left*), to target Aβ and promote its clearance from the brain (*right*), with the goal of reversing the neuropathology that leads to cognitive dysfunction

and gliosis. Furthermore, immunization of older PDAPP mice, which had already developed amyloid plaques, markedly reduced the extent of plaques and the progression of the AD-like neuropathology. Therefore, the efficacy of immunization with the synthetic $Aβ_{1-42}$ in the PDAPP model of AD (confirmed in other APP transgenic mouse lines) provided the initial evidence that this approach is a potentially disease-modifying therapeutic strategy for patients with AD [26].

The precise mode of action of Aβ immunization is not known, but based on further experiments performed in PDAPP and other transgenic mice, the effect is clearly mediated by anti-Aβ antibodies that are highly specific towards Aβ epitopes and do not bind other brain or systemic proteins. Further experiments with peripheral antibody administration in PDAPP mice showed that these antibodies can enter the central nervous system (~0.3 %), bind to amyloid plaques, significantly reduce both plaque and neuritic burdens and gliosis, and prevent loss of synaptophysin, a classical marker of synaptic integrity [30]. Antibodies directed at the N-terminus of the $Aβ_{42}$ peptide are thought to act in multiple ways, including direct capture and neutralization of soluble Aβ monomers and oligomers as well as disruption and clearance of parenchymal and vascular Aβ deposits by either direct dissolution of fibrillar material or Fc-mediated phagocytosis (principally via microglia) of amyloid deposits [30, 34–36].

2.2 AN1792 Clinical Experience

Following on the promising preclinical results, AN1792, a synthetic beta-amyloid 1–42 peptide, was the first active amyloid immunotherapy tested in clinical trials [37, 38]. Immunization of subjects with mild-to-moderate AD with AN1792 resulted in an antibody response that was predominantly raised against the dominant epitope located at or near the N-terminus of $Aβ_{1-42}$ [39] in ~53 % (Phase 1; [37]) and 19.7–20 % (Phase 2; (39)) of immunized subjects. However, the AN1792 clinical program had to be halted due to the occurrence of meningoencephalitis in approximately 6 % of subjects in the Phase 2 trial who were immunized with the active product [40]. Most patients who experienced this adverse event developed progressive confusion, lethargy, and headache. Yet other patients reported signs and symptoms such as fever, nausea, vomiting, seizures, and focal neurologic signs. Recovery was reported in 12 of the 18 patients, while 6 patients were noted to have persistent sequelae at the conclusion of the trial. No additional cases of meningoencephalitis were reported over a 4.6-year follow-up study of subjects previously enrolled in the Phase 2 trial [41]. Further investigations indicated the AN1792-associated meningoencephalitis as an event caused by an Aβ-directed proinflammatory cytotoxic T-cell response to a major T-cell antigenic epitope within the carboxyl portion of $Aβ_{1-42}$ [42]. Neuropathologic examination of one case of meningoencephalitis revealed a perivascular T-cell infiltrate with a lack of B lymphocytes, as well as microglial activation and multinucleated giant cells [43].

Nevertheless, results from these initial studies suggested the potential of immunotherapy for the treatment of AD. Results from these early immunotherapy trials with AN1792 showed potential benefit on certain cognitive and functional outcome measures [37, 38, 41] and a significant reduction in t-tau protein levels in the CSF [38] but a paradoxical greater atrophy rate of certain brain regions [44]. Further, observations on approximately a dozen subjects of the AN1792 trials (Phase 1 and 2) who have come to autopsy indicate that this active immunotherapeutic approach results in removal of amyloid plaques from brains of AD subjects [43, 45–48] and an amelioration of plaque-associated neuritic and glial abnormalities [49]. However, in this small group of subjects who died, brain amyloid removal apparently did not result in improved survival or in an improvement in the time to severe dementia [47]. Whether the effects of immunotherapy on AD pathology and neurofibrillary dysfunction will ultimately translate to clinical benefit and a delayed disability is being evaluated with next-generation immunotherapy programs.

3 Clinical Programs with Amyloid-β Immunotherapy

Several next-generation Aβ active immunotherapies are currently under evaluation (Table 1). These newer Aβ active immunotherapies seek to avoid the T-cell response observed with AN1792, and are designed to elicit a strong B-cell response and carrier-induced T-cell response without activating an Aβ-specific proinflammatory T-cell response. These therapeutic vaccines are typically constructed with short Aβ peptides, fragmented peptides, or peptide mimetics conjugated with a carrier backbone and administered with an adjuvant, the latter two of which are used to bolster the natural immune response [50, 51].

3.1 ACC-001

Vanutide cridificar (ACC-001) is a conjugate of multiple copies of $A\beta_{-7}$ peptide linked to a nontoxic variant of diphtheria toxin (CRM197) which is administered intramuscularly with or without the adjuvant QS-21 [52]. QS-21, a naturally occurring saponin (triterpene glycoside) molecule purified from the South American tree *Quillaja saponaria Molina*, is an adjuvant known to promote both humoral and cellular immune response against a number of antigens in various species. Preclinical data indicate that vanutide cridificar generates N-terminal anti-beta-amyloid antibodies without inducing a beta-amyloid-directed T-cell response and that it reverses cognitive impairment in murine models of AD [53]. Vanutide cridificar phase 2 clinical trials in mild-to-moderate AD (NCT01284387 [US]; NCT00479557 [EU]; NCT00955409

Table 1
List of anti-Aβ active immunotherapy compounds that have reached clinical development

Compound	Sponsor	Phase of development	Epitope/carrier/adjuvant	Route of administration	Population
ACC-001	Pfizer Inc. and Janssen R & D	2	$Aβ_{1-7}$/nontoxic diphtheria toxin (CRM197)/QS-21	i.m.	Mild-to-moderate AD Early AD
AD-02	Affiris	2	$Aβ_{1-6}$ mimetic/KLH/ aluminum	s.c.	Mild-to-moderate AD Early AD
ACI-24	AC Immune	1/2	Tetra-palmitoylated $Aβ_{1-15}$/ reconstituted in liposome	s.c.	Mild-to-moderate AD
CAD-106	Novartis	2	$Aβ_{1-6}$/bacteriophage Qβ coat protein	i.m./s.c.	Mild-to-moderate AD
Lu AF20513	Lundbeck	1	$Aβ_{1-12}$ + 2 foreign T-helper epitopes (P30/P2) from tetanus toxoid	Not known	Mild AD
UB-311	United Biomedical	2	2-UBITh® synthetic peptide coupled to $Aβ_{1-14}$/CpG oligonucleotide	i.m.	Mild-to-moderate AD
V950	Merck	1 (discontinued)	Multivalent Aβ peptide/ ISOCOMATRIX™	i.m.	Mild-to-moderate AD

[EU extension]; NCT00498602 [US]; NCT00960531 [US extension]; NCT00752232 [Japan]; NCT00959192 [Japan]; NCT01238991 [Japan extension]) and early AD (NCT01227564) have been completed.

Data from a study in Japanese patients with mild-to-moderate AD (NCT00752232; [54]) demonstrated that repeated i.m. administration of vanutide cridificar at three different dose levels (3, 10, and 30 μg) with QS-21 (50 μg) at 3-month intervals up to 1 year elicited high antibody titers and sustained anti-Aβ IgG responses, but only after the second immunization and with no difference between the doses. The addition of QS-21 was essential to stimulate high titer responses. Vanutide cridificar at all doses with or without QS-21 was generally safe and well tolerated. Contrary to that reported from other trials evaluating anti-amyloid therapies in AD [55], no ARIA-E or ARIA-H was observed in this study. No significant differences between vanutide cridificar and placebo were observed in cognitive evaluations, but this may be due to the small sample size and interpatient variability [54].

The completed Phase 2 ACCTION study (NCT01284387; [56]) is among the first AD studies to use amyloid PET imaging as an enrichment strategy to increase diagnostic certainty after observations that a fraction of clinically diagnosed AD patients do not have pathological amyloid burden by in vivo PET imaging [57]. This study evaluated the effect of ACC-001 with 50 μg QS-21 adjuvant on brain fibrillar amyloid burden as measured by amyloid imaging using ^{18}F-AV-45 (florbetapir) positron emission tomography (PET) in mild-to-moderate AD patients [58]. Exploratory endpoints included safety, immunogenicity, and cognitive and functional efficacy. 125 subjects aged 50–89 with baseline mini mental status examination (MMSE) scores of 18–26 were randomized in a 1:1:1 ratio to receive 3 μg or 10 μg of ACC with QS-21, or placebo, stratified by APOEε4 status. ACC-001 with QS-21 was given by six intramuscular injections over 18 months at weeks 0, 4, 12, 26, 52, and 78, with follow-up through week 104. The primary endpoint of change in PET global cortical average (GCA) standardized value uptake ratio (SUVr) was not statistically significantly different between the two ACC-001 with QS-21 treatment groups compared to placebo, but the changes were numerically consistent with a dose response. ACC-001 was immunogenic with anti-Aβ IgG titers modestly higher in the 10 μg group than the 3 μg group, but the proportion of responders (defined as a titer ≥300 U/mL) was similar in both groups. The only safety signal noted with ACC-001 + QS-21 was a 5.8 % incidence of asymptomatic amyloid-related imaging abnormalities with edema/effusion (ARIA-E), not seen with placebo, and an increase in injection reactions (7.7 % vs. 47.7 %), the majority of which were mild and transient. The plasma Aβ levels increased in parallel with peak anti-Aβ titers after each injection. In the subset with CSF assessments, CSF p-tau changes from baseline in both active treatment groups were not statistically different from placebo but were numerically consistent with a dose response. Volumetric brain MRI showed incrementally greater treatment-related decrease in brain volume which was statistically significant in the 10 μg group ($p = 0.023$) compared with placebo. Decline in CDR-SB was typical for the study patient population. A baseline imbalance may have accounted for a somewhat slower decline in the placebo arm. Given the small size of this trial and the small biomarker effects, a lack in clinical efficacy outcomes was expected [58].

3.2 AD01–04

The AFFITOPE family of vaccines is designed to target aggregated Aβ, the purported toxic species in the genesis of AD [59], by using peptide mimics of the N-terminus of Aβ conjugated to keyhole limpet hemocyanin [60]. It is hypothesized that this approach may have a favorable safety profile since the vaccine lacks the common

T cell epitope that is associated with a pro-inflammatory TH1 response [42] and their controlled specificity allows the production of anti-Aβ antibodies while preventing cross-reactivity with the amyloid precursor protein. The first generation of these vaccines (AD01, AD02) administered with an adjuvant (Alum) was shown to elicit antibody titers to a similar degree as the control $Aβ_{1-6}$ KLH + alum conjugate vaccine in Tg2576 mice. These elicited antibodies have higher reactivity to oligomers and fibrils vs. monomers, recognized Aβ deposits in mouse and human brain sections, and reduced brain amyloid levels in Tg2576 mice without inducing CAA and microhemorrhages [61].

Three Phase 1 clinical trials with AD01 (NCT00495417, NCT00711139, NCT01225809), three Phase 1 trials with AD02 (NCT00633841, NCT00711321, NCT01093664), and a Phase 1 trial with AD03 (NCT01309763) in mild-to-moderate AD patients have been completed. A Phase 2 trial with AD02 in patients with early AD (NCT01117818) has been completed and a Phase 2 (NCT02008513) to evaluate continued administration with AD02 was terminated. The data from Phase 1 studies showed a favorable safety profile with AD02 and AD01 at 1 year [62]. No data is available from the completed Phase 1 study with AD03.

In the double-blind, placebo-controlled, randomized, multi-center, AD02 trial with early AD patients, two dose levels of AD02 were evaluated in combination with one of the two adjuvant formulations vs. placebo (placebo formulation 1, placebo formulation 2, 25 μg AD02 + formulation 1, 25 μg AD02 + formulation 2, 75 μg AD02 + formulation 2). 333 subjects with early AD aged 50–80 years were enrolled and received four monthly injections of the study drug followed by two booster immunizations at months 9 and 15. Surprisingly, only the placebo formulation 2 group showed clinical stabilization and reduced hippocampal atrophy. Affiris, the company developing these compounds, has renamed placebo formulation 2 as "AD04" but no further information is currently available (06 Jun2014: http://www.alzforum.org/news/research-news/surprise-placebo-not-av-vaccine-said-slow-alzheimers; 4 June 2014 PressConference:http://webtv.braintrust.at/affiris/2014-06-04/).

3.3 ACI–24

ACI-24 is a liposome-based vaccine in which two terminal palmitoylated lysine residues are covalently linked at each end of $Aβ_{1-15}$ to anchor the peptide into the liposome [63]. Administration of ACI-24 in double-transgenic APPxPS-1 mice elicited antibody responses mainly of the IgG isotype (IgG1, IgG2b, IgG3) that are either associated with non-inflammatory TH2 or T-cell-independent responses. Further, ACI-24 immunization did not result in significant increases of inflammatory cytokines (IL-1β, IL-6, IFN-γ, or TNF-α) or microglial activation/astrogliosis. APPxPS-1 mice treated with six inoculations of ACI-24 over 3 months showed improvements over control-treated mice in a hippocampal-dependent novel object recognition test. ACI-24 is currently being evaluated in a Phase 1/2, double-blind, randomized, placebo-controlled trial in patients with mild-to-moderate AD (EudraCT 2008-006257-40). Enrolled subjects must be 40–90 years of age, have an MMSE between 18 and 28, and have evidence of brain amyloid burden by amyloid PET imaging. The main objectives of this study are to evaluate the safety, tolerability, immunogenicity, and efficacy of ACI-24 in a 52-week period. Assessments of cognition, function, and fluid/imaging biomarkers are performed.

3.4 CAD106

CAD106 is composed of multiple copies of $A\beta_{1-6}$ conjugated to a carrier, viruslike particle (VLP), derived from *Escherichia coli* RNA bacteriophage $Q\beta$ [64, 65]. Preclinical data [64] showed that CAD106 induced $A\beta$ antibody titers which reduced brain amyloid accumulation in two APP transgenic mouse lines without any increase in microhemorrhages or inflammatory reactions. CAD106 elicited production of antibodies of different IgG subclasses and thus has the potential for different effector functions. Antibody production was similarly elicited by CAD106 in rhesus monkeys and these antibodies were shown to protect from $A\beta$ toxicity in vitro. A case of meningitis was observed in one of the 77 monkeys that were treated with CAD106 with no relation to titers and no occurrence of encephalitis [65].

One Phase 1 study (NCT00411580), two Phase 2 studies (NCT00733863, NCT007795418), and their corresponding extension studies (NCT00956410, NCT01023685) have completed [65]. The Phase 1 study evaluated safety, tolerability, and immunogenicity of CAD106 administered subcutaneously over 52 weeks. This study included 58 patients with mild-to-moderate AD in two cohorts: 50 μg CAD106 or placebo administered at weeks 0, 6, and 18 (cohort 1); or 150 μg CAD106 or placebo at weeks 0, 2, and 6 (cohort 2). Most AEs were mild, with injection-site erythema as the most frequent effect (4 % in cohort I; 64 % in cohort II), while serious AEs were considered unrelated to study medication. CAD106 was associated with an antibody response in 67 % of treated patients in cohort 1 and 82 % patients in cohort 2. These results are consistent with CAD106 only eliciting B-cell and $Q\beta$-related T-cell responses.

In two 52-week, Phase 2a, studies in 58 patients with mild AD, 150 μg CAD106 was administered subcutaneously at weeks 0, 6, and 12 (study 1), or either subcutaneously or intramuscularly at weeks 0, 2, and 6 (study 2). The results of study 1 showed antibody response in 20/22 patients. Because the results indicated that the week 2 injection did not enhance antibody response, a 0/6/12-week regimen was selected for further study. In addition, a Phase 2 study investigating repeated administration of CAD106 intramuscularly has completed (NCT01097096). This study evaluated CAD106 at two doses (150 μg or 450 μg) or placebo at a

7:1 randomization ratio in mild AD patients (MMSE 20–26). Subjects received up to seven injections of CAD106 or placebo over 60 weeks with a follow-up at 78 weeks. One hundred twenty-one patients were enrolled with 106 receiving CAD106 and 15 receiving placebo. Two-thirds of the CAD106-treated patients were classified as strong serological responders. CAD106 was generally safe and well tolerated with four cases of asymptomatic ARIA (3 ARIA-H and 1 ARIA-E) reported. In biomarker substudies, strong serological responders demonstrated reduced brain amyloid load on Florbetapir PET and decreased P-Tau levels in CSF as compared to controls [67]. A large Phase 2/3 prevention trial in persons at risk of developing AD due to APOEε4 homozygote status is planned (NCT02565511).

3.5 Lu AF20513

Lu AF20513 is a therapeutic vaccine constructed of three copies of the B-cell epitope of $A\beta_{42}$ ($A\beta_{1-12}$) attached to P30 and P2 T-helper epitopes from tetanus toxoid (TT), which replaces the T-helper epitopes of $A\beta_{42}$. This construct is intended to reduce the potential for proinflammatory responses and to improve the ability of the elderly to mount an effective immune response by stimulation of pre-existing memory T-helper cells from previous exposure to the TT vaccine [68]. Co-administration of Lu AF20513 with an adjuvant (either CFA/IFA or Quil-A, which has a human use version, QS-21) in an AD transgenic mouse model, Tg2576, induced robust anti-Aβ IgG titers, which are functionally potent based on in vitro assay results. Treatment with Lu AF21503 reduced brain amyloid plaque burden as well as soluble $A\beta_{40}$ and $A\beta_{42}$ in Tg2576 mice brain. Finally, Lu AF21503 reduced glial activation without increasing cerebral amyloid angiopathy or microhemorrhages. Currently, a Phase 1 open-label, dose-escalation, multiple immunization study (NCT02388152; EudraCT 2014-001797-34) is being conducted to evaluate the safety, tolerability, and immunogenicity of Lu AF21503 in patients with mild AD.

3.6 UB-311

The UB-311 immunotherapeutic vaccine consists of the $A\beta_{1-14}$ peptide coupled to the UBITh® helper T-cell epitope. UB-311 is designed for minimization of inflammatory reactivity through the use of a proprietary vaccine delivery system that biases T-helper type 2 regulatory responses in preference to T-helper type 1 pro-inflammatory responses [69]. A Phase 1 open-label clinical trial in mild-to-moderate AD patients (NCT00965588) to evaluate safety, tolerability, and immunogenicity of intramuscularly administered UB-311 at weeks 0, 4, and 12 has been completed. In addition, an observational extension study (NCT01189084) to monitor long-term immunogenicity in subjects enrolled in the original Phase 1 therapeutic trial has also completed. While no data has been posted or published, the company website (United Biomedical, Inc.) stated that UB-311 was safe and well tolerated in the Phase 1 study and that a Phase 2 study is being initiated.

3.7 V950

V950 is a multivalent Aβ compound [70]. Preclinical studies have shown that administration of V950 results in the production of anti-Aβ antibodies in the serum, and CSF that recognizes pyroglutamate-modified and other N-terminally truncated Aβ fragments [70]. A Phase 1 study of V950 in patients with AD has been completed and results are available (www.clinicaltrials.gov; NCT00464334). This study evaluated safety, tolerability, and immunogenicity of i.m. administered V950 formulated with aluminum adjuvant with or without ISCOMATRIX at 0, 2, and 6 months. Four dose levels of V950 (placebo to 0.5, 0.5, 5, or 50 mg) were tested in combination with four dose levels of ISCOMATRIX (0, 16, 47, 94 μg). Subjects were on average 74.2 (± 8.85) years old and 45/86 were female. Anti-Aβ antibody titers measured 1 month post the third immunization ranged from less than baseline or only approximately 2.7-fold higher than baseline. No additional studies have been initiated.

3.8 DNA Amyloid-β Immunotherapy

While still in preclinical evaluations, DNA Aβ vaccines represent the next generation of immunotherapies for AD [71–73]. Since its introduction in the early 1990s as a way to deliver immunogens via genetically engineered DNA, investigators have made much progress on optimizing this platform for eliciting higher antibody responses which are more consistent and sustained [74]. Progress in other disease areas (infectious diseases, HIV, and oncology) has recently led to development of DNA Aβ vaccines for AD. The two main approaches include utilizing viral vectors (either live attenuated or non-live) or naked DNA plasmids and in-tandem fusion of one or multiple copies of the full-length Aβ$_{42}$ (e.g., [75, 76]) or N-terminal Aβ peptides without the T-helper epitope (e.g., [77–79]). The shorter N-terminal peptide DNA vaccines also typically include fusions with a sequence for an immune modulator, such as PADRE (pan human leukocyte antigen DR-binding peptide) that provides a non-self T-helper cell epitope. Immunization with these constructs as seen in other disease areas does not translate to high titers in nonhuman primates or in humans [74]. Large efforts to improve antibody production with different dosing regimen, prime-boost strategies, and optimized delivery methods (e.g., electroporation) are under way (e.g., [80–82]; reviewed in [71–73]) before clinical testing is likely to begin.

4 Benefits and Challenges with Active Immunotherapy

Active immunotherapy offers several advantages over the passive approach. It has the potential of generating persistent therapeutic antibody titers over a longer time period, which obviates the need for frequent re-administration that is required of passive immunotherapy. This simpler mode of administration is appealing in light of the possible need to treat AD early in the disease course and for years thereafter. The antibodies raised with active immunotherapy are likely to be polyclonal responses against different epitopes and IgG subtypes, thus having the potential for greater efficacy against multiple amyloid beta species versus the monoclonal approach with passive immunotherapy. Due to the slow rise to peak titers and the route of administration (intramuscular or subcutaneous), active immunotherapy may also provide a better safety profile compared with monoclonal antibodies, which are typically administered by intravenous infusion that reaches the maximum concentration rapidly post-infusion.

However, as active immunotherapy relies on the patient's own immune response, the extent and nature of anti-Aβ antibody production are likely to vary substantially among individuals. For this reason, some patients may not be able to mount an efficacious antibody titer level, especially in the immunosenescent elderly population [83]. The reduced predictability and control over antibody titers elicited have implications for the number of individuals who would benefit from treatment. Nonresponders would need to be accurately identified and offered other treatment regimens. The time lag to maximum titers also means that it may take a longer time for the onset of therapeutic benefit. Further, if there is an antibody-related safety issue observed once a response is elicited, it would not be easy to turn off an immune system that is already primed to produce antibodies. Finally, the optimum dose regimen needed to achieve the beneficial antibody titers is also an evolving science that will need to be empirically evaluated.

5   Conclusion

The search for the next-generation therapeutics for AD continues despite the lack of success for the last 10 or more years [24, 25, 84, 85]. Active immunotherapy with therapeutic vaccines targeted against the Aβ molecule represents one promising avenue of drug development. Initial experience with AN1792 led to the development of second-generation vaccines that allow for B-cell-generated specific Aβ antibodies that circumvents the T-helper cell-induced proinflammatory responses associated with the safety events observed with AN1792. The optimum titer required to generate a therapeutic benefit is presently not known and will likely relate to the choice of constructs, formulations, and combinations of adjuvant immunomodulators. The dose regimen to obtain such optimum titers is also under evaluation.

Finally, in recognition that AD begins 10–20 years or more before the earliest clinical symptoms appear and prior to dementia onset, there is a growing consensus in the field that intervention at earlier stages of AD may be more impactful [84–87]. To date, most programs for active immunotherapy against Aβ have evaluated patient populations at the mild or mild-to-moderate AD stage, whereas more recent programs are moving towards intervention at a stage before widespread neurodegeneration has occurred. In fact, active immunotherapy may be especially suited for long-term treatment of predementia AD patients who are younger, more active, and healthier than those who have already progressed to the dementia stage.

References

1. Bachman DL, Wolf PA, Linn R et al (1992) Prevalence of dementia and probable senile dementia of the Alzheimer type in the Framingham Study. Neurology 42:115–119
2. Rocca WA, Hofman A, Brayne C et al (1991) Frequency and distribution of Alzheimer's disease in Europe: a collaborative study of 1980-1990 prevalence findings. Ann Neurol 30(3):381–390
3. Cummings JL, Cole G (2002) Alzheimer disease. JAMA 287:2335–2338
4. Cummings JL (2004) Alzheimer's disease. N Engl J Med 351:56–67
5. Brookmeyer R, Johnson E, Zieger-Graham K et al (2007) Forecasting the global burden of Alzheimer's disease. Alzheimers Dement 3:186–191
6. Alzheimer' s Association (2015) Alzheimer's disease facts and figures. Alzheimers Dement 11(3):332
7. Hardy J, Selkoe DJ (2002) The amyloid hypothesis of Alzheimer's disease: progress and problems on the road to therapeutics. Science 297:353–356
8. Selkoe D (2011) Resolving controversies on the path to Alzheimer's therapeutics. Nat Med 17(9):1060–1065
9. Citron M, Oltersdorf T, Haass C et al (1992) Mutation of the J-amyloid precursor protein in familial Alzheimer's disease increases J-protein production. Nature 360:672–674
10. Scheuner D, Eckman C, Jensen M et al (1996) Secreted amyloid beta-protein similar to that in the senile plaques of Alzheimer's disease is increased in vivo by the presenilin 1 and 2 and APP mutations linked to familial Alzheimer's disease. Nat Med 2:864–870
11. Citron M, Westaway D, Xia W et al (1997) Mutant presenilins of Alzheimer's disease increase production of 42-residue amyloid beta-protein in both transfected cells and transgenic mice. Nat Med 3(1):67–72
12. Mawuenyega K, Sigurdson W, Oyod V et al (2010) Decreased clearance of CNS beta amyloid in AD. Science 330(6012):1774
13. Holtzman DM, Morris JC, Goate AM (2011) Alzheimer's disease: the challenge of the second century. Sci Transl Med 3:77sr1
14. Bertram L, Tanzi RE (2012) The genetics of Alzheimer's disease. Prog Mol Biol Transl Sci 107:79–100
15. Jonsson T, Atwal J, Steinberg S et al (2012) A mutation in APP protects against Alzheimer's disease and age-related cognitive decline. Nature 488:96–99
16. Grimmer T, Tholen S, Yousefi BH et al (2010) Progression of cerebral amyloid load is associated with the apolipoprotein E ε-4 genotype in Alzheimer's disease. Biol Psychiatry 68:879–884
17. Castellano JM, Kim JS, Stewart FR et al (2011) Human apoE isoforms differentially regulate brain amyloid-β peptide clearance. Science Translational Medicine 9(89):89ra57. doi:10.1126/scitranslmed.3002156
18. Caccamo A, Oddo S, Sugarman MC et al (2005) Age- and region-dependent alterations in Abeta-degrading enzymes: implications for Abeta-induced disorders. Neurobiol Aging 26(5):645–654
19. Jin M, Shepardson N, Yang T et al (2011) Soluble amyloid beta-protein dimers isolated from Alzheimer cortex directly induce Tau hyperphosphorylation and neuritic degeneration. PNAS 108(14):5819–5824
20. Braak H, Thal DR, Ghebremedhin E et al (2011) Stages of the pathologic process in Alzheimer's disease: age categories from 1 to 100 years. J Neuropathol Exp Neurol 70(11):960–969
21. Knapp MJ, Knopman DS, Solomon PR et al (1994) A 30-week randomized controlled trial of high-dose tacrine in patients with

Alzheimer's disease. The Tacrine Study Group. JAMA 271:985–991

22. Rogers SL, Doody RS, Mohs RC (1998) Donepezil improves cognition and global function in Alzheimer disease: a 15-week, double-blind, placebo-controlled study. Donepezil Study Group. Arch Intern Med 158:1021–1031

23. Trinh NH, Hoblyn J, Mohanty S et al (2003) Efficacy of cholinesterase inhibitors in the treatment of neuropsychiatric symptoms and functional impairment in Alzheimer disease. JAMA 289:210–216

24. Schneider L, Mangialasche F, Andreasen N et al (2014) Clinical trials and late-stage drug development for Alzheimer's disease: an appraisal from 1984 to 2014. J Intern Med 275(3):251–283

25. Cummings JL, Morstorf T, Zhong K (2014) Alzheimer's disease drug-development pipeline: few candidates, frequent failures. Alzheimers Res Ther 6:37

26. Schenk D, Barbour R, Dunn W et al (1999) Immunization with amyloid-β attenuates Alzheimer disease-like pathology in the PDAPP mouse. Nature 400:173–177

27. Town T (2009) Alternative Aβ immunotherapy approaches for Alzheimer's disease. CNS Neurol Disord Drug Targets 8(2):114–127

28. Fu HJ, Liu B, Frost JL, Lemere CA (2010) Amyloid-β immunotherapy for Alzheimer's disease. CNS Neurol Disord Drug Targets 9(2):197–206

29. Schenk D, Basi GS, Pangalos MN (2012) Treatment strategies targeting amyloid β-protein. Cold Spring Harb Perspect Med 2:a006387

30. Bard F, Cannon C, Barbour R et al (2000) Peripherally administered antibodies against amyloid β peptide enter the central nervous system and induce pathology in a mouse model of Alzheimer disease. Nature 6:916–919

31. Bacskai BJ, Hickey GA, Skoch J et al (2003) Four-dimensional multiphoton imaging of brain entry, amyloid binding, and clearance of an amyloid-beta ligand in transgenic mice. Proc Natl Acad Sci U S A 100(21):12462–7

32. Games D, Adams D, Alessandrini R et al (1995) Alzheimer-type neuropathology in transgenic mice overexpressing V717F β-amyloid precursor protein. Nature 373:523–527

33. Wisniewski T, Boutajangout A (2010) Immunotherapeutic approaches for Alzheimer's disease in transgenic mouse models. Brain Struct Funct 214:201–218

34. Schenk D, Hagen M, Seubert P (2004) Current progress in β-amyloid immunotherapy. Curr Opin Immunol 16:599–606

35. Shankar GM, Li S, Mehta TH et al (2008) Amyloid-beta protein dimers isolated directly from Alzheimer's brains impair synaptic plasticity and memory. Nat Med 14(8):837–42

36. Zago W, Buttini M, Comery TA et al (2012) Neutralization of soluble, synaptotoxic amyloid β species by antibodies is epitope specific. J Neurosci 32(8):2696–2702

37. Bayer A, Bullock R, Jones RW et al (2005) Evaluation of the safety and immunogenicity of synthetic Aβ42 (AN1792) in patients with AD. Neurology 64:94–101

38. Gilman S, Koller M, Black RSK et al (2005) Clinical effects of Abeta immunization (AN1792) in patients with AD in an interrupted trial. Neurology 64:1553–1562

39. Lee M, Bard F, Johnson-Wood K et al (2005) Aβ42 immunization in Alzheimer's disease generates Aβ N-terminal antibodies. Ann Neurol 58:430–435

40. Orgogozo JM, Gilman S, Dartigues JF et al (2003) Subacute meningoencephalitis in a subset of patients with AD after Abeta42 immunization. Neurology 61:46–54

41. Vellas B, Black R, Thal LJ et al (2009) Long-term follow-up of patients immunized with AN1792: reduced functional decline in antibody responders. Curr Alzheimer Res 6:144–151

42. Pride M, Seubert P, Grundman M et al (2008) Progress in the active immunotherapeutic approach to Alzheimer's disease: clinical investigations into AN1792-associated meningoencephalitis. Neurodegener Dis 5:194–196

43. Ferrer I, Rovira MB, Guerra MLS et al (2004) Neuropathology and pathogenesis of encephalitis following amyloid-β immunization in Alzheimer's disease. Brain Pathol 14:11–20

44. Fox NC, Black RS, Gilman S et al (2005) Effects of Abeta immunization (AN1792) on MRI measures of cerebral volume in Alzheimer disease. Neurology 64:1563–1572

45. Nicoll JAR, Wilkinson D, Homes C et al (2003) Neuropathology of human Alzheimer disease after immunization with amyloid-β peptide: a case report. Nat Med 9:448–452

46. Masliah E, Hansen L, Adame A et al (2005) Abeta vaccination effects on plaque pathology in the absence of encephalitis in Alzheimer disease. Neurology 64:129–131

47. Holmes C, Boche D, Wilkinson D et al (2008) Long-term effects of Aβ42 immunization in Alzheimer's disease: follow-up of a randomized,

placebo-controlled phase 1 trial. Lancet 372:216–223

48. Boche D, Denham N, Holmes C et al (2010) Neuropathology after active Aβ42 immuno-therapy: implications for Alzheimer's disease pathogenesis. Acta Neuropathol 120:369–384

49. Serrano-Pozo A, William CM, Ferrer I et al (2010) Beneficial effect of human anti-amy-loid-b active immunization on neurite mor-phology and tau pathology. Brain 133:1312–1327

50. Lobello K, Ryan JM, Liu E et al (2012) Targeting beta amyloid: a clinical review of immunotherapeutic approaches in Alzheimer's disease. Int J Alzheimers Dis 2012:628070. doi:10.1155/2012/628070

51. Winblad B, Graf A, Riviere ME et al (2014) Active immunotherapy options for Alzheimer's disease. Alzheimers Res Ther 6:7

52. Hagen M, Seubert P, Jacobsen S et al (2011) The Aβ peptide conjugate vaccine, Acc-001, generates N-terminal anti-Aβ antibodies in the absence of Aβ directed T-cell responses [abstract]. Alzheimers Dement 7:S460–S461

53. Basi GS, Feinberg H, Oshidari F et al (2010) Structural correlates of antibodies associated with acute reversal of amyloid-related behav-ioral deficits in a mouse model of Alzheimer's disease. J Biol Chem 285(5):3417–3427. doi:10.1074/jbc.M109.045187

54. Arai H, Suzuki H, Yoshiyama T (2015) Vanutide cridificar and the QS-21 adjuvant in Japanese subjects with mild to moderate Alzheimer's disease: Results from two Phase 2 studies. Curr Alzheimer Res 12:242–254

55. Sperling RA, Jack CR, Black SE et al (2011) Amyloid related imaging abnormalities (ARIA) in amyloid modifying therapeutic trials: recom-mendations from the Alzheimer's Association Research Roundtable Workgroup. Alzheimers Dement 7(4):367–385

56. Margolin R, Ketter N, Guthrie S et al. (2013) Biomarker strategy for enrichment and assess-ment of biological effect in a Phase 2 study of ACC-001, an anti-Aβ vaccine for Alzheimer's disease. Poster presentation. July 2013 AAIC Boston, MA USA

57. Salloway S, Sperling R, Gregg K et al. (2013) Characterization of the clinical course of placebo-treated amyloid-negative subjects with mild-moderate Alzheimer's disease (AD): results from the Phase 3 PET sub-studies of bapineuzumab and solanezumab. Poster presentation. July 2013 AAIC Boston, MA USA

58. Ketter N, Liu E, Di J, et al (2014) A phase 2 randomized double-blind placebo-controlled study of Vanutide Cridificar vaccine (ACC-001) in patients with mild-to-moderate Alzheimer's disease. Poster presentation at 7th Clinical Trials Conference on Alzheimer's disease, Philadelphia, PA, November 20–22, 2014

59. Mucke L, Selkoe DJ (2012) Neurotoxicity of amyloid β-protein: synaptic and network dys-function. Cold Spring Harb Perspect Med 2:a006338

60. Schneeberger A, Mandler M, Otawa O et al (2009) Development of AFFITOPE vaccines for Alzheimer's disease (AD) –from concept to clinical testing. J Nutr Health Aging 3:264–267

61. Mandler M, Santic R, Gruber P et al (2015) Tailoring the antibody response to aggregated Aβ using novel Alzheimer vaccines. PLoS ONE. doi:10.1371/journal.pone.0115237

62. Mandler M, Santic R, Weninger H et al (2009) The MimoVax vaccine: a novel Alzheimer treatment strategy targeting truncated Aβ40/42 by active immunization [abstract]. Alzheimers Dement 5:114

63. Muhs A, Hickman DT, Pihlgren M et al (2007) Liposomal vaccines with conformation-specific amyloid peptide antigens define immune response and efficacy in APP transgenic mice. PNAS 104(23):9810–9815

64. Wiessner C, Wiederhold K-H, Tissot AC et al (2011) The second generation active Aβ immunotherapy CAD106 reduces amyloid accumulation in APP transgenic mice while minimizing potential side effects. J Neurosci 31(25):9323–9331

65. Winblad B, Andreasen N, Minthon L et al (2012) Safety, tolerability, and antibody response of active Aβ immunotherapy with CAD106 in patients with Alzheimer's disease: randomised, double-blind, placebo-controlled, first-in-human study. Lancet Neurol 11:597–604

66. Farlow MR, Andreasen N, Riviere M-E et al (2015) Long-term treatment with active Aβ immunotherapy with CAD106 in mild Alzheimer's disease. Alzheimers Res Ther 7:23. doi:10.1186/s13195-015-0108-3

67. Graf A, Riviere ME, Caputo A et al (2014) Active Aβ immunotherapy CAD106 Phase II dose-adjuvant finding study: safety and CNS biomarkers. Alzheimers Dement 10(4):274. doi:http://dx.doi.org/10.1016/j.jalz.2014.04.448

68. Davtyan H, Ghochikyan A, Petrushina I et al (2013) Immunogenicity, efficacy, safety, and mechanism of action of epitope vaccine (Lu AF20513) for Alzheimer's disease: prelude to a clinical trial. J Neurosci 33:4923–4934

69. Wang CY, Finstad CL, Walfield AM et al (2007) Site-specific UBITh amyloid-beta vaccine for immunotherapy of Alzheimer's disease. Vaccine 25:3041–3052

70. Savage MJ, Wu G, McCampbell A et al (2010) A novel multivalent Abeta peptide vaccine with preclinical evidence of a central immune response that generates antisera recognizing a wide range of Abeta peptide species. [abstract]. Alzheimers Dement 6(4):S142

71. Cribbs DH (2010) Abeta DNA vaccination for Alzheimer's disease: focus on disease prevention. CNS Neruol Disord Drug Targets 9(2):207–216

72. Alves RPS, Yang MJ, Batista MT et al (2014) Alzheimer's disease: is a vaccine possible? Braz J Med Biol Res 47(6):438–444

73. Kudrna JJ, Ungen KE (2015) Gene-based vaccines and immunotherapeutic strategies against neurodegenerative diseases: Potential utility and limitations. Hum Vaccin Immunother 11(8):1921–1926

74. Kutzler MA, Weiner DB (2008) DNA vaccines: ready for prime time? Nat Rev Genet 9(10):776–788

75. Matsumoto Y, Niimi N, Kohyama K (2013) Development of a new DNA vaccine for Alzheimer's disease targeting a wide range of Aβ species and amyloidogenic peptides. PLoS One e75203. doi:10.1371/journal.pone.0075203

76. Lambracht-Washington D, Rosenberg RN (2012) Active DNA Aβ42 vaccination as immunotherapy for Alzheimer's disease. Transl Neurosci 3(4):307–313

77. Agadjanyan MG, Ghochikyan A, Petrushina I et al (2005) Prototype Alzheimer's disease vaccine using the immunodominant B cell epitope from beta-amyloid and promiscuous T cell epitope pan HLA DR-binding peptide. J Immunol 174:1580–1586

78. Movsesyan N, Ghochikyan A, Mkrtichyan M et al (2008) Reducing AD-like pathology in 3xTg-AD mouse model by DNA epitope vaccine – a novel immunotherapeutic strategy. PLoS One 3:e2124

79. Guo W, Sha S, Jiang T, Xing X, Cao Y et al (2013) A new DNA vaccine fused with the C3d-p28 induces a Th2 immune response against amyloid-beta. Neural Regen Res 8(27):2581–2590

80. Lambracht-Washington D, Qu B-X, Fu M et al (2013) A peptide prime-DNA boost immunization protocol provides significant benefits as a new generation Aβ42 DNA vaccine for Alzheimer's disease. J Neuroimmunol 254:63–68

81. Liu S, Shi DY, Wang HC et al (2014) Co-immunization with DNA and protein mixture: a safe and efficacious immunotherapeutic strategy for Alzheimer's disease in PDAPP mice. Sci Rep 5:7771. doi:10.1038/srep0777

82. Wang S, Yu Y, Geng S et al (2013) A coimmunization vaccine of Aβ42 ameliorates cognitive deficits without brain inflammation in an Alzheimer's disease model. Alzheimers Res Ther 6:26

83. Grubeck-Loebenstein B, Della Bella S, Iorio AM et al (2009) Immunosenescence and vaccine failure in the elderly. Aging Clin Exp Res 21:201–209

84. Salloway S, Sperling R, Fox NC et al (2014) Two phase 3 trials of bapineuzumab in mild-to-moderate Alzheimer's disease. N Engl J Med 370(4):322–33

85. Doody RS, Thomas RG, Farlow M et al (2014) Phase 3 trials of solanezumab for mild-to-moderate Alzheimer's disease. N Engl J Med 370(4):311–21

86. Sperling RA, Rentz DM, Johnson KA et al (2014) The A4 study: stopping AD before symptoms begin? Sci Transl Med 6(228):228fs13. doi:10.1126/scitranslmed.3007941

87. Mattsson N, Carrillo MC, Dean RA et al (2015) Revolutionizing Alzheimer's disease and clinical trials through biomarkers. Alzheimers Dement (Amst) 1:412–419

Chapter 3

Immunotherapy Against N-Truncated Amyloid-β Oligomers

Thomas A. Bayer and Oliver Wirths

Abstract

Immunotherapy against aggregated proteins has received considerable attention in the field of neurodegenerative disorders, especially true for Alzheimer's disease (AD), which is characterized by the presence of extracellular amyloid-Aβ plaques and intraneuronal neurofibrillary tangles consisting of tau protein. Numerous studies have demonstrated that the amyloid cascade triggers tau pathology, with tau being intimately involved in the molecular mechanisms leading to neuron death in AD. We and others therefore believe that Aβ is the trigger and tau is the executer of neurodegeneration. The nature of neurotoxic Aβ is still enigmatic, because amyloid-plaque structures that harbor high levels of Aβ are not correlating with the symptoms of AD, nor do they trigger neuron loss. New hypotheses have emerged trying to explain this conundrum. One is that amyloid plaques, although built as a consequence of high Aβ levels in brain, are acting as a waste bin, thereby keeping toxic Aβ aggregates locally fixed in a nontoxic form. Another hypothesis claims that intraneuronal Aβ aggregation triggers neuron loss and lastly many researchers believe that soluble Aβ aggregates of full-length $A\beta_{1-42}$ are the major trigger for the amyloid cascade of pathological events. On the other side, $A\beta_{1-42}$ has consistently been shown to aggregate fast into amyloid fibrils that are the building blocks of amyloid plaques while it should not be forgotten that full-length $A\beta_{1-42}$ is a physiological peptide produced throughout our life-span. There is now increasing evidence that N-truncated Aβ variants represent better drug targets than full-length Aβ. Full-length Aβ peptides start with an aspartate at position 1 (Asp-1) and end with alanine at position 42 (Ala-42). In AD brain, two N-truncated species are especially highly abundant: Pyroglutamate $A\beta_{3-42}$ ($A\beta_{pE3-42}$) starts with a transformation of Glu to pyroglutamate at position three (pyroGlu-3), and $A\beta_{4-42}$ starts with Phe at position four (Phe-4). In contrast to pan-Aβ antibodies or antibodies that recognize all forms of pyroglutamate $A\beta_{3-42}$ those antibodies that recognize exclusively oligomeric forms of pyroglutamate $A\beta_{3-42}$ and/or $A\beta_{4-42}$ have a low tendency to detect amyloid plaques. Both variants form soluble aggregates, have a high aggregation propensity, and have toxic properties in cell culture assays. Once expressed in neurons in transgenic mouse brain, they induce massive neuron loss associated with behavioral deficits. Interestingly, only minor plaque load is seen in these models arguing for a toxic mechanism of soluble aggregates of pyroglutamate $A\beta_{3-42}$ and $A\beta_{4-42}$. Therefore, we believe that these oligomer-specific antibodies will provide excellent tools for drug development to fight AD.

Key words Transgene model, Plaques, Pyroglutamate Abeta, Abeta 4–42, Neurodegeneration, Neuropathology, Neuron loss

Martin Ingelsson and Lars Lannfelt (eds.), *Immunotherapy and Biomarkers in Neurodegenerative Disorders*, Methods in Pharmacology and Toxicology, DOI 10.1007/978-1-4939-3560-4_3, © Springer Science+Business Media New York 2016

1   Introduction

Alzheimer's disease (AD) is a progressive neurodegenerative disorder characterized by the presence of extracellular amyloid plaques composed of amyloid-β (Aβ) surrounded by dystrophic neurites and neurofibrillary tangles. Aβ is produced by proteolytic cleavage of the larger β-amyloid precursor protein (APP) [1]. The correlation of mutant genes present in early-onset familial forms of AD together with enhanced production of Aβ peptides led to the hypothesis that amyloidogenic Aβ is closely involved in the AD pathogenic process [2]. In addition to full-length Aβ peptides starting with aspartate at position one of the Aβ sequence, a variety of N-terminally truncated and/or posttranslationally modified Aβ peptides have been described in the literature (reviewed in [3]). These modifications include isomerization [4] which has been shown to enhance Aβ peptide aggregation and the formation of fibrils [5] or other modifications like phosphorylation [6] or metal-induced oxidation [7]. In recent years, pyroglutamate-modified Aβ peptides have gained considerable attention, as augmented toxicity and aggregation propensity, together with increased stability and high abundance in AD brain, have been repeatedly described for such species (reviewed in [8]).

There is accumulating evidence that pyroGlu-modified Aβ peptides might represent a worthwhile target for immunotherapy approaches [3, 9]. In current therapeutic phase III clinical trials, the effects of passive immunotherapy against Aβ have been tested [10, 11] or are currently ongoing.

2   Evidence from Postmortem Human Brain

Three recent reviews already covered the potential role of N-truncated Aβ peptides in AD pathology in detail [3, 8, 9]. Although a vast heterogeneity of N-terminal truncations of Aβ peptides extracted from amyloid plaques from sporadic and familial AD cases was reported by several groups, there is increasing knowledge that the two variants $A\beta_{4-x}$ (Phe-4) and pyroglutamate $A\beta_{pE3-x}$ (pyroGlu-3) are those with the highest abundance [3] (Fig. 1). N-truncated Aβ peptides have already been discovered in 1985 by Masters et al. [12]. It could be demonstrated that the majority of peptides extracted from sporadic AD cases and of patients with Down's syndrome started with Phe-4 while full-length Aβ beginning with Asp-1 was the main peptide in vascular deposits as shown by Glenner and Wong [13]. Shortly thereafter Selkoe and co-workers [14] reported that the plaque core was unsequenceable, although by using pyroglutamate amino peptidase the same group reported that the N-terminus could be de-blocked, leading to the

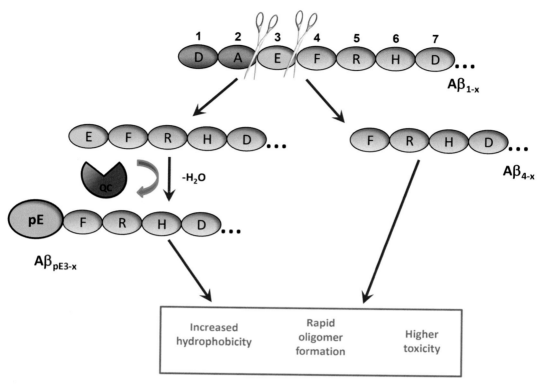

Fig. 1 N-truncation of Aβ peptides leading to pyroglutamate $Aβ_{3-x}$ and $Aβ_{4-x}$ (adapted from and reviewed in [8]). For the generation of pyroglutamate $Aβ_{3-x}$ the first step is the cleavage of the two N-terminal amino acid residues by unknown protease(s). Next, enzymatic catalysis by glutaminyl cyclase (QC) transforms N-terminal glutamate (E) into pyroglutamate (pE). The generation of $Aβ_{4-x}$ does not require a posttranslational modification. The first three N-terminal amino acid residues are cleaved by unknown protease(s) directly generating $Aβ_{4-x}$

discovery of pyroGlu-3 in AD plaques [15]. By applying different techniques, several groups corroborated these results in the brain of patients with sporadic and inherited forms of AD and verified that the N-terminus of plaque-Aβ is quite heterogeneous, bearing high levels of pyroglutamate $Aβ_{3-42}$ and $Aβ_{4-42}$ [2, 16–29]. A final conclusion on the exact levels of the various N-truncated Aβ variants is challenging [3], which is mainly due to different methods, tools, and brain samples that have been used to extract the various Aβ pools. There are numerous factors that can influence the respective analysis, ranging from variations in antibody specificities and sensitivities used for immunostaining, Western blotting, or immunoprecipitation, as well as extraction protocols and brain areas studied [3]. Most consistently, high amounts of N-truncated Aβ starting with Phe-4 and pyroGlu-3 were reported. In presymptomatic AD cases, Phe-4 has been demonstrated to represent the N-truncated variant appearing initially [24].

Most of the abovementioned studies have analyzed the brains with biochemical techniques. However, the use of conformation-specific

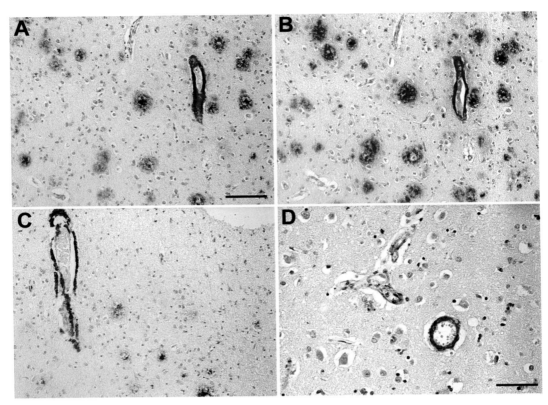

Fig. 2 Comparative immunostaining against pan-Aβ and N-truncated Aβ peptides Aβ$_{pE3-X}$ and Aβ$_{4-X}$ in the brain of patients with sporadic Alzheimer's disease. Staining was performed with antibodies 4G8 ((**a**), epitope Aβ$_{17-24}$), 1-57 ((**b**), against Aβ$_{pE3-X}$; Synaptic Systems [30]), 9D5 ((**c**), against oligomeric Aβ$_{pE3-X}$; Synaptic Systems [108]), and NT4X-167 ((**d**), against oligomeric Aβ$_{4-X}$; [32]). Scale bar: (**a**)–(**c**) = 100 μm, (**d**) = 50 μm

antibodies is important to better understand the spatial and cellular distribution of those peptides in brain. While antibodies directed against all aggregates ranging from monomers to high-molecular-weight aggregates of pyroGlu Aβ detect virtually all amyloid plaques in AD brain [30], those that recognize only oligomeric forms like the 9D5 antibody do only rarely stain plaques (Fig. 2) [31]. The same staining pattern is seen with antibodies against oligomeric Aβ4-X like the NT4X antibody (Fig. 2) [32].

3   Pyroglutamate-Aβ in Transgenic Mouse Models of AD

While the presence of pyroGlu-modified and other N-terminal truncated Aβ peptides has been described in human AD patients since many years, there is more recently also a growing body of literature on the identification of these peptides in various transgenic mouse models of AD. One major difference between human brains and these animal models is the relative amount of pyroGlu-modified Aβ peptides, as well as of N-terminal truncated Aβ peptides in general. It has been demonstrated that Aβ$_{pE3-42}$ comprised ~25 % of the overall amount of Aβ peptides in plaques of AD brains [33] with ~80 % of all peptides showing N-truncations. The levels in, e.g., the widely used Tg2576 model are far lower, with some reports indicating an absence of pyroGlu-modified peptides [34] whereas other studies show that even in very old Tg2576 mice at 23 months of age only 5 % of all Aβ peptides harbor an N-terminal truncation [35]. The widely used APP23 mouse model [36] also harbors only small amounts of Aβ$_{pE3}$ in aged animals [28] and the scarcity of these peptides has been attributed to the rather narrow life-span of these animals in comparison to the human situation where development of the full-blown disease might take decades [37]. Some mouse models expressing mutant human presenilin 1 (PSEN1) in addition to human mutant amyloid precursor protein (APP) have been demonstrated to harbor considerable amounts of pyroGlu-modified and other N-truncated Aβ peptides. In a recent comparative study investigating an array of different mouse lines, Aβ$_{pE3}$-positive amyloid deposits have been demonstrated by immunohistochemistry in all models analyzed (among them, e.g., 3×Tg, APP/PS1ΔE9, and TgCRND8), although in varying amounts [38].

In APP/PS1KI mice, expressing human mutant APP on a mutant PS1 knock-in background, a variety of N-truncated Aβ peptides have been identified by 2D-gel electrophoresis in combination with mass spectrometry. Different time points have been analyzed and, e.g., Aβ$_{4/5-x}$ could be detected already at 2.5 months of age and Aβ$_{pE3}$ at 6 months of age [39]. Ensuing immunohistochemical studies corroborated the presence of Aβ$_{pE3}$-positive deposits at 6 months of age and led to the identification of intraneuronal Aβ$_{pE3}$immunoreactivity at already 2 months of age in motor neurons of the spinal cord [40], as well as in the CA1 pyramidal neurons of the hippocampus preceding neuron loss in this brain region [41]. Analysis of cortical Aβ$_{pE3}$ deposits revealed an interesting finding: while Aβ$_{pE3}$-positive amyloid plaques increased significantly with aging, plaques with immunoreactivity for full-length Aβ starting with aspartic acid at position 1 showed a concomitant decrease in abundance, although the overall plaque load was unchanged. This leads to the assumption that the formation of pyroGlu-modified extracellular deposits is a rather late phenomenon that depends on rearrangements of pre-existing plaques [30]. A further double-transgenic model showing fast disease progression with ample distribution in the research community is the 5XFAD model [42]. This model also develops an abundant age-dependent deposition of pyroGlu-modified Aβ peptides in extracellular plaques, with behavioral deficits and cortical neuron loss at later stages [43]. In order to investigate the effect of increased Aβ$_{pE3}$ formation in more detail, 5XFAD mice were crossed with mice overexpressing glutaminyl cyclase (QC) under the control of the neuron-specific Thy1 promotor. The resulting 5XFAD/QC mice showed significantly higher levels of soluble and insoluble $A\beta_{pE3-42}$ peptides, an increased plaque load, as well as an aggravated behavioral phenotype [44]. In addition, the influence of endogenous QC was investigated and 5XFAD/QC-knockout mice that lacked endogenous QC in a homozygous manner were generated. In accordance with an important role of QC in pyroGlu formation, 5XFAD/QC-KO mice showed a drastic reduction in $A\beta_{pE3-42}$ levels, a reduced extracellular amyloid plaque load, and a rescue of the behavioral deficit [44], clearly proving that QC is an essential enzyme in the generation of pyroGlu-modified $A\beta$ peptides.

As almost all of the currently used mouse models of AD express mutant human APP and/or mutant human PSEN1, they only represent useful models for the early onset, very rare familial forms of AD (FAD). Recently, novel transgenic models have been described that express only N-truncated $A\beta$ peptides in the absence of human APP overexpression and without the use of FAD-related mutations. The TBA2 [45], TBA2.1 [46], and TBA42 [47] models overexpress a transgenic construct comprising the thyrotropin-releasing hormone (TRH) signal peptide fused to $A\beta_{Q3-42}$ under the control of the murine Thy1 promotor. The N-terminal glutamine (Q) residue at position 3 of $A\beta$ facilitates the conversion to $A\beta_{pE3-42}$ and represents a proper substrate for QC that catalyzes this reaction [48]. Heterozygous TBA2 mice as well as homozygous TBA2.1 revealed an abundant neuron loss in the Purkinje cell layer of the cerebellum and the hippocampus, respectively, and disclosed $A\beta_{pE3}$-positive intraneuronal immunoreactivity [45, 46]. The influence of $A\beta_{pE3-42}$ on full-length $A\beta$ with regard to a potential seeding effect has been investigated by crossing 5XFAD and TBA42 mice. At the age of 6 months, amyloid plaque load and soluble and insoluble $A\beta$ levels were analyzed in the resulting FAD42 mice. ELISA measurements as well as plaque load analysis revealed an increased $A\beta_{pE3-x}$ level; however, mass spectrometry analysis did not detect any major changes in $A\beta_{x-42}$ or other $A\beta$ species. Nevertheless an aggravated behavioral phenotype compared to the single transgenic parental 5XFAD and TBA42 lines was evident [47]. The data suggests that although $A\beta_{pE3-x}$ is still only present in minor amounts compared to $A\beta_{1-42}$, even small increases in $A\beta_{pE3-x}$ might have considerable effects.

We have recently developed the novel transgenic mouse model Tg4-42 that resembles sporadic AD as it develops a hippocampus neuron loss associated with spatial reference memory deficits [49]. Tg4–42 mice express wild-type human $A\beta_{4-42}$ in the CA1 neurons of the hippocampus. Detailed behavioral and neuropathological analyses revealed that aged Tg4-42 mice show an abundant neuron loss in the CA1 region of the hippocampus together with severe deficits in spatial reference memory. Breeding these mice to homozygosity led to a shift in these pathological alterations toward an earlier onset [49, 50]. Moreover, the antibody NT4X, specific for the N-terminus of $A\beta_{4-x}$, showed prominent staining of intraneuronal $A\beta$ in young 5XFAD mice which might indicate an early risk factor for neuronal loss [32]. Intraneuronal accumulation of pyro-Glu $A\beta$ was not found in young 5XFAD mice.

4 Evidence from In Vitro Studies

There is also evidence from cell culture experiments that N-truncation of $A\beta$ leads to increased toxicity. N-truncated $A\beta_{x-40}$ peptides exhibited an enhanced aggregation and neurotoxicity in comparison to full-length $A\beta_{1-40}$ in vitro, while no difference was reported between full-length $A\beta_{1-42}$ and the other truncated $A\beta_{x-42}$ peptides [51]. $A\beta$ starting with Asp-1, Phe-4, Ser-8, Val-12, and Lys-17 were compared. The authors concluded that N-terminal deletions enhance aggregation of $A\beta$ into neurotoxic, β-sheet fibrils and suggested that such peptides may initiate and/or nucleate the pathological deposition of $A\beta$ into plaques. Others reported that pyroGlu-3 was found to be more neurotoxic as compared to full-length $A\beta$ [52]. PyroGlu-3-modified $A\beta$ peptides displayed dramatically accelerated initial formation of aggregates compared to unmodified full-length $A\beta$ [53]. The N-terminal pyroGlu-3 and pyroGlu-11 modifications revealed a decrease of solubility which was accompanied by an increase in hydrophobicity [54]. There is increasing evidence that soluble small and diffusible $A\beta$ oligomers represent the earliest and most toxic assemblies in AD [55] and it has been demonstrated that soluble $A\beta_{1-42}$ and $A\beta_{pE3-42}$ oligomers induced neuronal cell death in primary neuron cultures [56].

Nussbaum et al. [57] reported that $A\beta_{pE3-42}$ and $A\beta_{1-42}$ form metastable, cytotoxic, hybrid oligomers possessing a prion-like activity and a recent study suggested that $A\beta_{pE3-42}$ undergoes faster formation of prefibrillar aggregates due to its increased hydrophobicity, thus shifting the initial stages of fibrillogenesis toward smaller hypertoxic oligomers of partial α-helical structure [58]. Bouter et al. [49] demonstrated that soluble aggregates of $A\beta_{4-42}$ and pyroGlu $A\beta_{pE3-42}$ are unstructured in the monomeric state. Following heating, both $A\beta$ variants showed a high propensity to form folded structures. Oligomeric $A\beta_{4-42}$ and $A\beta_{pE3-42}$ were rapidly converted to soluble aggregated species under consumption of their respective monomers. These soluble aggregates were capable of converting into ThT-reactive fibrillar aggregates with $A\beta_{4-42}$ and $A\beta_{pE3-42}$ showing significant ThT reactivity already during the nucleation phase of aggregation. Like $A\beta_{1-42}$ and $A\beta_{pE3-42}$, $A\beta_{4-42}$ peptides also possessed neurotoxic properties in cell-based assays.

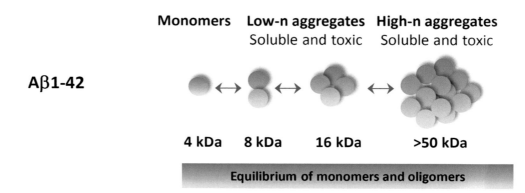

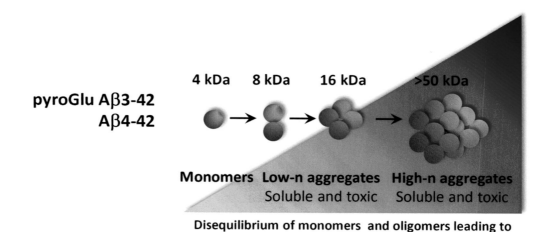

Fig. 3 N-truncated pyroglutamate Aβ$_{3-42}$ and Aβ$_{4-42}$ are more toxic as compared to full-length Aβ$_{1-42}$ due to enhanced levels of soluble oligomers. *Upper graph*: Monomers and low- and high-molecular-weight aggregates of **Aβ1_42** are in **equilibrium**. As Aβ$_{1-42}$ is a physiological peptide, which is continuously generated also in healthy individuals, the level of oligomeric Aβ$_{1-42}$ is tightly regulated. *Lower graph*: Soluble monomers, low- and high-molecular-weight aggregates of N-truncated **pyroglutamate Aβ3_42 and Aβ4_42** are in **disequilibrium**. The level of soluble oligomeric aggregates of N-truncated Aβ variants increases over time, thereby triggering in AD pathology (adapted from [3])

The novel antibody NT4X specific for oligomeric Aβ$_{4-42}$ rescued toxicity of Aβ$_{4-42}$ in vitro, but not that of full-length Aβ$_{1-42}$ [32].

A scheme of the different pathological features of full-length Aβ$_{1-42}$ on one side and the two truncated versions Aβ$_{4-42}$ and Aβ$_{pE3-42}$ on the other side is shown in Fig. 3.

5 Evidence from Preclinical Trials

In recent years, immunotherapy approaches by using either active or passive immunization strategies received considerable attention in the AD research field. Initial pioneering preclinical studies in the PDAPP mouse model using active immunization with the full-length $A\beta_{1-42}$ peptide revealed a prevention of amyloid plaque formation in young animals, while treatment of aged mice reduced the progression of AD-related pathological changes [59]. Subsequent clinical trials have been conducted, which however had to be stopped after a substantial number of patients developed adverse reactions in terms of meningoencephalitis [60]. This has been mainly attributed to the presence of T-cell epitopes in the mid- and C-terminal portion of $A\beta_{1-42}$ [61].

Passive immunization using $A\beta$ antibodies also showed promising results in preclinical studies using transgenic AD mouse models [62, 63] and therefore clinical trials were conducted shortly thereafter. However, passive immunization approaches also bear the risk of undesired side effects as, e.g., cerebral hemorrhages have been reported as a consequence of the clearance of vascular $A\beta$ deposits [64, 65]. Recently, the results of several large phase III passive immunization trials employing more than 2000 mild-to-moderate AD patients using bapineuzumab, the first humanized antibody in clinical studies, have been disclosed. Although treatment differences in biomarkers were detected in ApoE4 carriers, no improvement in clinical outcomes was noted among AD patients [11]. The same holds true for two trials investigating the effects of solanezumab in mild-to-moderate AD patients, which as well showed no significant improvement in the primary outcome measures when analyzed independently [10]. However, analysis of pooled data from both trials showed a significant reduction in cognitive decline in mild AD patients but these results rose questions whether the concept of the amyloid cascade hypothesis is still valid [66].

Analyses of naturally occurring antibodies in the plasma of AD patients and non-demented control individuals have revealed the presence of autoantibodies against a variety of $A\beta$ species. In one study, reactivity against oligomeric assemblies of $A\beta$ peptides was found to decline with progression of AD, as well as with age [67], which is in good agreement with a decrease in the plasma levels of IgM autoantibodies against pyroGlu-modified $A\beta$ species [68].

N-truncated $A\beta$ species, including those detecting pyroGlu-modified or $A\beta_{4-x}$ variants, gained increasing interest as targets of immunotherapy, as they might reflect pathological correlates compared to full-length $A\beta_{1-42}$ which is also believed to act as a physiological peptide, e.g., in the regulation of the sleep-wake cycle or in synaptic transmission by regulating long-term depression [3, 69, 70].

Several preclinical studies using passive immunization with antibodies against $A\beta_{pE3}$ in transgenic AD mouse model have been conducted. Weekly intraperitoneal injections of mAb07/1 against the N-terminus of $A\beta_{pE3}$ in either a preventative setting (from 5.8 to 13.8 months) or as a therapeutic regimen (from 23 to 24.7 months) have been carried out in the APP/PS1ΔE9 model. A significant reduction in the amount of $A\beta_{pE3}$-positive plaques was detected in the cerebellum and the hippocampus (preventative trial) or the cerebellum alone (therapeutic trial), while insoluble Aβ levels were not significantly different in brain homogenates between immunized and control mice [71]. In a different study, a monoclonal antibody against AβpE3 (mE8) was described, which lowered $A\beta_{1-42}$ levels in cortex and hippocampus in aged PDAPP mice (27 months) after a 3-month treatment period. The murine equivalent of bapineuzumab, the monoclonal antibody 3D6 recognizing the N-terminus (Aβ1-5) of Aβ peptides, was used as a control antibody and did not show any effects after a 3-month immunization period in mice treated from 9 to 12 or 18 to 21 months of age [72]. The discrepant effects in terms of Aβ reduction were attributed to differences in antibody target engagement. While mE8 crossed the blood-brain barrier and bound to Aβ deposits, 3D6 showed a lack of plaque binding which could be due to a saturation process with soluble Aβ species in the brain. In addition, immunization with 3D6 caused an extensive increase in microbleedings, in contrast to mE8 which did not show any such effects [72]. In addition to antibodies detecting linear epitopes of $A\beta_{pE3-x}$, conformation-specific antibodies (9D5 and 8C4) have been described that detect low-molecular-weight species of pyroGlu-modified Aβ species [31]. In in vitro assays, the 9D5 antibody efficiently reduced the formation of higher molecular aggregates when added to monomeric preparations of $A\beta_{pE3-42}$ while it showed no interference with $A\beta_{1-42}$ aggregation. In addition, 9D5 did not interfere with $A\beta_{1-42}$ toxicity in SH-SY5Y neuroblastoma cells but was able to abolish the detrimental effects of $A\beta_{pE3-42}$ peptides. In a pilot study using weekly intraperitoneal injections of 9D5 in 4.5-month-old 5XFAD mice for 6 weeks, a reduced Aβ plaque load and a stabilization of the anxiety phenotype were detected [31]. Immunohistochemical staining using 9D5 in brain specimen from sporadic AD patients revealed that only a minor portion of the overall plaque deposits showed immunoreactivity [73]. In a subfraction of AD patients, a vascular staining pattern was detected which was significantly reduced compared to the vascular staining intensity using other Aβ antibodies [74]. This suggests that antibodies detecting oligomeric $A\beta_{pE3}$ species could represent useful therapeutic agents, as they might yield fewer side effects due to lower probability of cerebral hemorrhages in sporadic AD patients.

In summary, we have discussed (1) that it is possible to identify novel structural epitopes using antibodies against the N-terminus of N-truncated Aβ species, (2) that some of these epitopes are not present in amyloid plaques, and finally (3) that antibodies directed against these epitopes rescue specific toxicities of N-truncated Aβ variants, but not that of full-length Aβ. Therefore, we believe to have presented evidence that these N-truncated Aβ species are suitable therapeutic targets for AD due to their significant biochemical and biophysical differences as compared to $Aβ_{1-42}$ (Fig. 3).

References

1. Selkoe DJ (2001) Alzheimer's disease: genes, proteins, and therapy. Physiol Rev 81(2):741–766
2. Selkoe DJ (1998) The cell biology of beta-amyloid precursor protein and presenilin in Alzheimer's disease. Trends Cell Biol 8(11):447–453
3. Bayer T, Wirths O (2014) Focusing the amyloid cascade hypothesis on N-truncated Abeta peptides as drug targets against Alzheimer's disease. Acta Neuropathol 127(6):787–801
4. Kuo YM, Webster S, Emmerling MR et al (1998) Irreversible dimerization/tetramerization and post-translational modifications inhibit proteolytic degradation of A beta peptides of Alzheimer's disease. Biochim Biophys Acta 1406(3):291–298
5. Shimizu T, Matsuoka Y, Shirasawa T (2005) Biological significance of isoaspartate and its repair system. Biol Pharm Bull 28(9):1590–1596
6. Kumar S, Rezaei-Ghaleh N, Terwel D et al (2011) Extracellular phosphorylation of the amyloid beta-peptide promotes formation of toxic aggregates during the pathogenesis of Alzheimer's disease. EMBO J 30(11):2255–2265
7. Dong J, Atwood CS, Anderson VE et al (2003) Metal binding and oxidation of amyloid-β within isolated senile plaque cores: Raman microscopic evidence†. Biochemistry 42(10):2768–2773
8. Jawhar S, Wirths O, Bayer TA (2011) Pyroglutamate Abeta - a hatchet man in Alzheimer disease. J Biol Chem 286(45):38825–38832
9. Perez-Garmendia R, Gevorkian G (2013) Pyroglutamate-modified amyloid beta peptides: emerging targets for Alzheimer s disease immunotherapy. Curr Neuropharmacol 11(5):491–498
10. Doody RS, Thomas RG, Farlow M et al (2014) Phase 3 trials of solanezumab for mild-to-moderate Alzheimer's disease. N Engl J Med 370(4):311–321
11. Salloway S, Sperling R, Fox NC et al (2014) Two Phase 3 trials of bapineuzumab in mild-to-moderate Alzheimer's disease. N Engl J Med 370(4):322–333
12. Masters CL, Simms G, Weinman NA et al (1985) Amyloid plaque core protein in Alzheimer disease and Down syndrome. Proc Natl Acad Sci 82:4245–4249
13. Glenner GG, Wong CW (1984) Alzheimer's disease: initial report of the purification and characterization of a novel cerebrovascular amyloid protein. Biochem Biophys Res Commun 120:885–890
14. Selkoe DJ, Abraham CR, Podlisny MB et al (1986) Isolation of low-molecular-weight proteins from amyloid plaque fibers in Alzheimer's disease. J Neurochem 46(6):1820–1834
15. Mori H, Takio K, Ogawara M et al (1992) Mass spectrometry of purified amyloid beta protein in Alzheimer's disease. J Biol Chem 267(24):17082–17086
16. Miller DL, Papayannopoulos IA, Styles J et al (1993) Peptide compositions of the cerebrovascular and senile plaque core amyloid deposits of Alzheimer's disease. Arch Biochem Biophys 301(1):41–52
17. Lewis H, Beher D, Cookson N et al (2006) Quantification of Alzheimer pathology in ageing and dementia: age-related accumulation of amyloid-β (42) peptide in vascular dementia. Neuropathol Appl Neurobiol 32(2):103–118
18. Teller JK, Russo C, DeBusk LM et al (1996) Presence of soluble amyloid beta-peptide precedes amyloid plaque formation in Down's syndrome. Nat Med 2(1):93–95
19. Scheuner D, Eckman C, Jensen M et al (1996) Secreted amyloid beta-protein similar to that in the senile plaques of Alzheimer's disease is increased in vivo by the presenilin 1 and 2 and APP mutations linked to familial Alzheimer's disease. Nat Med 2(8):864–870

20. Citron M, Westaway D, Xia W et al (1997) Mutant presenilins of Alzheimer's disease increase production of 42-residue amyloid beta-protein in both transfected cells and transgenic mice. Nat Med 3(1):67–72

21. Saido TC, Iwatsubo T, Mann DM et al (1995) Dominant and differential deposition of distinct beta-amyloid peptide species, Abeta N3(pE), in senile plaques. Neuron 14(2):457–466

22. Russo C, Saido TC, DeBusk LM et al (1997) Heterogeneity of water-soluble amyloid beta-peptide in Alzheimer's disease and Down's syndrome brains. FEBS Lett 409(3):411–416

23. Russo C, Schettini G, Saido TC et al (2000) Presenilin-1 mutations in Alzheimer's disease. Nature 405(6786):531–532

24. Sergeant N, Bombois S, Ghestem A et al (2003) Truncated beta-amyloid peptide species in pre-clinical Alzheimer's disease as new targets for the vaccination approach. J Neurochem 85(6):1581–1591

25. Miravalle L, Calero M, Takao M et al (2005) Amino-terminally truncated Abeta peptide species are the main component of cotton wool plaques. Biochemistry 44(32):10810–10821

26. Güntert A, Dobeli H, Bohrmann B (2006) High sensitivity analysis of amyloid-beta peptide composition in amyloid deposits from human and PS2APP mouse brain. Neuroscience 143(2):461–475

27. Portelius E, Bogdanovic N, Gustavsson MK et al (2010) Mass spectrometric characterization of brain amyloid beta isoform signatures in familial and sporadic Alzheimer's disease. Acta Neuropathol 120(2):185–193

28. Schieb H, Kratzin H, Jahn O et al (2011) Beta-amyloid peptide variants in brains and cerebrospinal fluid from amyloid precursor protein (APP) transgenic mice: comparison with human Alzheimer amyloid. J Biol Chem 286(39):33747–33758

29. Moore BD, Chakrabarty P, Levites Y et al (2012) Overlapping profiles of abeta peptides in the Alzheimer's disease and pathological aging brains. Alzheimers Res Ther 4(3):18

30. Wirths O, Bethge T, Marcello A et al (2010) Pyroglutamate Abeta pathology in APP/PS1KI mice, sporadic and familial Alzheimer's disease cases. J Neural Transm 117(1):85–96

31. Wirths O, Erck C, Martens H et al (2010) Identification of low molecular weight pyroglutamate Abeta oligomers in Alzheimer disease: a novel tool for therapy and diagnosis. J Biol Chem 285(53):41517–41524

32. Antonios G, Saiepour N, Bouter Y et al (2013) N-truncated Abeta starting with position four: early intraneuronal accumulation and rescue of toxicity using NT4X-167, a novel monoclonal antibody. Acta Neuropathol Commun 1(1):56. doi:10.1186/2051-5960-1-56

33. Harigaya Y, Saido TC, Eckman CB et al (2000) Amyloid beta protein starting pyroglutamate at position 3 is a major component of the amyloid deposits in the Alzheimer's disease brain. Biochem Biophys Res Commun 276(2):422–427

34. Kalback W, Watson MD, Kokjohn TA et al (2002) APP transgenic mice Tg2576 accumulate Abeta peptides that are distinct from the chemically modified and insoluble peptides deposited in Alzheimer's disease senile plaques. Biochemistry 41(3):922–928

35. Kawarabayashi T, Younkin L, Saido T et al (2001) Age-dependent changes in brain, CSF, and plasma amyloid (beta) protein in the Tg2576 transgenic mouse model of Alzheimer's disease. J Neurosci 21(2):372–381

36. Sturchler-Pierrat C, Abramowski D, Duke M et al (1997) Two amyloid precursor protein transgenic mouse models with Alzheimer disease-like pathology. Proc Natl Acad Sci U S A 94(24):13287–13292

37. Kuo YM, Kokjohn TA, Beach TG et al (2001) Comparative analysis of amyloid-beta chemical structure and amyloid plaque morphology of transgenic mouse and Alzheimer's disease brains. J Biol Chem 276(16):12991–12998

38. Frost JL, Le KX, Cynis H et al (2013) Pyroglutamate-3 amyloid-β deposition in the brains of humans, non-human primates, canines, and Alzheimer disease–like transgenic mouse models. Am J Pathol 183(2):369–381

39. Casas C, Sergeant N, Itier JM et al (2004) Massive CA1/2 neuronal loss with intraneuronal and N-terminal truncated Abeta42 accumulation in a novel Alzheimer transgenic model. Am J Pathol 165(4):1289–1300

40. Wirths O, Weis J, Kayed R et al (2007) Age-dependent axonal degeneration in an Alzheimer mouse model. Neurobiol Aging 28(11):1689–1699

41. Breyhan H, Wirths O, Duan K et al (2009) APP/PS1KI bigenic mice develop early synaptic deficits and hippocampus atrophy. Acta Neuropathol 117(6):677–685

42. Oakley H, Cole SL, Logan S et al (2006) Intraneuronal beta-amyloid aggregates, neurodegeneration, and neuron loss in transgenic mice with five familial Alzheimer's disease mutations: potential factors in amyloid plaque formation. J Neurosci 26(40):10129–10140

43. Jawhar S, Trawicka A, Jenneckens C et al. (2012) Motor deficits, neuron loss, and reduced anxiety coinciding with axonal degeneration and intraneuronal Abeta aggregation in the 5XFAD mouse model of Alzheimer's disease. Neurobiol Aging 33(1). doi:196.e29-196.e40

44. Jawhar S, Wirths O, Schilling S et al (2011) Overexpression of glutaminyl cyclase, the enzyme responsible for pyroglutamate abeta

formation, induces behavioral deficits, and glutaminyl cyclase knock-out rescues the behavioral phenotype in 5XFAD mice. J Biol Chem 286(6):4454–4460

45. Wirths O, Breyhan H, Cynis H et al (2009) Intraneuronal pyroglutamate-Abeta 3-42 triggers neurodegeneration and lethal neurological deficits in a transgenic mouse model. Acta Neuropathol 118:487–496

46. Alexandru A, Jagla W, Graubner S et al (2011) Selective hippocampal neurodegeneration in transgenic mice expressing small amounts of truncated A{beta} is induced by pyroglutamate-A{beta} formation. J Neurosci 31(36):12790–12801

47. Wittnam JL, Portelius E, Zetterberg H et al (2012) Pyroglutamate amyloid β (Aβ) aggravates behavioral deficits in transgenic amyloid mouse model for Alzheimer disease. J Biol Chem 287(11):8154–8162

48. Cynis H, Schilling S, Bodnar M et al (2006) Inhibition of glutaminyl cyclase alters pyroglutamate formation in mammalian cells. Biochim Biophys Acta 1764(10):1618–1625

49. Bouter Y, Dietrich K, Wittnam JL et al (2013) N-truncated amyloid beta (Abeta) 4-42 forms stable aggregates and induces acute and long-lasting behavioral deficits. Acta Neuropathol 126(2):189–205

50. Bouter Y, Kacprowski T, Weissmann R et al (2014) Deciphering the molecular profile of plaques, memory decline and neuron loss in two mouse models for Alzheimer's disease by deep sequencing. Front Aging Neurosci 6:75. doi:10.3389/fnagi.2014.00075

51. Pike CJ, Overman MJ, Cotman CW (1995) Amino-terminal deletions enhance aggregation of beta-amyloid peptides in vitro. J Biol Chem 270(41):23895–23898

52. Russo C, Violani E, Salis S et al (2002) Pyroglutamate-modified amyloid -peptides - AbetaN3(pE) - strongly affect cultured neuron and astrocyte survival. J Neurochem 82(6):1480–1489

53. Schilling S, Lauber T, Schaupp M et al (2006) On the seeding and oligomerization of pGlu-amyloid peptides (in vitro). Biochemistry 45(41):12393–12399

54. Schlenzig D, Manhart S, Cinar Y et al (2009) Pyroglutamate formation influences solubility and amyloidogenicity of amyloid peptides. Biochemistry 48(29):7072–7078

55. Walsh DM, Klyubin I, Fadeeva JV et al (2002) Naturally secreted oligomers of amyloid beta protein potently inhibit hippocampal long-term potentiation in vivo. Nature 416(6880):535–539

56. Youssef I, Florent-Béchard S, Malaplate-Armand C et al (2008) N-truncated amyloid-β oligomers induce learning impairment and neuronal apoptosis. Neurobiol Aging 29(9):1319–1333

57. Nussbaum JM, Schilling S, Cynis H et al (2012) Prion-like behaviour and tau-dependent cytotoxicity of pyroglutamylated amyloid-beta. Nature 485(7400):651–655

58. Matos JO, Goldblat G, Jeon J et al (2014) Pyroglutamylated amyloid-β peptide reverses cross β-sheets by a prion-like mechanism. J Phys Chem B 118(21):5637–5643

59. Schenk D, Barbour R, Dunn W et al (1999) Immunization with amyloid-beta attenuates Alzheimer-disease-like pathology in the PDAPP mouse. Nature 400(6740):173–177

60. Orgogozo JM, Gilman S, Dartigues JF et al (2003) Subacute meningoencephalitis in a subset of patients with AD after Abeta42 immunization. Neurology 61(1):46–54

61. Monsonego A, Imitola J, Petrovic S et al (2006) Aβ-induced meningoencephalitis is IFN-γ-dependent and is associated with T cell-dependent clearance of Aβ in a mouse model of Alzheimer's disease. Proc Natl Acad Sci U S A 103(13):5048–5053

62. Bard F, Barbour R, Cannon C et al (2003) Epitope and isotype specificities of antibodies to β-amyloid peptide for protection against Alzheimer's disease-like neuropathology. Proc Natl Acad Sci 100(4):2023–2028

63. Bard F, Cannon C, Barbour R et al (2000) Peripherally administered antibodies against amyloid beta-peptide enter the central nervous system and reduce pathology in a mouse model of Alzheimer disease. Nat Med 6(8):916–919

64. Burbach GJ, Vlachos A, Ghebremedhin E et al (2007) Vessel ultrastructure in APP23 transgenic mice after passive anti-Aβ immunotherapy and subsequent intracerebral hemorrhage. Neurobiol Aging 28(2):202–212

65. Pfeifer M, Boncristiano S, Bondolfi L et al (2002) Cerebral hemorrhage after passive anti-Aβ immunotherapy. Science 298(5597):1379

66. Tayeb HO, Murray ED, Price BH et al (2013) Bapineuzumab and solanezumab for Alzheimer's disease: is the 'amyloid cascade hypothesis' still alive? Expert Opin Biol Ther 13(7):1075–1084

67. Britschgi M, Olin CE, Johns HT et al (2009) Neuroprotective natural antibodies to assemblies of amyloidogenic peptides decrease with normal aging and advancing Alzheimer's disease. Proc Natl Acad Sci U S A 106(29):12145–12150

68. Marcello A, Wirths O, Schneider-Axmann T et al (2011) Reduced levels of IgM autoantibodies against N-truncated pyroglutamate Abeta in plasma of patients with Alzheimer's disease. Neurobiol Aging 32(8):1379–1387

69. Roh JH, Huang Y, Bero AW et al. (2012) Disruption of the sleep-wake cycle and diurnal fluctuation of beta-amyloid in mice with Alzheimer's disease pathology. Sci Transl Med 4(150):150ra122

70. Snyder EM, Nong Y, Almeida CG et al (2005) Regulation of NMDA receptor trafficking by amyloid-beta. Nat Neurosci 8(8):1051–1058

71. Frost JL, Liu B, Kleinschmidt M et al (2012) Passive immunization against pyroglutamate-3 amyloid-beta reduces plaque burden in Alzheimer-like transgenic mice: a pilot study. Neurodegener Dis 10(1-4):265–270

72. Demattos RB, Lu J, Tang Y et al (2012) A plaque-specific antibody clears existing beta-amyloid plaques in Alzheimer's disease mice. Neuron 76(5):908–920

73. Venkataramani V, Wirths O, Budka H et al (2012) Antibody 9D5 recognizes oligomeric pyroglutamate amyloid-beta in a fraction of amyloid-beta deposits in Alzheimer's disease without cross-reactivity with other protein aggregates. J Alzheimers Dis 29: 361–371

74. Wirths O, Hillmann A, Pradier L et al (2013) Oligomeric pyroglutamate amyloid-beta is present in microglia and a subfraction of vessels in patients with Alzheimer's disease: implications for immunotherapy. J Alzheimers Dis 35:741–749

Chapter 4

Immunotherapy Against Amyloid-β Protofibrils: Opportunities and Challenges

Lars Lannfelt

Abstract

Immunotherapy has emerged as a promising treatment option for Alzheimer's disease (AD). Although many challenges still remain, data from drug programs within the immunotherapy area indicate that targeting amyloid β peptide (Aβ) with monoclonal antibodies might lead to positive treatment effects. Antibodies can be made highly specific for their target and monoclonal antibodies usually have a more favorable safety profile as compared to small molecules. Results from previous immunotherapy trials have indicated the importance of targeting early AD. Some of the anti-Aβ immunotherapy studies indicate that positive effects in the clinic are possible, which is encouraging for continued research. Promisingly, the monoclonal antibody aducanumab had dose-dependent effects both on cognitive measures and on amyloid PET imaging following 12 months of treatment. This is the first time a candidate drug targeting Aβ has shown a clinical effect. Our finding of the *Arctic* AD mutation in the amyloid β precursor protein (AβPP) gene led us to consider large soluble oligomers, i.e., protofibrils, of Aβ as particularly toxic and a promising target for immunotherapy. Furthermore, both preclinical and clinical data suggest that Aβ protofibrils have particular neurotoxic properties. Our research efforts lead to the isolation of mAb158, an antibody highly selective for these Aβ species. However, several of the antibodies in clinical trials have caused amyloid-related imaging abnormalities (ARIAs), side effects that pose a problem for the development of this class of drugs. BAN2401 is the humanized version of mAb158 and the antibody is now in a large phase 2b trial. The safety profile has so far been satisfactory.

Key words Alzheimer's disease, Amyloid-β, Aβ, Protofibril, Oligomer, Immunotherapy, BAN2401, mAb158, ARIA

List of Abbreviations

A4	Anti-amyloid treatment in Alzheimer's disease prevention trial
Aβ	Amyloid β
AD	Alzheimer's disease
API	Alzheimer's prevention initiative
ARIA-E	Amyloid-related imaging abnormalities with edema
ARIA-H	Amyloid-related imaging abnormalities with microhemorrhages
BACE	Beta-secretase
CSF	Cerebrospinal fluid
DIAN	Dominantly inherited Alzheimer network trial

Martin Ingelsson and Lars Lannfelt (eds.), *Immunotherapy and Biomarkers in Neurodegenerative Disorders*, Methods in Pharmacology and Toxicology, DOI 10.1007/978-1-4939-3560-4_4, © Springer Science+Business Media New York 2016

1   Introduction

Immunotherapy has emerged as an encouraging treatment possibility for Alzheimer's disease (AD), after decades of academic research on AD pathogenesis and major efforts from the pharmaceutical industry. Although many challenges still remain, data from drug programs indicate that targeting amyloid β (Aβ) with monoclonal antibodies might lead to positive treatment effects, providing hope for new generations of therapies in the future.

1.1   Aβ in the Disease Process

According to the amyloid hypothesis, the Aβ peptide, which is the main constituent of extracellular plaques found in the AD brain [1], initiates the disease process and is therefore an attractive target for intervention [2, 3]. This hypothesis has been supported by the findings of several mutations in the Aβ region of the amyloid β precursor protein (AβPP) gene as well as in other genes in families with autosomal dominant, early-onset AD [4–8]. The mutations have been shown to increase the production of Aβ in vitro as well as in vivo [9]. The *Arctic AβPP* mutation indicates that large, soluble Aβ oligomers, i.e., protofibrils, are toxic and are driving the disease process. We found that the *Arctic* Aβ peptide had a propensity to form large soluble Aβ protofibrils [8] and later studies on AD cases with the *Arctic* mutation indeed showed that they were negative for fibrillized amyloid, as measured by the brain retention of the amyloid ligand Pittsburgh compound B (^{11}C-PIB) with positron emission tomography (PET) [10]. However, in the most prevalent form of the disease, late-onset sporadic AD, decreased Aβ clearance rather than increased production is most likely initiating the disease process [11].

1.2   Aβ Immunotherapy

Biopharmaceuticals are drugs that have developed rapidly during the last decade. Immunotherapy targeting Aβ has emerged as an attractive approach for disease intervention in AD. Aβ immunotherapy confers a lower risk of side effects in a vulnerable patient population during long-term treatment as compared to small-molecule anti-Aβ therapy. Antibodies can be made highly specific for their target and monoclonal antibodies usually have a more favorable safety profile as compared to small molecules. Importantly—in spite of their overall failures—some late-phase anti-Aβ immunotherapy trials have indicated that positive effects in the clinic are possible, which is encouraging for continued research.

The development of the active vaccine AN1792 by Elan started when it was observed that immunization of transgenic mice with fibrillar Aβ resulted in anti-Aβ antibody-mediated clearance of existing amyloid deposits and prevention of plaque formation [12]. AN1792 was halted in phase 2 due to aseptic meningoencephalitis in 6 % of the treated patients [13]. In a follow-up study performed approximately 5 years after the immunizations were conducted in the phase 2 study, previously identified antibody responders were compared to placebo-treated patients [14]. The antibody responders demonstrated significantly reduced cognitive decline compared to placebo-treated patients and maintained a low antibody titer, supporting the hypothesis that Aβ immunotherapy may have long-term effects.

Active immunization, such as AN1792, has certain disadvantages. The number of responders to the vaccine in an elderly population is low, dose adjustments are hard to make, and it is difficult to target a certain Aβ species and also to halt treatment, as antibody titers might persist for a long time. Thus, the main focus of the last decade has been passive immunotherapy directed toward different forms of Aβ.

1.3   Bapineuzumab

Bapineuzumab (Elan/Pfizer/Johnson & Johnson) is a monoclonal antibody directed against Aβ1-5, targeting fibrillar Aβ. The development was stopped in 2012 after the drug failed to reach the clinical endpoint in a phase 3 clinical trial. Interestingly, bapineuzumab treatment leads to a small but significant reduction of total tau as well as of phospho-tau in cerebrospinal fluid (CSF) [15]. However, the CSF Aβ levels did not differ between bapineuzumab and placebo-treated patients. In a separate study the amyloid load was found to be reduced in the brains of patients treated with bapineuzumab, as measured by binding of ^{11}C-PIB to brain amyloid with PET [16]. Moreover, bapineuzumab treatment was associated with vasogenic edema called amyloid-related imaging abnormalities with edema (ARIA-E), as well as intracerebral microhemorrhages (ARIA-H). The adverse event profile resulted in a lowering of the dose and the desired clinical effect was not achieved [17]. This led to the termination of the i.v. program.

1.4   Solanezumab

Solanezumab (Eli Lilly) was developed to target the mid-region of soluble, monomeric Aβ. In a phase 2 study of solanezumab in mild-to-moderate AD a dose-dependent increase in CSF $Aβ_{42}$ was observed. No effect was found on CSF tau, amyloid PET, hippocampal volume, or ADAS-Cog [18]. In two phase 3 studies, solanezumab failed to meet primary clinical endpoints [19]. It was discovered that a high proportion of study subjects did not have amyloid in the brain, which has led to the addition of positive amyloid PET or pathological CSF biomarkers in the inclusion criteria in further clinical studies. However, when data from the two studies were pooled, a positive pattern emerged revealing a slowing of cognitive decline in the subgroup of mild AD [20]. Furthermore, an open-label extension study in patients who completed the phase 3 trial suggests that patients who received solanezumab during the double-blind studies had a cognitive benefit consistent with a treatment effect that changes the underlying pathology of AD. A new phase 3 study in mild AD patients is now being performed and the antibody has also been selected for evaluation in prodromal familial AD within the Dominantly Inherited Alzheimer Network Trial (DIAN) and Anti-Amyloid Treatment in Alzheimer's Disease Prevention Trial (A4) trials.

1.5   Gantenerumab

Gantenerumab (Roche) targets a combination of the N-terminal and mid-regions of Aβ and preferentially binds to aggregated Aβ. The antibody is intended for use in prodromal AD and is also being evaluated as part of the DIAN trial. Gantenerumab showed a negative outcome on all endpoints in the clinical trial against prodromal AD. The incidence of ARIAs was found to be rather high (up to 14 %) and was correlated to both drug dose and the patient's number of APOE ε4 alleles. The phase 2/3 of clinical development was halted in December 2014, but the antibody is still included in the DIAN trial.

1.6   Crenezumab

Crenezumab (Genentech/Roche) targets oligomeric and fibrillar Aβ and was developed by AC Immune and licensed by Genentech. Crenezumab is currently in phase 2 of clinical development for mild-to-moderate AD, as well as being part of the Alzheimer's Prevention Initiative (API) in which subjects at risk are being subjected to preventive immunotherapy. Furthermore, the antibody is in a trial that will test the effect of the drug on 300 presymptomatic individuals in Colombia with a presenilin 1 mutation. In November 2014 at the CTAD conference in Philadelphia, phase 2 results for the crenezumab study were presented and showed that the drug failed to meet the primary endpoints. With biomarker endpoints it also did not show any significant difference of amyloid PET between treatment group and placebo. Similarly, volumetric MRI, CSF tau, and FDG PET showed no significant differences between the groups. However, a positive trend in cognition was observed in individuals with mild disease.

1.7   Aducanumab

Aducanumab (Biogen/Neurimmune) binds equally well to Aβ fibrils and Aβ protofibrils/oligomers, but has a low affinity to Aβ monomers. Aducanumab was given in five doses, from 1 to 10 mg/kg, in addition to a placebo arm in a small clinical study. The included population consisted of subjects with prodromal and mild AD with MMSE ≥20 who were on stable concomitant medication with regular AD therapy. A dose-dependent effect was seen on Mini Mental State Examination (MMSE) and Clinical Dementia Rating (CDR) following 12 months of treatment. Moreover, a dose-dependent effect could also be seen with amyloid PET imaging. This is the first disease-modifying therapy that has had a positive effect on cognition in AD patients. Clearly, the aducanumab study gives optimism for the future of Aβ immunotherapy. One problem might be the relatively high incidence of ARIA-E in the study.

2   Immunotherapy Targeting Amyloid β Protofibrils

2.1   Development of the Antibody BAN2401, Selectively Targeting Toxic Aβ

The *Arctic Aβ* peptide has a propensity to form large soluble Aβ protofibrils [8] and studies on Alzheimer cases with the *Arctic* mutation indeed showed that they were negative for fibrillized amyloid [10]. Thus, amyloid plaques containing mainly fibrillized Aβ are probably not what is driving the disease process and likely not the most suitable target for disease intervention. Protofibrils have been shown to be toxic to neurons, and should thus constitute an attractive target for immunotherapy. BAN2401 (Eisai/ BioArctic Neuroscience) selectively targets soluble Aβ protofibrils and is currently in phase 2b, having shown a favorable safety profile in earlier studies [21, 22].

2.2   The Role of Aβ Protofibrils in Disease Development

2.2.1   Soluble Aβ Correlates with Disease Severity

Amyloid β has remained in the focus of AD research since the peptide was found to be the main constituent of senile plaques. However, it has been shown that the amyloid plaque density in brain does not correlate with the severity of dementia [23–27]. Several research groups showed that neuronal injury instead can be caused by soluble aggregated Aβ [28, 29] and such species should thus be an interesting target for AD disease-modifying treatment. However, as soluble Aβ can be anything from monomers to large protofibrils, correct target identification requires an understanding of Aβ toxicity.

2.2.2   Aβ Protofibrils as a Target for AD Immunotherapy

During the aggregation of monomeric Aβ to insoluble fibrils, intermediate species called protofibrils are formed, which was first described by Walsh and colleagues in 1997 [30]. Using synthetic Aβ peptides, protofibrils have been defined as large (>100 kDa), soluble oligomeric species appearing as a peak in the void volume of a size-exclusion chromatography (SEC) with a Sephadex G75 column [8]. Such large oligomers have been shown to induce electrophysiological changes and cause neurotoxicity in rat cortical neurons [31], as well as inhibit long-term potentiation in mouse hippocampus [32]. In addition, $Aβ_{42}$ protofibrils have been shown to induce an inflammatory process through microglial activation, an effect not seen by insoluble fibrils [33].

2.2.3   The Arctic Mutation

The sizes and assembly states of the soluble protofibrils and oligomers of various sizes have been identified in human brains and in brains from AβPP transgenic mice [34–38]. The *Arctic* mutation ($AβPP_{E693G}$), causing early-onset familial AD, has been shown to specifically increase the rate of formation of Aβ protofibrils [8, 39]. By combining the *Arctic* and *Swedish* [5] mutations a transgenic mouse model was developed, with early plaque pathology and with Aβ plaques as difficult to dissolve as those in the human AD brain, a model of high value for research [40]. Furthermore, these mice display early intraneuronal Aβ accumulation and protofibril formation, followed by plaque formation [41]. In the *ArcSwe* mice, cognitive deficits were shown to occur concomitantly with the formation of intracellular Aβ deposits but before plaque formation [42]. The levels of Aβ protofibrils in brain, but not the levels of total Aβ, correlated with spatial learning, adding further evidence to the theory of soluble protofibrils being a toxic Aβ species [41]. The pool of soluble toxic Aβ was shown to consist of molecules in the size range of 80–500 kDa [38]. Such species were selectively detected by mAb158, a protofibril-selective antibody with low binding to monomers and aggregated insoluble Aβ fibrils [37, 43].

2.2.4   Effect of mAb158 in Transgenic Mice

When *ArcSwe* transgenic mice were treated with mAb158 the levels of insoluble Aβ in the brains of plaque-bearing mice were not affected. Instead, the antibody could prevent plaque formation if the treatment began before the appearance of plaques. In both cases, soluble Aβ protofibril levels were diminished [44], showing that mAb158 can selectively reduce the levels of protofibrils in vivo. A humanized version of mAb158—BAN2401, developed by BioArctic Neuroscience—has binding characteristics essentially indistinguishable from mAb158 with at least a 1000-fold higher selectivity for protofibrils as compared to monomers and at least 15 times lower binding to fibrils [43]. BAN2401 is now studied in a clinical phase 2b trial in early AD, as described below.

2.2.5   Target for AD Immunotherapy

Based on the available knowledge of the underlying mechanisms of AD, Aβ has become an appealing target for immunotherapy. Many studies have shown that soluble aggregated Aβ, and specifically Aβ protofibrils, is neurotoxic. This is particularly interesting, as protofibril levels have been shown to correlate with spatial learning in a transgenic mouse model [42]. In addition, the murine equivalent of BAN2401, mAb158, has been shown to significantly reduce protofibril levels both in brain and CSF from transgenic mice after chronic treatment [45].

2.3   BAN2401 in Clinical Development

Aβ immunotherapy has gained a lot of attention and has emerged as one of the most attractive approaches for disease intervention in AD. As neurotoxicity has been suggested to be caused by soluble Aβ aggregates rather than insoluble fibrils, soluble protofibrils could be highlighted as a suitable target for immunotherapy. Moreover, preclinical and clinical data on mAb158/BAN2401 suggest that the antibody targets an Aβ species found to be toxic in a clinical setting as well as in preclinical experiments. Results from previous immunotherapy trials have indicated the importance of targeting early AD, and CSF biochemical markers or amyloid PET are therefore used in the ongoing BAN2401 phase 2b trial to identify an early patient population with a pathology consistent with AD. When aiming at a chronic treatment regimen for a vulnerable patient population, safety and convenience will be key.

3 Major Side Effects in Clinical Trials with Aβ Immunotherapy: Amyloid-Related Imaging Abnormalities (ARIAs)

The major side effect with passive immunotherapy against Aβ, ARIA-E, is a poorly understood type of edema. Most of these adverse events have been seen at an early treatment stage, especially with higher antibody doses and in carriers of the APOE $\varepsilon 4$ allele. However, the edema sometimes occurs late in the treatment, at lower doses, and in non-carriers of the APOE $\varepsilon 4$ allele.

Alzheimer patients usually have a significant amount of Aβ in the small vessel walls of the brain, a condition known as congophilic amyloid angiopathy (CAA). The angiopathy is in close proximity to the blood–brain barrier (BBB). Anti-Aβ antibodies with high binding to CAA give rise to a reaction in the BBB which can result in damage and subsequent edema, i.e., ARIA-E. The underlying mechanisms are incompletely understood, but could be the result of antibodies binding and dissolving aggregated Aβ in the intima of the blood vessel walls, where a local reaction may lead to impairment of the BBB. In theory, antibodies avoiding fibrillized Aβ1-40 should be less prone to cause CAA, as the Aβ deposits in the vessel mainly consist of fibrillized Aβ1-40 (Table 1).

In the clinical studies with bapineuzumab the frequency of these adverse events led to a dose reduction and limited the possibilities to fully explore the potential effect of bapineuzumab. In APOE $\varepsilon 4$ heterozygotes ARIA-E was reported in 11.4 % of cases and in APOE $\varepsilon 4$ homozygotes the frequency was 27.3 % with the 0.5 mg/kg dose. In non-$\varepsilon 4$-carriers ARIA was also seen: in the 0.5 mg/kg group it was 4.2 %, in the 1.0 mg/kg group it was 9.4 %, and in the 2.0 mg/kg group it was 14.2 %. Severe problems with ARIA-E have also been seen with gantenerumab, which has delayed its development.

In addition, ARIA-E was common in the phase 1b trial of aducanumab. In APOE $\varepsilon 4$ carriers, the incidence of ARIA-E was 5 % in the 1 and 3 mg/kg groups, 43 % in the 6 mg/kg group, and 55 % in the 10 mg/kg group. In non-carriers, it was 9 % in the 3 mg/kg, 22 % in the 6 mg/kg, and 17 % in the 10 mg/kg group. One-third of ARIA-E cases were symptomatic and resolved spontaneously, whereas the remainder of the cases were asymptomatic and could only be detected on MRI.

A much lower incidence of ARIA-E has been reported for crenezumab, an IgG4 antibody. Only one single case of ARIA-E was found during the phase 1 and 2 studies. In the phase 3 study with solanezumab, the incidence of ARIA-E was not different from placebo. A possible explanation for the lower incidence of side effects with solanezumab might be that the antibody binds specifically to the nontoxic monomeric form of Aβ via a mid-region

Table 1
Aβ antibodies used in clinical trials for AD: Antibodies are ranked after the approximate amount of associated ARIA-E

Antibody	Corresponding mouse antibody	Company	Stage	Subclass	ARIA-E
Bapineuzumab	3D6	Janssen/Pfizer	Failed	IgG1	+++
Aducanumab[a]	-	Biogen/Neurimmune	Phase 3	IgG1	+++
Gantenerumab[a]	-	Roche	Phase 3	IgG1	+++
BAN2401	mAb158	Eisai/BioArctic	Phase 2b	IgG1	+
Crenezumab	?	Genentech/Roche	Phase 2b	IgG4	0
Solanezumab	m266	Lilly	Phase 3	IgG1	0
SAR228810	13C3	Sanofi	Phase 1	IgG4	?

[a]Not developed from mouse hybridoma antibodies

epitope, and not at all to aggregated Aβ forms. With BAN2401, ARIA-E has been reported to be <5 % in the first clinical trial [22].

A mechanism for the reported adverse events is the well-known effect of IgG1 and IgG3 antibodies to activate the immune system, including the microglial cells via binding to the Fcγ receptors, and complement activation via C1q. This may result in a proinflammatory response leading to ARIA-E. The IgG4 antibodies do not activate this cascade and thus avoid the problem. Sanofi states that this is the reason why their SAR228810 antibody against Aβ protofibrils was developed to be a human IgG4. However, the disadvantage with using IgG4 antibodies is that they might be less effective in removing Aβ with their lower effector function.

4 Conclusions

Immunotherapy has emerged as a promising treatment option for AD, after decades of academic research and efforts in the pharmaceutical industry. Data from drug programs indicate that targeting Aβ with monoclonal antibodies might lead to positive treatment effects, providing hope for new generations of therapies in the future. Especially, the aducanumab study gives optimism for the future. This is the first time a disease-modifying therapy against Aβ is giving a clear positive signal on cognition. The *Arctic* mutation points to large, soluble Aβ oligomers, i.e., protofibrils, to be toxic and driving the disease process. Thus, targeting this Aβ species should be a viable treatment option. BAN2401 is thus a promising candidate for such a therapy.

Acknowledgements

Hans Basun, Gunilla Osswald, Christer Möller, Dag Sehlin, and Anna Lord for helpful comments on the manuscript.

Competing Interests:

Lars Lannfelt is co-founder of BioArctic Neuroscience AB.

References

1. Glenner GG, Wong CW (1984) Alzheimer's disease and Down syndrome: sharing of a unique cerebrovascular amyloid fibril protein. Biochem Biophys Res Commun 122(3):1131–1135

2. Hardy J, Selkoe DJ (2002) The amyloid hypothesis of Alzheimer's disease: progress and problems on the road to therapeutics. Science 297:353–356

3. Golde T (2005) The Abeta hypothesis: leading us to rationally-designed therapeutic strategies for the treatment or prevention of Alzheimer disease. Brain Pathol 15:84–87

4. Chartier-Harlin M-C, Crawford F, Houlden H (1991) Early-onset alzheimer's disease caused by mutations at codon 717 of the beta-amyloid precursor protein gene. Nature 353:844–846

5. Mullan M, Crawford F, Axelman K et al (1992) A pathogenic mutation for probable Alzheimer's disease in the APP gene at the N-terminus of beta-amyloid. Nat Genet 1:345–347

6. Citron M, Oltersdorf T, Haass C et al (1992) Mutation of the beta-amyloid precursor protein in familial Alzheimer's disease increases beta-protein production. Nature 360:672–674

7. Scheuner D, Eckman CB, Jensen M et al (1996) Secreted amyloid beta-protein similar to that in senile plaques of Alzheimer's disease is increased in vivo by the presenilin 1 and 2 and APP mutations linked to familial Alzheimer's disease. Nat Med 2(8):864–870

8. Nilsberth C, Westlind-Danielsson A, Eckman CB et al (2001) The 'Arctic' APP mutation (E693G) causes Alzheimer's disease by enhanced Abeta protofibril formation. Nat Neurosci 4:887–893

9. Bouwers N, Sleegers K, Van Broeckhoven C (2008) Molecular genetics of Alzheimer's disease: an update. Ann Med 40(8):562–583

10. Schöll M, Wall A, Thordardottir S et al (2012) Low PiB PET retention in presence of pathologic CSF biomarkers in Arctic APP mutation carriers. Neurology 79(3):229–236

11. Mawuenyega KG, Sigurdson W, Ovod V et al (2010) Decreased clearance of CNS beta-amyloid in Alzheimer's disease. Science 330:1774

12. Schenk D, Barbour R, Dunn W et al (1999) Immunization with amyloid-beta attenuates Alzheimer-disease-like pathology in the PDAPP mouse. Nature 400(6740):173–177

13. Gilman S, Koller M, Black R et al (2005) Clinical effects of Abeta immunization (AN1792) in patients with AD in an interrupted trial. Neurology 64(9):1553–1562

14. Vellas B, Black R, Thal LJ et al (2009) Long-term follow-up of patients immunized with AN1792: reduced functional decline in antibody responders. Curr Alzheimer Res 6:144–151

15. Blennow K, Zetterberg H, Rinne J et al (2012) Effect of immunotherapy with bapineuzumab on cerebrospinal fluid biomarker levels in patients with mild to moderate Alzheimer disease. Arch Neurol 69(8):1002–1010

16. Rinne J, Brooks D, Rossor M et al (2010) 11C-PiB PET assessment of change in fibrilla amyloid-beta load in patients with Alzheimer's disease treated with bapineuzumab: a phase 2, double-blind, placebo-controlled, ascending dose study. Lancet Neurol 9(4):363–372

17. Salloway S, Sperling R, Fox NC et al (2014) Two phase 3 trials of bapineuzumab in mild-to-moderate Alzheimer's disease. N Engl J Med 370(4):322–333

18. Farlow M, Arnold SE, van Dyck CH et al (2012) Safety and biomarker effects of solanezumab in patients with Alzheimer's disease. Alzheimers Dement 8:261–271

19. Lilly. Alzheimer Research Forum 24 August, 2012. www.alzforum.org

20. Doody RS, Thomas RG, Farlow M et al (2014) Phase 3 trials of solanezumab for mild-to-moderate Alzheimer's disease. N Engl J Med 370(4):311–321

21. Lannfelt L, Relkin NR, Siemers ER (2014) Amyloid-beta directed immunotherapy for Alzheimer's disease. J Intern Med 275(3):284–295

22. Logovinsky V, Satlin A, Lai R, Swanson C, Kaplow J, Osswald G, Basun B, Lannfelt L. (in press) Safety and tolerability of BAN2401—a clinical study in Alzheimer´s disease with a protofibril selective Aβ antibody. Alzheimer Res Ther.

23. Katzman R (1986) Alzheimer's disease. N Engl J Med 314:964–973

24. Terry RD, Masliah E, Salmon DP et al (1991) Physical basis of cognitive alterations in Alzheimer's disease: synapse loss is the major correlate of cognitive impairment. Ann Neurol 30:572–580

25. Dickson DW, Chrystal HA, Bevona C et al (1995) Correlations of synaptic and pathological markers with cognition of the elderly. Neurobiol Aging 16:285–298

26. Näslund J, Haroutunian V, Mohs R et al (2000) Correlation between elevated levels of amyloid beta-peptide in the brain and cognitive decline. JAMA 283(12):1571–1577

27. Ingelsson M, Fukumoto H, Newell KL et al (2004) Early Abeta accumulation and progressive synaptic loss, gliosis, and tangle formation in AD brain. Neurology 62(6):925–931

28. Pike CJ, Walancewics AJ, Glabe CG et al (1991) In vitro aging of beta-amyloid protein causes peptide aggregation and neurotoxicity. Brain Res 563:311–314

29. Busciglio J, Lorenzo A, Yankner B (1992) Methodological variables in the assessment of beta-amyloid neurotoxicity. Neurobiol Aging 13:609–612

30. Walsh DM, Hartley DM, Kusumoto Y et al (1997) Amyloid beta-protein fibrillogenesis. J Biol Chem 272(35):22364–22372

31. Hartley DM, Walsh DM, Ye CP et al (1999) Protofibrillar intermediates of amyloid beta-protein induce acute electrophysiological changes and progressive neurotoxicity in cortical neurons. J Neurosci 19(20):8876–8884

32. O'Nuallain B, Freir DB, Nicoll AJ et al (2010) Amyloid beta-protein dimers rapidly form stable synaptotoxic protofibrils. J Neurosci 30(43):14411–14419

33. Paranjape GS, Gouwens LK, Osborn DC et al (2012) Isolated amyloid-beta(1-42) protofibrils, but not isolated fibrils, are robust stimulators of microglia. ACS Chem Neurosci 3(4):302–311

34. McLean C, Cherny R, Fraser F et al (1999) Soluble pool of Abeta amyloid as a determinant of severity of neurodegeneration in Alzheimer's disease. Ann Neurol 46:860–866

35. Johansson AS, Berglind-Dehlin F, Karlsson G et al (2006) Physiochemical characterization of the Alzheimer's disease-related peptides A beta 1-42Arctic and A beta 1-42wt. FEBS J 273(12):2618–2630

36. Lesne S, Koh MT, Kotilinek L et al (2006) A specific amyloid-beta protein assembly in the brain impairs memory. Nature 440(7082):352–357

37. Englund H, Sehlin D, Johansson AS et al (2007) Sensitive ELISA detection of amyloid-beta protofibrils in biological samples. J Neurochem 103(1):334–345

38. Sehlin D, Englund H, Simu B et al (2012) Large aggregates are the major soluble Abeta species in AD brain fractionated with density gradient ultracentrifugation. PLoS One 7(2), e32014

39. Sahlin C, Lord A, Magnusson K et al (2007) The Arctic Alzheimer mutation favors intracellular amyloid-beta production by making amyloid precursor protein less available to alpha-secretase. J Neurochem 101(3):854–862

40. Philipson O, Hammarstrom P, Nilsson KP et al (2009) A highly insoluble state of Abeta similar to that of Alzheimer's disease brain is found in Arctic APP transgenic mice. Neurobiol Aging 30(9):1393–1405

41. Lord A, Kalimo H, Eckman CB et al (2006) The Arctic Alzheimer mutation facilitates early intraneuronal Abeta aggregation and senile plaque formation in transgenic mice. Neurobiol Aging 27:67–77

42. Lord A, Englund H, Soderberg L et al (2009) Amyloid-beta protofibril levels correlate with spatial learning in Arctic Alzheimer's disease transgenic mice. FEBS J 276(4):995–1006

43. Magnusson K, Sehlin D, Syvanen S et al (2013) Specific uptake of an amyloid-beta protofibril-binding antibody-tracer in AbetaPP transgenic mouse brain. J Alzheimers Dis 37(1):29–40

44. Lord A, Gumucio A, Englund H et al (2009) An amyloid-beta protofibril-selective antibody prevents amyloid formation in a mouse model of Alzheimer's disease. Neurobiol Dis 36(3):425–434

45. Tucker S, Möller C, Tegerstedt K et al (2015) The murine version of BAN2401 (mAb158) selectively reduces amyloid-β protofibrils in brain and cerebrospinal fluid of tg-ArcSwe mice. J Alzheimers Dis 43:575–588

Part II

Immunotherapy in Other Neurodegenerative Disorders

Chapter 5

Immunotherapy Against α-Synuclein Pathology

Elvira Valera and Eliezer Masliah

Abstract

Immunotherapy is one of the most promising disease-modifying alternatives for the treatment of Parkinson's disease (PD), a neurodegenerative disorder that affects approximately 1.5 million people in the USA and 1 % of people over 60 years old. Both vaccination and passive immunization approaches with antibodies targeting alpha-synuclein (α-syn) have been extensively explored, especially since the discovery that this protein may propagate from cell to cell and be accessible to antibodies when embedded into the plasma membrane or in the extracellular space. Moreover, developing immunotherapies that discriminate abnormal conformations of α-syn using either monoclonal antibodies or single-chain variable fragments is a top priority in this field. Finally, research on intracellular antibodies (intrabodies) has shown promise for their use as novel therapeutic tools. In this chapter we provide an overview on the most relevant immunotherapeutic advances targeting α-syn in PD and related disorders, including the current Phase I clinical trials exploring this type of approach for PD patients.

Key words Immunotherapy, Vaccines, Antibodies, Intrabodies, Alpha-synuclein, Parkinson's disease

1 Introduction

Disorders with parkinsonism and dementia affect over ten million people worldwide, and within this group Parkinson's disease (PD) is the second most common neurodegenerative disease in the elderly after Alzheimer's disease (AD) [1]. Behaviorally, and from a diagnostic point of view, PD is characterized by non-motor and motor symptoms, including tremors, rigidity, bradykinesia, impaired posture and gait, loss of sense of smell, constipation, REM behavior disorder, orthostatic hypotension and mood changes, among others [2]. Neuropathologically, PD, and related disorders are characterized by accumulation of protease-resistant α-synuclein (α-syn) in synapses and axons, formation of neuronal inclusions known as Lewy bodies, and degeneration of selected neuronal populations in the neocortex, limbic, and striato-nigral systems, accompanied with neuroinflammation [3–5]. The heterogeneous group of disorders characterized by the abnormal accumulation of α-syn within brain cells is known as synucleinopathies,

Martin Ingelsson and Lars Lannfelt (eds.), *Immunotherapy and Biomarkers in Neurodegenerative Disorders*, Methods in Pharmacology and Toxicology, DOI 10.1007/978-1-4939-3560-4_5, © Springer Science+Business Media New York 2016

and includes idiopathic PD, PD dementia, dementia with Lewy bodies (DLB) [6], and multiple system atrophy (MSA).

Alpha-syn is a protein involved in synaptic transmission and vesicle release and is specifically upregulated in a discrete population of presynaptic terminals during acquisition-related synaptic rearrangement [7–9]. Alpha-syn was initially identified in AD brains associated with plaque formation and neurodegeneration [10, 11]. The abnormal aggregation and accumulation of α-syn are correlated to the neuropathological changes observed in PD and other synucleinopathies [12–14]; inhibiting these processes would therefore be a key mechanism for preventing its toxicity.

Currently, the lack of disease-modifying alternatives for neurodegenerative diseases in general, and, for PD in particular, is one of the major obstacles for significantly improving and extending the lives of the millions of patients that suffer from these disorders. Therefore developing effective therapies that are able to stop or slow down the progression of the disease is a major research and clinical priority. Due to the fact that α-syn is at the core of the pathological changes that affect the PD brain, this protein has become the target of most disease-modifying efforts. These include treatment with antisense RNAs, autophagy inducers, α-syn degrading enzymes, chaperones, stabilizers and anti-aggregation agents, therapies that are aimed at inhibiting α-syn expression, aggregation, accumulation, and/or toxic propagation. Among these therapeutic alternatives, immunotherapy has been prominently featured in the past few years in several preclinical and clinical studies. In this chapter we focus on the past and present advances in the field of immunotherapy against α-syn and provide the reader with future directions and considerations for this type of approaches.

2 Immunotherapy Against α-syn as Disease-Modifying Alternative for PD and Other Synucleinopathies

One of the most promising disease-modifying alternatives for PD targeting α-syn is immunotherapy, and based on strong preclinical evidence there are currently four Phase I clinical trials devoted to assess the safety of this approach for PD patients. Immunotherapy is a therapeutic strategy based on humoral immunity that focuses on stimulating or restoring the ability of the adaptive immune system to fight a disease. Humoral immunization against α-syn can be provided in an active or in a passive form. Active immunization (also known as *vaccination*) stimulates the immune system to produce specific antibodies against an antigen, such as toxic α-syn conformations. Passive immunization involves the direct administration of anti-α-syn antibodies—which has been generated in another organism—to the patient, thus conferring temporary protection against its toxic effects. Finally, cell-mediated immunity involving the activation of phagocytes, natural killer cells, antigen-specific cytotoxic T lymphocytes, and the release of various cytokines in response to an antigen has also been explored for the potential treatment of synucleinopathies [15, 16].

It is important to note that while vaccination confers a long-lasting protection against pathological α-syn conformations that could potentially be used as a preventive measure for PD in pre-symptomatic patients, the beneficial effects of passive immunother-apy are temporary by nature. However, passive immunotherapy may target highly specific conformations and epitopes of α-syn and could also circumvent prominent side effects of vaccination, such as the T-cell autoimmune responses and meningoencephalitis that were observed in 6 % of the participants in the first active immuno-therapy trials against amyloid-beta using the synthetic peptide AN1792 [17].

3   Active Immunization with α-syn and α-syn-Mimicking Peptides

The first preclinical vaccination approaches for synucleinopathies were performed using the full human α-syn protein sequence [18]. In this transgenic (tg) model, active immunization with α-syn decreased accumulation of aggregated α-syn in neurons and reduced neurodegeneration [18]. Furthermore, the antibodies that were produced by the immunized mice bound and promoted the intra-cellular degradation of α-syn aggregates via lysosomal pathways [18], probably after interaction with oligomers in the plasma mem-brane and subsequent internalization. Interestingly, epitope map-ping showed that the antibodies generated after the immunization targeted the C-terminus of α-syn. These results provided the first evidence that vaccination can effectively reduce the accumulation of α-syn within neurons and that this approach might prove efficacious for the treatment of PD and other synucleinopathies.

More recent active immunization approaches have used small peptides that mimic abnormal conformations of α-syn (AFFITOPEs®) in animal models of PD and MSA [19, 20]. AFFITOPEs® are short immunogenic peptides that are too small for inducing a T-cell response and do not carry the native epitope, but rather a sequence that mimics the conformation of the original epitope (e.g., oligomeric α-syn) [21]. The rationale for developing these mimics instead of using the native α-syn sequence is that actively immunizing patients with abnormal conformations of an endogenous protein could induce the production of autoanti-bodies leading to undesired autoimmune reactions. However, these polyclonal antibody responses might target not only abnor-mal conformational epitopes of toxic α-syn aggregates, but also innocuous parts of the protein, leading to reduced efficacy of the active immunotherapy [21]. AFFITOPEs® induce the generation of long-term and more specific antibody responses for the treatment of synucleinopathies such as PD. Interestingly, AFFITOPEs® that mimic the C-terminus region of α-syn are able to elicit an immune response specific to α-syn oligomers [20]. Immunization with AFFITOPEs® induces high antibody titers against α-syn aggregates, reduces the levels of α-syn oligomers and tyrosine hydroxylase fibers, and minimizes motor and memory deficits in two α-syn tg models [20]. Furthermore, AFFITOPEs® also reduce neurodegeneration and demyelination in neocortex, striatum, and corpus callosum in a tg model of MSA [19]. Microglial activation, increased anti-inflammatory cytokine production, and reduced spreading of α-syn to astroglial cells are the suggested mechanisms for α-syn clearance following immunization with this AFFITOPE® [19, 20]. Taken together, the results obtained with AFFITOPE® vaccination in mouse models suggest that this type of active immunotherapy could help ameliorate the neurodegenerative pathology in synucleinopathies. Based on those results, two Phase I clinical trials with the AFFITOPEs® PD01A and PD03A for PD and MSA are currently ongoing. For further information on the AFFITOPE strategy and the ongoing clinical trials, please see Chap. 8 of this book (Immunotherapy of Parkinson's disease, Schneeberger et al.).

4   Passive Immunization with Monoclonal Antibodies Against α-syn Toxic Conformations

Despite the promising results obtained in preclinical active immunotherapy studies, the direct administration of monoclonal antibodies designed to bind very specific conformational epitopes of abnormal α-syn aggregates provides with a much more targeted therapy against α-syn that could be potentially used as disease-modifying alternative. In this sense, antibodies that recognize an epitope in the C-terminus of α-syn seem to be more effective at ameliorating the pathology in some tg mouse models of PD, as they clear intracellular aggregates, inhibit α-syn propagation, and prevent C-terminus cleavage of the protein that may lead to increased aggregation [22–25]. Interestingly, the C-terminus of α-syn is the region of the protein believed to be exposed following its insertion in the plasma membrane [26], suggesting that using antibodies against C-terminal epitopes would facilitate the recognition and binding of extracellular antibodies and subsequent internalization. However, other studies have also reported that antibodies against the N-terminus are effective at clearing α-syn aggregates in different tg models, reducing their propagation and diminishing motor dysfunctions [27, 28]. As the N-terminus of α-syn is involved in membrane interaction and formation of amphipathic helices, the authors hypothesized that targeting this part of the protein would inhibit fibrillization and thereby the toxicity of α-syn.

The strong preclinical evidence supporting the therapeutic value of antibodies directed against α-syn for PD has translated into the clinic, and in this sense the C-terminus antibody PRX002 (Prothena Biosciences) and the N-terminus antibody BIIB054 (Biogen) are currently the focus of two Phase I clinical trials. Importantly, for their transition to clinic the antibodies have been humanized by replacing the hypervariable loops of a fully human antibody with the hypervariable loops of the murine antibody that was tested in animal models. Humanized antibodies possess a human Fc portion, which makes them considerably less immunogenic in humans and allows them to interact with human effector cells and the complement cascade [29].

5 Intrabodies and Single-Chain Antibodies: Gene Therapy with Antibody Fragments

Immunoglobulins are voluminous proteins ($\approx$150 kDa) containing numerous disulfide bonds and posttranslational modifications that do not easily cross the blood–brain barrier (BBB) and recognize a limited variety of epitopes. Therefore, recent strategies have focused on using antibody fragments such as single-chain variable fragments (scFvs), fusion proteins of the variable domains of the heavy and light chains linked by a flexible linker and that retain antigen-binding properties. Interestingly, scFvs can be further modified to increase BBB penetrability and facilitate the clearance of α-syn. A fusion protein comprising an scFv against α-syn (clone D5) plus the LDL domain of apolipoprotein B (apoB) was recently studied in a tg model of DLB. The fusion antibody easily crosses the BBB aided by the apoB domain and gets internalized by neurons using the endosomal sorting complexes required for transport (ESCRT) pathway for enhanced degradation of α-syn aggregates [30], thus attenuating neuronal degeneration in vivo. In a similar manner, a fusion protein comprising an scFv and a specific protease could further aid in the clearance of aggregation-prone proteins [31]. Moreover, scFvs that detect individual conformational species of α-syn have been identified [30, 32, 33], and could be potentially used to discriminate among protein conformers [34] for the differential treatment of synucleinopathies or for diagnostic purposes.

Recently, gene therapy with intracellular scFv (intrabodies) has shown promising anti-aggregation and neuroprotective effects against misfolded α-syn aggregates [35–37]. An advantage to the use of intrabodies versus extracellular antibodies is that they can target antigens present in various subcellular locations such as the cytosol, nucleus, endoplasmic reticulum, mitochondria, peroxisomes, and plasma membrane [29, 38], thus being able to easily access intracellular α-syn aggregates. However, intrabodies require to be directly expressed in target cells by means of gene therapy; they have low stability and poor solubility [39]. Despite these disadvantages, a stable cell line expressing the anti-α-syn intrabody NAC32 showed highly significant reductions in abnormal α-syn aggregation in two in vitro models [36]. Moreover, fusion of a proteasome-targeting PEST motif to poorly soluble anti-α-syn intrabodies can significantly increase their solubility and enhance degradation of the target protein [37], thus supporting the versatility of this type of approach.

6   Proposed Mechanisms of Action of Antibodies Against α-syn

Regardless of the origin (active or passive), immunotherapy stimulates or directly provides a humoral protection (antibodies) against toxic α-syn conformations. The mechanisms by which antibodies against α-syn work at ameliorating the pathology are multiple (Fig. 1). Anti-α-syn antibodies are able to reduce aggregation, prevent cell-to-cell propagation of α-syn [24, 25, 27], and thus facilitate the clearance of extracellular α-syn (Fig. 1). Furthermore, antibodies may also inhibit extracellular α-syn C-terminal cleavage [24] and bind and inactivate toxic conformations of the protein (Fig. 1). Both aggregation and cell-to-cell propagation are intimately related to the toxicity of α-syn and PD pathology, suggesting that these processes are promising therapeutic targets for immunotherapy. Moreover, it has been observed that antibodies are able to penetrate cells expressing α-syn, probably thanks to their binding to α-syn oligomers in the plasma membrane [40] followed by interaction of the constant domain of IgG with Fcγ receptors and receptor-mediated endocytosis [41]. Fcγ receptors are expressed on a wide variety of cell types including microglia and neurons [42–44]. Although the activation of Fcγ receptors can result in a pro-inflammatory response including the release of cytokines and other mediators [43, 45], there is evidence suggesting that both active and passive immunization against α-syn can modify the microglial phenotype into one with a greater propensity for phagocytosing α-syn and reduced inflammatory responses [19, 20, 24]. In neurons, antibodies can be imported through the ESCRT pathway, leading to lysosomal degradation of α-syn aggregates [30]. Moreover, antibodies against α-syn may also reduce its oligomerization and fibrillization in living cells, thus ameliorating the pathology in cell and mouse models of PD [20, 46, 47] (Fig. 1). Finally, in addition to central effects, potential peripheral actions of immunotherapy, including a peripheral sink effect on α-syn, have also been hypothesized [48].

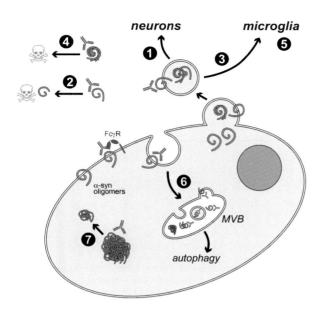

Mechanisms mediating the effects of anti-α-syn antibodies

Extracellular

① Block cell-to-cell propagation

② Block toxic extracellular cleavage (calpain 1)

③ Induce α-syn uptake by phagocytic cells (Fcγ receptors, microglia)

④ Reduce toxicity of small aggregates (oligomers, protofibrils)

⑤ Regulate cytokine response

Intracellular

⑥ Induce α-syn clearance (ESCRT-autophagy, lysosome)

⑦ Inhibit seeding/dissociate existing aggregates

Fig. 1 Mechanisms mediating the effects of anti-α-syn antibodies. Antibodies against α-syn may exert both extracellular and intracellular actions, including stimulating α-syn clearance, blocking α-syn propagation and toxicity, and reducing α-syn pro-inflammatory actions. *ESCRT* endosomal sorting complexes required for transport. *FcγR* Fcγ receptors, *MVB* multivesicular body

7 Conclusions and Future Directions

Developing safe and improved next-generation immunization therapies for the treatment of PD is the main focus of current clinical studies. However, one of the most relevant current challenges of immunotherapies for neurodegenerative disorder remains the diminished efficacy of the therapy in humans when compared to preclinical results obtained in mouse models, as it has been observed with several immunotherapeutic approaches against neurotoxic protein aggregates such as amyloid-beta [49]. In order to develop effective therapies, active or passive strategies that are effective in animal models must be carefully adapted and optimized to the human disease, and more research is needed regarding mechanisms of action that are specific to the human pathology. Targeting α-syn conformers that are specific to PD and making use of the existing knowledge on the different disease stages and windows of therapeutic opportunity would most likely improve the outcome of the immunotherapy. In this sense, it is important to consider that immunotherapeutic approaches would be more effective at pre-symptomatic or early symptomatic stages, before α-syn accumulation is widespread. Finally it is worth mentioning that PD, a complex disorder that progresses through several stages, might require an equally complex therapeutic approach in order to obtain disease-modifying results. In this respect, the effectiveness of therapies such as immunotherapy against α-syn, aimed at reducing α-syn accumulation and cell-to-cell transfer, could be increased if this approach were combined with complementary treatment(s) targeting other aspects of the disease (e.g., neuroinflammation, neuronal loss).

Acknowledgements

Supported by National Institutes of Health (NIH) grants AG18440, AG022074, and NS044233.

References

1. Savica R, Grossardt BR, Bower JH et al. (2013) Incidence and pathology of synucleinopathies and tauopathies related to parkinsonism. JAMA Neurol70(7):859-866

2. Jankovic J (2008) Parkinson's disease: clinical features and diagnosis. J Neurol Neurosurg Psychiatry 79(4):368–376

3. Dickson DW (2001) Alpha-synuclein and the Lewy body disorders. Curr Opin Neurol 14(4): 423–432

4. Spillantini MG, Schmidt ML, Lee VM et al (1997) Alpha-synuclein in Lewy bodies. Nature 388(6645):839–840

5. Takeda A, Hashimoto M, Mallory M et al (1998) Abnormal distribution of the non-Abeta component of Alzheimer's disease amyloid precursor/alpha-synuclein in Lewy body disease as revealed by proteinase K and formic acid pretreatment. Lab Invest 78(9): 1169–1177

6. McKeith IG, Dickson DW, Lowe J et al (2005) Diagnosis and management of dementia with Lewy bodies: third report of the DLB Consortium. Neurology 65(12):1863–1872

7. Fortin DL, Nemani VM, Voglmaier SM et al (2005) Neural activity controls the synaptic accumulation of alpha-synuclein. J Neurosci 25(47):10913–10921

8. George JM, Jin H, Woods WS et al (1995) Characterization of a novel protein regulated during the critical period for song learning in the zebra finch. Neuron 15(2):361–372

9. Iwai A, Masliah E, Yoshimoto M et al (1995) The precursor protein of non-A beta component of Alzheimer's disease amyloid is a presynaptic protein of the central nervous system. Neuron 14(2):467–475

10. Uéda K, Fukushima H, Masliah E et al (1993) Molecular cloning of cDNA encoding an unrecognized component of amyloid in Alzheimer disease. Proc Natl Acad Sci U S A 90(23):11282–11286

11. Masliah E, Iwai A, Mallory M et al (1996) Altered presynaptic protein NACP is associated with plaque formation and neurodegeneration in Alzheimer's disease. Am J Pathol 148(1): 201–210

12. Lashuel HA, Petre BM, Wall J et al (2002) Alpha-synuclein, especially the Parkinson's disease-associated mutants, forms pore-like annular and tubular protofibrils. J Mol Biol 322(5):1089–1102

13. Tsigelny IF, Bar-On P, Sharikov Y et al (2007) Dynamics of alpha-synuclein aggregation and inhibition of pore-like oligomer development by beta-synuclein. FEBS J 274(7):1862–1877

14. Braak H, Del Tredici K, Rub U et al (2003) Staging of brain pathology related to sporadic Parkinson's disease. Neurobiol Aging 24(2): 197–211

15. Reynolds AD, Banerjee R, Liu J et al (2007) Neuroprotective activities of CD4+CD25+ regulatory T cells in an animal model of Parkinson's disease. J Leukoc Biol 82(5): 1083–1094

16. Reynolds AD, Stone DK, Hutter JA et al (2010) Regulatory T cells attenuate Th17 cell-mediated nigrostriatal dopaminergic neurodegeneration in a model of Parkinson's disease. J Immunol 184(5):2261–2271

17. Orgogozo JM, Gilman S, Dartigues JF et al (2003) Subacute meningoencephalitis in a subset of patients with AD after Abeta42 immunization. Neurology 61(1):46–54

18. Masliah E, Rockenstein E, Adame A et al (2005) Effects of alpha-synuclein immunization in a mouse model of Parkinson's disease. Neuron 46(6):857–868

19. Mandler M, Valera E, Rockenstein E et al (2015) Active immunization against alpha-synuclein ameliorates the degenerative pathology and prevents demyelination in a model of multiple system atrophy. Mol Neurodegener 10(1):10

20. Mandler M, Valera E, Rockenstein E et al (2014) Next-generation active immunization approach for synucleinopathies: implications for Parkinson's disease clinical trials. Acta Neuropathol 127(6):861–879

21. Schneeberger A, Mandler M, Mattner F et al (2010) AFFITOME® technology in neurodegenerative diseases: the doubling advantage. Hum Vaccin 6(11):948–952

22. Valera E, Masliah E (2013) Immunotherapy for neurodegenerative diseases: Focus on α-synucleinopathies. Pharmacol Ther 38(3):311–22

23. Masliah E, Rockenstein E, Mante M et al (2011) Passive immunization reduces behavioral and neuropathological deficits in an alpha-synuclein transgenic model of Lewy body disease. PLoS One 6(4):e19338

24. Games D, Valera E, Spencer B et al (2014) Reducing C-terminal-truncated alpha-synuclein by immunotherapy attenuates neurodegeneration and propagation in Parkinson's disease-like models. J Neurosci 34(28):9441–9454

25. Bae EJ, Lee HJ, Rockenstein E et al (2012) Antibody-aided clearance of extracellular alpha-synuclein prevents cell-to-cell aggregate transmission. J Neurosci 32(39):13454–13469

26. Bartels T, Ahlstrom LS, Leftin A et al (2010) The N-terminus of the intrinsically disordered protein alpha-synuclein triggers membrane binding and helix folding. Biophys J 99(7):2116–2124

27. Tran HT, Chung CH, Iba M et al (2014) Alpha-synuclein immunotherapy blocks uptake and templated propagation of misfolded alpha-synuclein and neurodegeneration. Cell Rep 7(6):2054–2065

28. Shahaduzzaman M, Nash K, Hudson C et al (2015) Anti-human alpha-synuclein N-terminal peptide antibody protects against dopaminergic cell death and ameliorates behavioral deficits in an AAV-alpha-synuclein rat model of Parkinson's disease. PLoS One 10(2), e0116841

29. Chames P, Van Regenmortel M, Weiss E et al (2009) Therapeutic antibodies: successes, limitations and hopes for the future. Br J Pharmacol 157(2):220–233

30. Spencer B, Emadi S, Desplats P et al (2014) ESCRT-mediated uptake and degradation of brain-targeted alpha-synuclein single chain antibody attenuates neuronal degeneration in vivo. Mol Ther 22(10):1753–1767

31. Boddapati S, Levites Y, Suryadi V et al (2012) Bispecific tandem single chain antibody simultaneously inhibits beta-secretase and promotes alpha-secretase processing of AbetaPP. J Alzheimers Dis 28(4):961–969

32. Emadi S, Liu R, Yuan B et al (2004) Inhibiting aggregation of alpha-synuclein with human single chain antibody fragments. Biochemistry 43(10):2871–2878

33. Emadi S, Barkhordarian H, Wang MS et al (2007) Isolation of a human single chain antibody fragment against oligomeric alpha-synuclein that inhibits aggregation and prevents alpha-synuclein-induced toxicity. J Mol Biol 368(4):1132–1144

34. Bousset L, Pieri L, Ruiz-Arlandis G et al (2013) Structural and functional characterization of two alpha-synuclein strains. Nat Commun 4:2575

35. Zhou C, Emadi S, Sierks MR et al (2004) A human single-chain Fv intrabody blocks aberrant cellular effects of overexpressed alpha-synuclein. Mol Ther 10(6):1023–1031

36. Lynch SM, Zhou C, Messer A (2008) An scFv intrabody against the nonamyloid component of alpha-synuclein reduces intracellular aggregation and toxicity. J Mol Biol 377(1):136–147

37. Joshi SN, Butler DC, Messer A (2012) Fusion to a highly charged proteasomal retargeting sequence increases soluble cytoplasmic expression and efficacy of diverse anti-synuclein intrabodies. MAbs 4(6)

38. Lo AS, Zhu Q, Marasco WA (2008) Intracellular antibodies (intrabodies) and their therapeutic potential. Handb Exp Pharmacol 181:343–373

39. Kvam E, Sierks MR, Shoemaker CB et al (2010) Physico-chemical determinants of soluble intrabody expression in mammalian cell cytoplasm. Protein Eng Des Sel 23(6):489–498

40. Stefanovic AN, Stockl MT, Claessens MM et al (2014) alpha-Synuclein oligomers distinctively permeabilize complex model membranes. FEBS J 281(12):2838–2850

41. Congdon EE, Gu J, Sait HB et al (2013) Antibody uptake into neurons occurs primarily via clathrin-dependent Fcgamma receptor endocytosis and is a prerequisite for acute tau protein clearance. J Biol Chem 288(49):35452–35465

42. Murinello S, Mullins RF, Lotery AJ et al (2014) Fcgamma receptor upregulation is associated

with immune complex inflammation in the mouse retina and early age-related macular degeneration. Invest Ophthalmol Vis Sci 55(1):247–258

43. Fuller JP, Stavenhagen JB, Teeling JL (2014) New roles for Fc receptors in neurodegeneration-the impact on Immunotherapy for Alzheimer's disease. Front Neurosci 8:235

44. Kam TI, Song S, Gwon Y et al (2013) FcgammaRIIb mediates amyloid-beta neurotoxicity and memory impairment in Alzheimer's disease. J Clin Invest 123(7): 2791–2802

45. Adolfsson O, Pihlgren M, Toni N et al (2012) An effector-reduced anti-β-amyloid (Aβ) antibody with unique aβ binding properties promotes neuroprotection and glial engulfment of Aβ. J Neurosci 32(28):9677–9689

46. Näsström T, Gonçalves S, Sahlin C et al (2011) Antibodies against alpha-synuclein reduce oligomerization in living cells. PLoS One 6(10):e27230

47. Lindstrom V, Fagerqvist T, Nordstrom E et al (2014) Immunotherapy targeting alpha-synuclein protofibrils reduced pathology in (Thy-1)-h[A30P] alpha-synuclein mice. Neurobiol Dis 69:134–143

48. Patrias LM, Klaver AC, Coffey MP et al (2010) Specific antibodies to soluble alpha-synuclein conformations in intravenous immunoglobulin preparations. Clin Exp Immunol 161(3): 527–535

49. Panza F, Logroscino G, Imbimbo BP et al (2014) Is there still any hope for amyloid-based immunotherapy for Alzheimer's disease? Curr Opin Psychiatry 27(2):128–137

Chapter 6

Extracellular α-Synuclein as a Target for Immunotherapy

Jun Sung Lee and Seung-Jae Lee

Abstract

Both genetic and pathological studies strongly suggest that α-synuclein is the main disease-causing molecule in Parkinson's disease (PD). Moreover, a growing body of evidence suggests that α-synuclein, an intra-neuronal protein, is exocytosed from neurons and that extracellular α-synuclein could mediate the major pathological changes in PD, such as neurodegeneration, neuroinflammation, and progressive spreading of protein inclusions. Here, we review the mechanism(s) involved in generation and clearance of extracellular α-synuclein and their pathophysiological implications in neurodegeneration and neuroinflammation. We also discuss extracellular α-synuclein as a therapeutic target for immunotherapy.

Key words Parkinson's disease, Lewy body, Alpha-synuclein, Protein aggregation, Microglia, Aggregate clearance, Lysosome

1 Introduction

The common pathological features of neurodegenerative diseases include abnormal deposition of specific proteins, chronic inflammation in particular brain regions, and selective loss of specific populations of neurons. Parkinson's disease (PD) is a progressive neurodegenerative disease, characterized by the presence of protein inclusions known as Lewy bodies (LBs) and Lewy neurites (LNs), neuroinflammation, and selective degeneration of dopaminergic neurons, mainly in the substantia nigra pars compacta (SNpc) [1]. These pathological changes in the SNpc contribute to motor symptoms, such as resting tremor, bradykinesia, and rigidity of muscle tone [2]. Patients with PD also manifest various non-motor abnormalities, including cognitive impairment, psychiatric symptoms, autonomic dysfunction, and sensory impairment [3]. Some of the non-motor symptoms, such as hyposmia, constipation, and RBD (rapid eye movement sleep behavior disorder), are described as "pre-motor symptoms" as they frequently predate—sometimes by decades—the onset of motor symptoms [4].

Martin Ingelsson and Lars Lannfelt (eds.), *Immunotherapy and Biomarkers in Neurodegenerative Disorders*, Methods in Pharmacology and Toxicology, DOI 10.1007/978-1-4939-3560-4_6, © Springer Science+Business Media New York 2016

The wide range of clinical symptoms could be attributable to the affliction of multiple brain systems. By analyzing the spatial patterns of α-synuclein deposition in *postmortem* brain tissues from PD patients, it was postulated that LBs propagate in a highly predictable manner as the disease progresses [5]. In the central nervous system (CNS), Lewy pathology and neuronal loss first appear in the lower brain stem and olfactory bulb, progressively ascend through the midbrain and mesocortex, and finally spread to wide areas of the neocortex. Furthermore, LB-like pathology was also shown in various peripheral neurons, including neurons in the enteric nervous system during the pre-motor stages of the disease [6]. Progression of the Lewy pathology in various regions outside the midbrain may account for the abundance of the non-motor symptoms commonly observed in PD patients.

The cause of PD still remains elusive. However, the involvement of α-synuclein in both familial and sporadic PD has been extensively demonstrated. α-synuclein is a 140-amino-acid-long protein with a natively unfolded structure [7]. It was identified that fibrillar aggregate of α-synuclein is a major component of LBs [8] and α-synuclein preparation spontaneously forms amyloid fibrils that are structurally related with the ones found in LBs. The involvement of α-synuclein in PD was also postulated by genetic studies. So far, five missense mutations (A53T, A30P, E46K, H50Q, and G51D) have been identified in the gene encoding α-synuclein (*SNCA*) in the inherited forms of parkinsonism [9–13]. All the mutant variants except H50Q were shown to accelerate either oligomerization or fibrillation [14–16]. In addition, multiplication mutations, such as duplication and triplication, in the genomic region including the *alpha-synuclein* gene were also observed in familial cases of PD [17–20]. Increase in α-synuclein protein levels by the multiplication mutations might also facilitate aggregation of this protein [21, 22]. Recently, genome-wide association studies suggested *alpha-synuclein* as a strong genetic risk factor for sporadic PD [23, 24]. The link between α-synuclein aggregation and neuronal toxicity was supported by animal model studies, in which overexpression of wild-type and mutant forms of α-synuclein led to neuronal loss and LB-like inclusion formation [25]. Collectively, these studies suggest that α-synuclein may be causally involved in the development of both familial and sporadic PD.

2   Generation and Physical Nature of Extracellular α-Synuclein

Alpha-synuclein is a cytosolic protein highly expressed in neurons of the neocortex, hippocampus, substantia nigra, thalamus, and cerebellum [26]. Monomeric and oligomeric forms of α-synuclein have also been found in human body fluids, such as plasma, cerebrospinal fluid (CSF) [27], and brain interstitial fluid [28] from both healthy individuals and PD patients. Recent studies provided evidence indicating that a small but significant amount of neuronal α-synuclein was released into the extracellular space. Extracellular α-synuclein was produced via unconventional exocytosis from neuron [29]. Although exophagy [30] and exosome-associated secretion [31] have been proposed as the mechanisms of unconventional exocytosis of α-synuclein, contribution of these mechanisms in producing extracellular α-synuclein has to be further validated.

Secretion of α-synuclein from neurons can be observed in healthy primary neurons in culture [32]. In addition, the presence of α-synuclein in human samples (e.g., plasma, CSF, and the interstitial fluid of brain parenchyma) from individuals without any neurological defects has been reported [27, 28]. These results indicate that secretion of α-synuclein is a naturally occurring phenomenon. Interestingly, secretion of α-synuclein was increased under various conditions leading to protein misfolding and failure of protein quality control [29, 33–35]. Based on these findings, we speculate that secretion of α-synuclein is a mechanism by which neuronal cells dispose of misfolded or damaged α-synuclein proteins. Supporting this idea, α-synuclein secreted from neuronal cells is more extensively oxidized and aggregated compared to the cytosolic α-synuclein [29, 36].

3   Neuronal Toxicity by Neuron-to-Neuron Transmission of α-Synuclein

Direct transfer of α-synuclein between neuronal cells has been shown in cell culture and rodent models [37–39]. In cultured neuronal cells, it was shown that neuron-released α-synuclein was taken up by neighboring neurons through endocytosis [38–40]. In the recipient cells, the transferred α-synuclein induced the formation of inclusion bodies that are positive for ubiquitin and thioflavin S, characteristic features of Lewy bodies [38]. Cell-to-cell transfer of α-synuclein was associated with cell death of recipient neurons. These findings suggest that α-synuclein aggregates produced in one neuron can be transmitted to neighboring neurons by sequential events of exocytosis and endocytosis. This would also explain the LB propagation from host to grafted tissues in patients with PD who received mesencephalic tissue transplants [41, 42]. More recently, when wild-type mice were injected intrastriatally with in vitro-generated, sonicated fibrils of α-synuclein, phosphorylated α-synuclein occurred throughout the brain, which was correlated spatiotemporally with progressive loss of dopaminergic neurons in the SNpc [43]. In terms of neuronal activity, application of oligomeric α-synuclein impaired long-term potentiation in the hippocampal slice preparations [44]. These studies indicate that α-synuclein transmission might be associated with neurodegeneration and synaptic dysfunction. Taken together, neuron-to-neuron transmission of α-synuclein aggregates and the associated neuronal cell death might be the underlying mechanism of the sequential propagation of LB lesions during PD progression [5].

4   Neuroinflammation by Activation of Astrocytes and Microglia

α-Synuclein is expressed almost exclusively in neuronal cells. In brain samples from patients with PD and dementia with Lewy bodies, however, deposition of α-synuclein aggregates has also been detected in glial cells, such as astrocytes [45, 46], indicating that α-synuclein released from neuronal cells can be transferred to glial cells. In cultured cells and a transgenic mouse model, it was shown that α-synuclein released from neuronal cells could be transferred to and accumulated in astrocytes. This induces the expression of genes that are associated with pro-inflammatory responses in astrocytes [47]. Robust transcriptional changes of genes related with proinflammatory cytokines and chemokines were observed when primary astrocytes were treated with α-synuclein secreted from a human dopaminergic neuronal cell line. On the other hand, anti-inflammatory molecules, such as TGFβ3, were reduced in astrocytes upon exposure to α-synuclein [48].

Cytokines and chemokines produced by astrocytes may act as autocrines to play a critical role in the activation, proliferation, and chemotaxis of astrocytes in the CNS [49]. These pro-inflammatory factors could also act as activators and chemo-attractants for microglia, which will lead to more robust and sustained inflammation.

Microglia are the main immune cells in the CNS. Microglia express cell surface receptors for various external and endogenous pathogens and induce the expression of a large variety of inflammatory cytokines and chemokines, affecting the parenchymal microenvironment in both auto- and paracrine fashions. Extracellular α-synuclein has been shown to activate microglia directly and stimulate inflammatory functions. The involvement of α-synuclein in microglia activation and induction of inflammatory responses were initially demonstrated with recombinant α-synuclein preparations [50, 51]. Recently, the molecular species of α-synuclein responsible for microglia activation and the identity of microglia cell surface receptor for extracellular α-synuclein were investigated in vitro and in vivo [36]. In this study, gene expression changes induced by extracellular α-synuclein and detailed signaling pathways related with immune response were analyzed. By using computational biology tools, the toll-like receptor 2 (TLR2) pathway, the Jak-Stat pathway, and the integrin pathway were suggested in various aspects in microglia activation. The following experimental studies demonstrated that the TLR2 pathway was responsible for the pro-inflammatory responses, while the integrin pathway was required for migration of microglia [36, 52]. It was also shown that the recognition of α-synuclein by TLR2 was conformation sensitive, so that only the oligomeric form(s) of α-synuclein was able to bind to TLR2 and trigger inflammatory responses in microglia. Taken together, these findings demonstrate that neuron-released extracellular α-synuclein provokes inflammatory microenvironment by activating astrocytes and microglia. Astrocytes are likely to act as an intermediary signal amplifier, sensing extracellular α-synuclein and relaying this information to microglia for robust inflammatory responses, and microglia respond more directly to neuron-derived α-synuclein oligomers.

Chronic inflammation such as increased levels of cytokines and chemokines in affected brain regions is often associated with neurodegenerative diseases. In PD patients, high levels of proinflammatory factors (TNFα, IL-1β, IL-2, IL-4, IL-6 TGFα, TGFβ1, and TGFβ2) and chemokines (CXCL12/CXCR4) have been detected in brain parenchyma and CSF [53, 54]. In addition, increased levels of cytokines (IL-1β, IFNγ, and TNFγ) and chemokines (CCL2, CCL3, CCL5, and CCL8) were observed in peripheral blood systems from PD patients [55]. The role of extracellular α-synuclein in chronic neuroinflammation needs further verification.

5   Clearance of Extracellular α-Synuclein

Extracellular α-synuclein can be removed either by uptake into neighboring cells or by proteolysis by extracellular proteases. Neuron-released α-synuclein can be taken up and degraded by neurons, astrocytes, and microglia [56, 57]. Among these, microglia are the principal scavengers for extracellular α-synuclein aggregates with the most efficient uptake and degradation. Internalized α-synuclein aggregates are delivered to lysosomes and degraded [40, 56]. Consistent with this, inhibition of lysosomal activity in cultured neurons and glia resulted in increased accumulation of internalized α-synuclein [38, 47].

Clearance of extracellular α-synuclein is also mediated by proteolytic enzymes in the extracellular space such as matrix metalloproteinases (MMP) [58], neurosin (kallikrein 6) [59], and plasmin [60]. Each of these three enzymes recognizes specific amino acid sequences, thus generating unique proteolytic fragments of α-synuclein. For example, MMP-3 cleaves sequences which are localized within or near the central non-Abeta component (NAC) region while neurosin, which is predominantly expressed in the CNS, cleaves residues located in the C-terminal region of α-synuclein. Plasmin was reported to cut the amino acids following lysine residues, which are mainly within the N-terminal and NAC regions in α-synuclein. Cleavage of α-synuclein by neurosin was confirmed in a study using a mouse model, where lentiviral expression of neurosin in α-synuclein transgenic mice resulted in reduced accumulation of α-synuclein and cellular toxicity [61]. In case of plasmin, it was demonstrated that α-synuclein fragments cleaved by plasmin lost their function as an inflammatory stimulator for astrocytes and microglia [60]. In contrast, proteolytic fragments of α-synuclein produced by MMP-3 showed enhanced aggregation in vitro and accordingly higher toxicity in cultured human neuroblastoma cell line [58]. Thus, extracellular proteolytic enzymes may either have a beneficial or a detrimental role and the contribution of these enzymes in the pathogenesis of PD needs to be further characterized [62, 63].

6   Extracellular α-Synuclein as a Target for Immunotherapy

In the last decade, immunotherapy using active or passive immunization has emerged as a promising tool to target and clear protein pathology in neurodegenerative diseases [64–67]. For PD, active immunization with α-synuclein in transgenic mice ameliorated behavioral deficits and α-synuclein deposition in the brain [68]. Likewise, decreased accumulation of α-synuclein aggregates as well as reduced behavioral deficits were reported after passive immunization with a monoclonal antibody in an α-synuclein transgenic mouse model [69]. Another study showed that administration of antibodies against α-synuclein oligomers reduced α-synuclein level in both of cell lysates and conditioned media [70].

The mechanisms underlying the therapeutic effects of immunization against α-synuclein remain elusive. It has become increasingly clear that extracellular α-synuclein is the molecule tightly related with the disease pathology, such as progressive spreading of α-synuclein aggregates, chronic neuroinflammation, neurodegeneration, and neuronal dysfunction [71]. This renders extracellular α-synuclein itself and cellular events involved in its generation and clearance as promising therapeutic targets for PD. In support of this, it was shown that antibody-mediated clearance of extracellular α-synuclein reduced neuronal and glial accumulation of α-synuclein and subsequently ameliorated neurodegeneration as well as behavioral deficits [57]. This was the first study demonstrating in vivo that administration of α-synuclein antibody prevents cell-to-cell transmission of α-synuclein by enhancing the clearance of extracellular α-synuclein by microglia.

In this study, the effects of monoclonal α-synuclein antibody (Ab274) on uptake and degradation of extracellular α-synuclein aggregates (both fibrils and oligomers) were analyzed in microglia, astrocytes, and neurons. Microglia were found to be much better scavengers for extracellular α-synuclein aggregates in the presence of the Ab274. The antibody-α-synuclein immune complexes entered microglia through the Fcγ receptors, which led to efficient

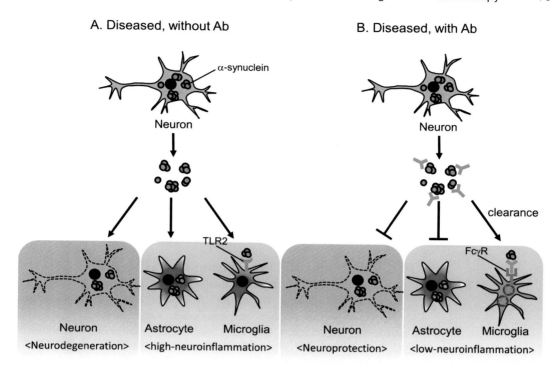

Fig. 1 Immunotherapeutic approach to target extracellular α-synuclein. (**a**) In the diseased brain, α-synuclein aggregates secreted from neurons can mediate aggregate propagation, neuronal death, and inflammatory responses in astrocytes and microglia through the TLR2 signaling pathway. Therefore, extracellular α-synuclein aggregates may be a suitable therapeutic target for PD and other synucleinopathy diseases. (**b**) Administration of antibodies against α-synuclein may have a beneficial effect by promoting clearance of extracellular α-synuclein through the Fcγ receptor-mediated endocytosis into microglia for subsequent lysosomal degradation. Accelerated clearance would prevent the pathogenic actions of extracellular α-synuclein on neurons and glia

delivery of these immune complexes to lysosomes, hence resulting in their degradation (Fig. 1). The role of Ab274 on cell-to-cell transmission of α-synuclein was investigated in a mouse model. When Ab274 was injected into the hippocampus of PDGFβ-α-synuclein tg mice, neuron-to-astrocyte transfer of α-synuclein was significantly reduced, while localization of α-synuclein and Ab274 in microglia was enhanced. These results suggest that Ab274 can prevent cell-to-cell transmission of α-synuclein by enhancing microglia-mediated clearance of extracellular α-synuclein.

Passive immunization of α-synuclein tg mice with Ab274 showed amelioration of neuronal loss, motor behavioral deficits, and production of pro-inflammatory cytokines. All these therapeutic effects occurred concomitantly with increased localization of α-synuclein in microglia, again suggesting that Ab274 works via enhancing the clearance of α-synuclein by microglia. More recently, another study showed that administration of α-synuclein monoclonal antibody blocked cell-to-cell transmission of α-synuclein by interfering with uptake of fibrils in neurons in culture. The same study also showed that systemic administration of the antibodies to mice reduced spreading of fibril-induced synucleinopathies in the brain and also decreased dopaminergic neuronal death, and motor dysfunctions [72]. This study, however, did not investigate the role of antibodies with respect to clearance of α-synuclein. Taken together, these studies suggest that immunotherapy targeted to α-synuclein probably works in multiple mechanisms, and clinical advantages might be expected if extracellular α-synuclein is selectively targeted by immunotherapy with the intra-neuronal α-synuclein being left intact.

7   Future Strategies for PD Immunotherapy

Evidence has been accumulating to support the notion that extra-cellular α-synuclein is a crucial factor mediating neurological changes in PD and perhaps also the other synuclein-related neuro-logical disorders. Moreover, evidence suggests that oligomeric forms of α-synuclein are responsible for inducing neurotoxicity and neuroinflammation [73]. Thus, immunotherapy specifically targeting α-synuclein oligomers might have additional advantages in terms of enhancing specificity for pathogenic species and mini-mizing interference with the physiological functions of the native α-synuclein. Therefore, generation of antibodies specific for patho-genic conformations of α-synuclein might be an effective strategy for immunotherapy against synucleinopathies. As an example, antibody specifically targeting cytotoxic protofibrils of α-synuclein (mAB47) was generated and could decrease the levels of protofi-brils in the Thy-1-h[A30P] mouse model [74]. In addition, an active immunization strategy which targets α-synuclein oligomers was performed in tg mouse models of PDGFβ- and mThy1-α-synuclein [75]. Vaccination with a short peptide (AFF1) induced the production of α-synuclein oligomer-specific antibodies and showed reduced accumulation of α-synuclein oligomers in neurons and increased the number of tyrosine hydroxylase-positive nerve terminals in the striatum. The vaccination was also shown to alleviate motor dysfunctions and memory deficits.

Another important issue is the delivery of antibodies into brain parenchyma through the blood–brain barrier. Recent studies made a significant improvement in developing antibody engineering techniques to produce the BBB-penetrating antibodies [76]. Improvements of antibodies in selectivity to the pathogenic forms and in BBB penetration ability should increase the chance for immunotherapy to become an effective strategy for PD and other synucleinopathies.

References

1. Forno LS (1996) Neuropathology of Parkinson's disease. J Neuropathol Exp Neurol 55:259–272
2. Fahn S, Sulzer D (2004) Neurodegeneration and neuroprotection in Parkinson disease. NeuroRx 1:139–154
3. Ferrer I (2011) Neuropathology and neurochemistry of nonmotor symptoms in Parkinson's disease. Parkinsons Dis 2011:708404
4. Langston JW (2006) The Parkinson's complex: parkinsonism is just the tip of the iceberg. Ann Neurol 59:591–596
5. Braak H, Del Tredici K (2008) Invited Article: Nervous system pathology in sporadic Parkinson disease. Neurology 70:1916–1925
6. Braak H, de Vos RA, Bohl J et al (2006) Gastric alpha-synuclein immunoreactive inclusions in Meissner's and Auerbach's plexuses in cases staged for Parkinson's disease-related brain pathology. Neurosci Lett 396:67–72
7. Weinreb PH, Zhen W, Poon AW et al (1996) NACP, a protein implicated in Alzheimer's disease and learning, is natively unfolded. Biochemistry 35:13709–13715
8. Spillantini MG, Schmidt ML, Lee VM et al (1997) Alpha-synuclein in Lewy bodies. Nature 388:839–840
9. Polymeropoulos MH, Lavedan C, Leroy E et al (1997) Mutation in the alpha-synuclein gene identified in families with Parkinson's disease. Science 276:2045–2047
10. Kruger R, Kuhn W, Muller T et al (1998) Ala30Pro mutation in the gene encoding alpha-synuclein in Parkinson's disease. Nat Genet 18:106–108
11. Zarranz JJ, Alegre J, Gomez-Esteban JC et al (2004) The new mutation, E46K, of alpha-synuclein causes Parkinson and Lewy body dementia. Ann Neurol 55:164–173
12. Appel-Cresswell S, Vilarino-Guell C, Encarnacion M et al (2013) Alpha-synuclein p.H50Q, a novel pathogenic mutation for Parkinson's disease. Mov Disord 28:811–813
13. Lesage S, Anheim M, Letournel F et al (2013) G51D alpha-synuclein mutation causes a novel Parkinsonian-pyramidal syndrome. Ann Neurol 73:459–471
14. Conway KA, Lee SJ, Rochet JC et al (2000) Accelerated oligomerization by Parkinson's disease linked alpha-synuclein mutants. Ann N Y Acad Sci 920:42–45
15. Greenbaum EA, Graves CL, Mishizen-Eberz AJ et al (2005) The E46K mutation in alpha-synuclein increases amyloid fibril formation. J Biol Chem 280:7800–7807
16. Ghosh D, Mondal M, Mohite GM et al (2013) The Parkinson's disease-associated H50Q mutation accelerates alpha-Synuclein aggregation in vitro. Biochemistry 52:6925–6927
17. Singleton AB, Farrer M, Johnson J et al (2003) Alpha-synuclein locus triplication causes Parkinson's disease. Science 302:841
18. Chartier-Harlin MC, Kachergus J, Roumier C et al (2004) Alpha-synuclein locus duplication as a cause of familial Parkinson's disease. Lancet 364:1167–1169
19. Ibanez P, Bonnet AM, Debarges B et al (2004) Causal relation between alpha-synuclein gene duplication and familial Parkinson's disease. Lancet 364:1169–1171
20. Ross OA, Braithwaite AT, Skipper LM et al (2008) Genomic investigation of alpha-synuclein multiplication and parkinsonism. Ann Neurol 63:743–750
21. Farrer M, Kachergus J, Forno L et al (2004) Comparison of kindreds with parkinsonism and alpha-synuclein genomic multiplications. Ann Neurol 55:174–179
22. Miller DW, Hague SM, Clarimon J et al (2004) Alpha-synuclein in blood and brain from familial Parkinson disease with SNCA locus triplication. Neurology 62:1835–1838
23. Satake W, Nakabayashi Y, Mizuta I et al (2009) Genome-wide association study identifies common variants at four loci as genetic risk factors for Parkinson's disease. Nat Genet 41:1303–1307
24. Simon-Sanchez J, Schulte C, Bras JM et al (2009) Genome-wide association study reveals genetic risk underlying Parkinson's disease. Nat Genet 41:1308–1312
25. Maries E, Dass B, Collier TJ et al (2003) The role of alpha-synuclein in Parkinson's disease: insights from animal models. Nat Rev Neurosci 4:727–738
26. Iwai A, Masliah E, Yoshimoto M et al (1995) The precursor protein of non-A beta component of Alzheimer's disease amyloid is a presynaptic protein of the central nervous system. Neuron 14:467–475
27. El-Agnaf OM, Salem SA, Paleologou KE et al (2003) Alpha-synuclein implicated in Parkinson's disease is present in extracellular biological fluids, including human plasma. FASEB J 17:1945–1947
28. Emmanouilidou E, Elenis D, Papasilekas T et al (2011) Assessment of alpha-synuclein secretion in mouse and human brain parenchyma. PLoS One 6:e22225

29. Jang A, Lee HJ, Suk JE et al (2010) Non-classical exocytosis of alpha-synuclein is sensitive to folding states and promoted under stress conditions. J Neurochem 113:1263–1274

30. Ejlerskov P, Rasmussen I, Nielsen TT et al (2013) Tubulin polymerization-promoting protein (TPPP/p25alpha) promotes unconventional secretion of alpha-synuclein through exophagy by impairing autophagosome-lysosome fusion. J Biol Chem 288:17313–17335

31. Emmanouilidou E, Melachroinou K, Roumeliotis T et al (2010) Cell-produced alpha-synuclein is secreted in a calcium-dependent manner by exosomes and impacts neuronal survival. J Neurosci 30:6838–6851

32. Lee HJ, Patel S, Lee SJ (2005) Intravesicular localization and exocytosis of alpha-synuclein and its aggregates. J Neurosci 25:6016–6024

33. Lee HJ, Baek SM, Ho DH et al (2011) Dopamine promotes formation and secretion of non-fibrillar alpha-synuclein oligomers. Exp Mol Med 43:216–222

34. Bae EJ, Ho DH, Park E et al (2013) Lipid peroxidation product 4-hydroxy-2-nonenal promotes seeding-capable oligomer formation and cell-to-cell transfer of alpha-synuclein. Antioxid Redox Signal 18:770–783

35. Lee HJ, Cho ED, Lee KW et al (2013) Autophagic failure promotes the exocytosis and intercellular transfer of alpha-synuclein. Exp Mol Med 45, e22

36. Kim C, Ho DH, Suk JE et al (2013) Neuron-released oligomeric alpha-synuclein is an endogenous agonist of TLR2 for paracrine activation of microglia. Nat Commun 4:1562

37. Danzer KM, Ruf WP, Putcha P et al (2011) Heat-shock protein 70 modulates toxic extracellular alpha-synuclein oligomers and rescues trans-synaptic toxicity. FASEB J 25:326–336

38. Desplats P, Lee HJ, Bae EJ et al (2009) Inclusion formation and neuronal cell death through neuron-to-neuron transmission of alpha-synuclein. Proc Natl Acad Sci 106:13010–13015

39. Hansen C, Angot E, Bergstrom AL et al (2011) Alpha-synuclein propagates from mouse brain to grafted dopaminergic neurons and seeds aggregation in cultured human cells. J Clin Invest 121:715–725

40. Lee HJ, Suk JE, Bae EJ et al (2008) Assembly-dependent endocytosis and clearance of extracellular alpha-synuclein. Int J Biochem Cell Biol 40:1835–1849

41. Kordower JH, Dodiya HB, Kordower AM et al (2011) Transfer of host-derived alpha synuclein to grafted dopaminergic neurons in rat. Neurobiol Dis 43:552–557

42. Li JY, Englund E, Holton JL et al (2008) Lewy bodies in grafted neurons in subjects with Parkinson's disease suggest host-to-graft disease propagation. Nat Med 14:501–503

43. Luk KC, Kehm V, Carroll J et al (2012) Pathological alpha-synuclein transmission initiates Parkinson-like neurodegeneration in non-transgenic mice. Science 338:949–953

44. Diogenes MJ, Dias RB, Rombo DM et al (2012) Extracellular alpha-synuclein oligomers modulate synaptic transmission and impair LTP via NMDA-receptor activation. J Neurosci 32:11750–11762

45. Wakabayashi K, Hayashi S, Yoshimoto M et al (2000) NACP/alpha-synuclein-positive filamentous inclusions in astrocytes and oligodendrocytes of Parkinson's disease brains. Acta Neuropathol 99:14–20

46. Halliday GM, Stevens CH (2011) Glia: initiators and progressors of pathology in Parkinson's disease. Mov Disord 26:6–17

47. Lee HJ, Suk JE, Patrick C et al (2010) Direct transfer of alpha-synuclein from neuron to astroglia causes inflammatory responses in synucleinopathies. J Biol Chem 285:9262–9272

48. Lee HJ, Kim C, Lee SJ (2010) Alpha-synuclein stimulation of astrocytes: potential role for neuroinflammation and neuroprotection. Oxid Med Cell Longev 3:283–287

49. Farina C, Aloisi F, Meinl E (2007) Astrocytes are active players in cerebral innate immunity. Trends Immunol 28:138–145

50. Zhang W, Wang T, Pei Z et al (2005) Aggregated alpha-synuclein activates microglia: a process leading to disease progression in Parkinson's disease. FASEB J 19:533–542

51. Reynolds AD, Glanzer JG, Kadiu I et al (2008) Nitrated alpha-synuclein-activated microglial profiling for Parkinson's disease. J Neurochem 104:1504–1525

52. Kim C, Cho ED, Kim HK et al (2014) Beta1-integrin-dependent migration of microglia in response to neuron-released alpha-synuclein. Exp Mol Med 46:e91

53. Mogi M, Harada M, Narabayashi H et al (1996) Interleukin (IL)-1 beta, IL-2, IL-4, IL-6 and transforming growth factor-alpha levels are elevated in ventricular cerebrospinal fluid in juvenile Parkinsonism and Parkinson's disease. Neurosci Lett 211:13–16

54. Savarin-Vuaillat C, Ransohoff RM (2007) Chemokines and chemokine receptors in neurological disease: raise, retain, or reduce? Neurotherapeutics 4:590–601

55. Reale M, Greig NH, Kamal MA (2009) Peripheral chemo-cytokine profiles in Alzheimer's

and Parkinson's diseases. Mini Rev Med Chem 9:1229–1241

56. Lee HJ, Suk JE, Bae EJ et al (2008) Clearance and deposition of extracellular alpha-synuclein aggregates in microglia. Biochem Biophys Res Commun 372:423–428

57. Bae EJ, Lee HJ, Rockenstein E et al (2012) Antibody-aided clearance of extracellular alpha-synuclein prevents cell-to-cell aggregate transmission. J Neurosci 32:13454–13469

58. Sung JY, Park SM, Lee CH et al (2005) Proteolytic cleavage of extracellular secreted {alpha}-synuclein via matrix metalloproteinases. J Biol Chem 280:25216–25224

59. Tatebe H, Watanabe Y, Kasai T et al (2010) Extracellular neurosin degrades alpha-synuclein in cultured cells. Neurosci Res 67:341–346

60. Kim KS, Choi YR, Park JY et al (2012) Proteolytic cleavage of extracellular alpha-synuclein by plasmin: implications for Parkinson disease. J Biol Chem 287:24862–24872

61. Spencer B, Michael S, Shen J et al (2013) Lentivirus mediated delivery of neurosin promotes clearance of wild-type alpha-synuclein and reduces the pathology in an alpha-synuclein model of LBD. Mol Ther 21:31–41

62. Levin J, Giese A, Boetzel K et al (2009) Increased alpha-synuclein aggregation following limited cleavage by certain matrix metalloproteinases. Exp Neurol 215:201–208

63. Sheehan JJ, Tsirka SE (2005) Fibrin-modifying serine proteases thrombin, tPA, and plasmin in ischemic stroke: a review. Glia 50:340–350

64. Atwal JK, Chen Y, Chiu C et al (2011) A therapeutic antibody targeting BACE1 inhibits amyloid-beta production in vivo. Sci Transl Med 3:84ra43

65. Delrieu J, Ousset PJ, Caillaud C et al (2012) 'Clinical trials in Alzheimer's disease': immunotherapy approaches. J Neurochem 120(Suppl 1):186–193

66. Gros-Louis F, Soucy G, Lariviere R et al (2010) Intracerebroventricular infusion of monoclonal antibody or its derived Fab fragment against misfolded forms of SOD1 mutant delays mortality in a mouse model of ALS. J Neurochem 113:1188–1199

67. Panza F, Frisardi V, Solfrizzi V et al (2012) Immunotherapy for Alzheimer's disease: from anti-beta-amyloid to tau-based immunization strategies. Immunotherapy 4:213–238

68. Masliah E, Rockenstein E, Adame A et al (2005) Effects of alpha-synuclein immunization in a mouse model of Parkinson's disease. Neuron 46:857–868

69. Masliah E, Rockenstein E, Mante M et al (2011) Passive immunization reduces behavioral and neuropathological deficits in an alpha-synuclein transgenic model of Lewy body disease. PLoS One 6:e19338

70. Nasstrom T, Goncalves S, Sahlin C et al (2011) Antibodies against alpha-synuclein reduce oligomerization in living cells. PLoS One 6:e27230

71. Lee HJ, Bae EJ, Lee SJ (2014) Extracellular alpha—synuclein-a novel and crucial factor in Lewy body diseases. Nat Rev Neurol 10:92–98

72. Tran HT, Chung CH, Iba M et al (2014) Alpha-synuclein immunotherapy blocks uptake and templated propagation of misfolded alpha-synuclein and neurodegeneration. Cell Rep 7:2054–2065

73. Du HN, Tang L, Luo XY et al (2003) A peptide motif consisting of glycine, alanine, and valine is required for the fibrillization and cytotoxicity of human alpha-synuclein. Biochemistry 42:8870–8878

74. Lindstrom V, Fagerqvist T, Nordstrom E et al (2014) Immunotherapy targeting alpha-synuclein protofibrils reduced pathology in (Thy-1)-h[A30P] alpha-synuclein mice. Neurobiol Dis 69:134–143

75. Mandler M, Valera E, Rockenstein E et al (2014) Next-generation active immunization approach for synucleinopathies: implications for Parkinson's disease clinical trials. Acta Neuropathol 127:861–879

76. Niewoehner J, Bohrmann B, Collin L et al (2014) Increased brain penetration and potency of a therapeutic antibody using a monovalent molecular shuttle. Neuron 81:49–60

Chapter 7

Immunotherapy of Parkinson's Disease

Achim Schneeberger, Suzanne Hendrix, and Markus Mandler

Abstract

Parkinson's disease (PD) is the second most common neurodegenerative disorder. It elicits a broad range of debilitating motor and as well as non-motor symptoms, both of which can lead to serious disability. There is currently no available agent with disease modifying properties. Immunotherapy is increasingly being investigated as a disease modifying treatment for PD based on our improved understanding of the pathophysiology of the disease. Current evidence points to a causal role of misfolded alpha-synuclein (α-syn) in the development and progression of PD and it has therefore become a primary focus for immunotherapy. Today, two principal approaches are being pursued: active and passive immunization. This chapter first addresses progress in active and passive immunotherapeutic approaches targeting α-syn for Parkinson's disease in animal models. We then discuss clinical progress of α-syn immunotherapy including ongoing clinical trials. Finally, we address challenges and future perspectives for PD immunotherapy.

Key words Alpha-synuclein, Parkinson's disease, Synucleinopathy, Clinical trial, AFFITOPE®, Passive immunotherapy, Vaccination

Abbreviations

α-syn	Alpha-synuclein
β-syn	Beta-synuclein
DA	Dopamine
DLB	Dementia with Lewy bodies
DOPAC	3,4-Dihydroxyphenylacetic acid
GCI	Glial cytoplasmatic inclusions
h	Human
HVA	Homovanillic acid
LB	Lewy body
mAb	Monoclonal antibody
MSA	Multiple system atrophy
PD	Parkinson's disease
PDD	Parkinson's disease dementia
REM	Rapid eye movement
MWM	Morris water maze

Martin Ingelsson and Lars Lannfelt (eds.), *Immunotherapy and Biomarkers in Neurodegenerative Disorders*, Methods in Pharmacology and Toxicology, DOI 10.1007/978-1-4939-3560-4_7, © Springer Science+Business Media New York 2016

1 Parkinson's Disease Is a Synucleinopathy

1.1 Parkinson's Disease

Parkinson's disease (PD) is the second most common neurodegenerative disorder [1, 2], affecting approximately 2 % of the population above 60 years of age in Western countries. Currently about five million people worldwide are affected by PD and its prevalence is rising as the world's population ages. The disease bears the name of James Parkinson, an English physician who first described the disease, which he termed the "shaking palsy" more than 200 years ago [3].

Increasing evidence points to a causal role of misfolded alpha-synuclein (α-syn) in the development and progression of the disease. Although traditionally considered a motor disease, PD is characterized by motor as well as non-motor features, both of which can cause significant disability. The cardinal motor symptoms of PD include resting tremor, bradykinesia, rigidity, and postural instability. Two forms of the disease are distinguished clinically: a tremor and an axial type of PD, depending on the predominance of symptoms. Motor symptoms begin insidiously and progress gradually over time. Non-motor features include neuropsychiatric (e.g., depression, REM sleep disorder), gastrointestinal (e.g., constipation), and autonomic symptoms. The most common disabling non-motor feature is dementia. Nonspecific, non-motor symptoms like hyposmia or constipation are typically the presenting sign and can precede motor signs by decades.

Today's treatments address the lack of dopamine and, thus, primarily the motor symptoms. They fall into different categories. Levodopa, the oldest agent used, is the precursor in the cascade of chemical reactions leading to the synthesis of dopamine. Monoamine oxidase inhibitors reduce dopamine degradation, while dopamine receptor agonists mimic receptor stimulation by dopamine. The common theme among these treatments is dopamine replacement and they are thus only symptomatic. Therefore, PD management faces several main challenges.

There is currently no agent with disease-modifying properties. As a result, it is not possible to halt disease progression. Moreover, currently available symptomatic drugs have limited activity, often leading to inadequate control of symptoms. Additionally, patients become more resistant to the symptomatic treatment as the disease progresses, which decreases the therapeutic effectivity and, ultimately, lead to their failure. Motor complications (e.g., dyskinesia) have also been associated with long-term use of symptomatic agents, in particular levodopa. Finally, measures to combat PD's non-motor symptoms are limited. An example to this is cognitive decline/dementia. There is no agent specifically addressing cognitive decline in PD. Donepezil, a cholinesterase inhibitor, originally licensed for Alzheimer's disease (AD), was an obvious candidate to test and potentially repurpose for use in PD patients also displaying dementia (PDD). Recently, however, Donepezil has been shown in a randomized clinical trial to possess only modest activity in PDD, primarily improving cognitive endpoints without detectable effects on the associated functional deficits [4].

1.2 Parkinson's Disease: A Synucleinopathy

The neuropathological hallmark of PD, beyond the degeneration of dopaminergic cells in the substantia nigra pars compacta and their projections to the caudate [5], is the Lewy body (LB). This eosinophilic cytoplasmic inclusion appears mainly in neurons and is predominantly composed of misfolded, fibrillar α-syn [6]. Dementia with Lewy bodies (DLB) is another disease characterized by the occurrence of such protein deposits. In contrast to PD, where LBs and Lewy neurites (LNs) are distributed in the mesencephalon, in the DLB brain they are also found in the cerebral cortex [7]. In multiple system atrophy (MSA), pathological α-syn is deposited within glial cytoplasmic inclusions (GCIs) in glial cells. PD, DLB, MSA, and other rare diseases (e.g., neurodegeneration with brain iron accumulation) are classified as synucleinopathies, reflecting the contribution of α-syn pathology to development and progression also of these disorders. Deposits of pathological α-syn are sometimes also present in AD, particularly in the amygdala and limbic structures [8, 9]. Hence, such cases can be said to have the Lewy body variant of AD.

1.3 Alpha-Synuclein

Alpha-synuclein is a 140-amino acid (aa), natively unfolded soluble protein localized in the presynaptic terminals and predominantly expressed in the neurons of the neocortex, hippocampus, substantia nigra, thalamus, and cerebellum [6, 10]. α-syn was first cloned from the neuromuscular junction of the electric eel *Torpedo Californica* [11] and could years later be identified in human brains as the precursor protein of the non-Aß component of amyloid plaques in AD [10, 12]. Under physiological conditions, α-syn is located in neuronal synaptic terminals and is specifically upregulated in a discrete population of presynaptic terminals during acquisition-related synaptic rearrangement and also appears to be involved in synaptic plasticity [13–15].

1.4 Role of Alpha-Synuclein in PD

There is mounting evidence for a causal and essential role of α-syn in PD pathogenesis (Table 1). Genetic studies revealed that certain dominantly inherited forms of PD are caused by mutations in, or duplications of, the α-syn gene [16]. Additionally, α-syn represents the major component of the disease's neuropathological signature lesions: LBs and LNs. Genome wide association studies (GWAS) have identified variants of the α-syn gene that pose the highest risk for the development of sporadic PD [17–20]. Moreover, overexpression of native, human α-syn recapitulates certain features of the disease in experimental animals. Finally, there is an overall correlation between α-syn pathology, with regard to its localization and

Table 1
Role for α-syn in Parkinson's disease

Indication for a central role of α-syn in PD	Analysis	References
α-syn is the major component of pathological hallmark lesions: Lewy bodies, Lewy neurites	Pathologic examination	[6, 33–36]
Point mutations in the α-syn gene (protein coding) cause familial PD forms	Genetic analyses	[35, 37]
Increase of cerebral α-syn (gene dose; a third copy of the wt gene is sufficient!) can cause familial PD forms	Genetic analyses	[21, 24, 38]
Specific α-syn gene variants confer risk of developing idiopathic PD	GWAS analysis (risk assessment)	[17–20]
Overexpression of human α-syn in experimental animals recapitulates key features of PD	Animal models	[39–43]
Pathologic α-syn can interfere with normal synapse function, dopamine transport, protein degradation and is neurotoxic	Animal models and tissue culture work	[25, 41, 44]
Distribution of α-syn pathology (central/peripheral) reflects clinical course/ expression of PD	Clinicopathological correlation analysis	[34, 45, 46]

distribution within the nervous system, and the type of clinical symptoms experienced by a given patient.

These studies highlight the importance of mutated and native α-syn for both genetic and sporadic forms of the disease. Less is known regarding the actual mechanisms of α-syn toxicity. Current understanding suggests that aggregated forms of α-syn are the most relevant toxic species. This is supported by several lines of evidence. Genetic studies demonstrate even moderate elevations of native α-syn to be associated with a higher risk for PD [21]. Similarly, Gaucher's disease, characterized by a defect in glucocerebrosidase that results in reduced clearance of proteins including α-syn, is also associated with a high frequency of PD [22]. High α-syn concentrations, occurring as a result of either overproduction or reduced clearance, lead to the formation of α-syn aggregates. Several studies consistently demonstrated that α-syn aggregates exert neurotoxic effects [23–26]. Therefore, lowering α-syn levels, which results in reduced aggregation/oligomerization and deposition into LBs might induce a beneficial, disease-modifying effect in PD patients.

While the accumulation and aggregation of α-syn appears to be the toxic culprit, downstream events such as inflammation, mitochondrial dysfunction and oxidative stress are likely to mediate and modulate its toxicity [27–29]. Emerging evidence points to a crucial role of inflammation in neurodegenerative disorders including PD [30]. Misfolded proteins, including α-syn, and nucleic acids released from dying cells have been shown to trigger inflammatory signaling pathways through specialized pattern recognition receptors (PRR) [31, 32]. Microglia is one cell type in the brain expressing PPRs. A working hypothesis is whether constant stimulation of microglia by pathological α-syn would divert them from their beneficial housekeeping functions turning them into cells that essentially contribute to the neurodegenerative processes by the sustained release of pro-inflammatory mediators.

1.5 Cell-to-Cell Propagation of Pathological α-syn is an Integral Element of PD Pathogenesis

Increasing evidence suggests propagation of pathological α-syn from cell-to-cell to be a central element of PD and other synucleinopathies [47]. The concept of cell-to-cell spreading of pathological α-syn was first put forward by Braak and colleagues [33]. These investigators described a stereotypical and topographical pattern of dissemination of α-syn aggregates in the nervous system of PD patients, which originates in the gut and ultimately spreads via the brain stem to cortical areas of the brain. Further evidence supporting a cell-to-cell transfer was provided by the demonstration of LBs in dopaminergic neurons, derived from "healthy" embryonic stem cells, that had been transplanted a decade before into the striatum of PD patients [48, 49].

Increasing data now support the notion that cell-to-cell transfer of pathological α-syn occurs in a prion like manner in PD. This includes the demonstration that intracerebral injection of purified α-syn fibrils results in the accumulation of α-syn aggregates in host neurons, transfer of aggregates from terminals to cell bodies and to anatomically related neurons [50–52]. Consistent with a prion process, this type of transfer of α-syn pathology has been observed in α-syn overexpressing mice, as well as in wild-type, but not in α-syn-null mice. Direct evidence that diseases like PD and MSA are prion-like disorders stems from the demonstration that inoculation of tissue homogenates derived from the brains of PD and MSA patients into the brain of experimental animals can trigger the formation of α-syn aggregates and their spread throughout the CNS of injected animals. Material inoculated was isolated from MSA [53] and PD [54] patients and found to cause pathology when injected intracerebrally into transgenic rodents heterozygous for the α-syn A53T mutation [53] as well as into wild-type mice and macaque monkeys [54].

2 Addressing Synucleinopathies by Immunological Means

2.1 Types of Specific Immunotherapy

The development and application of immunotherapeutic approaches for the treatment of synucleinopathies has been bolstered by the recent discovery that the intracellular protein α-syn can be secreted by neuronal cells and is subsequently also transmitted in a prion-like

fashion from cell-to-cell leading to spreading of pathologic alterations in the brain.

Two principal approaches are being pursued: active and passive
immunization. Active immunization, i.e., vaccination, involves the
administration of an antigen formulated in a manner that allows
the exposed organism to elicit a specific immune response directed
towards the antigen. In contrast, passive immunization refers to
the administration of in vitro generated antibodies (Abs) specific
for a given target. A common feature of these two approaches is
their high target specificity, although they differ on a number of
important aspects. Active immunization relies on the immune system of the vaccinated individual to activate/generate the intended
effector cells/molecules. While it is possible to establish dose-
response relationships for a cohort of patients, predicting the
response of a given patient is not yet possible. A new generation of
vaccines, typically based on short antigenic sequences, can target
self-antigens without imposing a risk of cellular autoimmunity.
Initial experience with vaccines targeting self-proteins, such as Aß,
demonstrated the feasibility of this approach in humans [55].
These previous studies also showed that the persistence of the Ab
response requires boost immunizations, presumably at 6–9 months
intervals. As for passive immunization, there is extensive experience for Aß in the case of AD [56, 57]. The respective clinical
programs demonstrate that Abs targeting the self-peptide Aß can
be safely administered to AD patients; Specific adverse events associated with Aß pathology/-immunotherapy include vasogenic
edema and increase in the number of microhemorrhages. Clinical
efficacy of Aß-specific Abs has yet to be proven. Ongoing programs
aim at administering respective Abs to cohorts of well-defined AD
patients (e.g., amyloid imaging positive; genetically defined populations) in early stages of their disease. In a phase II clinical trial
with AFFITOPE® AD02, a peptide-KLH conjugate vaccine targeting Aß developed by AFFiRiS, was found to be generally well tolerated. The most common local reactions were erythema, swelling,
warmth, induration, pain, and pruritus (Schneeberger et al., in
preparation).

Especially important to targeting α-syn, a regulator of synaptic
function, is the prevention of adverse effects of a given immunotherapeutic approach with regard to interference with the physiological functions of α-syn. The current thinking is that this can be
achieved by focusing on pathological variants of the molecule.
Prime targets are aggregated and post-translationally modified
forms of α-syn. Another aspect to keep in mind is the question as
to whether vaccination-induced effector mechanisms would result
in a general state of neuroinflammation, potentially aggravating
the clinical phenotype of the disease. The last decade experienced
preclinical evaluation of various active and passive vaccination
strategies [58–65] that support their use in PD treatment.

Active or passive immunization against α-syn both increase the clearance of toxic aggregates, which can occur due to an Fc receptor dependent and independent manner including macrophage activation or by autophagy. The therapies may also reduce extracellular α-syn propagation and thus promote neuroprotection. In addition, direct uptake of α-syn specific Abs in neurons and concomitant α-syn binding could trigger lysosomal α-syn degradation and reduction of toxic α-syn species intraneuronally.

2.2 Active Immunotherapy Targeting α-syn for Parkinson's Disease

Masliah and colleagues from the University of California San Diego were the first to provide experimental evidence supporting the concept of reducing α-syn by immunological means. They used mice overexpressing human α-syn under the control of the platelet-derived growth factor-β (PDGF-β) promoter and immunized them with a vaccine based on full-length α-syn admixed with Freund's adjuvant (complete for the first shot, incomplete form for the following administrations) [59, 63, 64].

Using the active immunotherapy approach mice immunized with full-length α-syn developed Abs with high relative affinity to α-syn. These animals showed decreased accumulation of aggregated human α-syn in neuronal cell bodies and synapses, which was associated with reduced neurodegeneration. With regard to their mode of action, experiments suggest that the Abs generated recognized abnormal human α-syn associated with the neuronal membrane and promoted the degradation of human α-syn aggregates, probably via lysosomal pathways. The therapeutic principle appeared to reside within the vaccine-induced Abs as suggested by the fact that similar effects were observed following the i.v. application of a fluorescein isothiocyanate (FITC)-tagged human α-syn-specific Ab. The authors conclude that vaccination is effective in reducing neuronal accumulation of human α-syn aggregates [63]. Importantly, in this model active immunization against α-syn did not trigger a detrimental neuroinflammatory response in immunized mice as evidenced by the evaluation of brains from immunized mice with microglial and astroglial markers [63].

The active vaccination experiments conducted by Masliah and colleagues demonstrated the feasibility of this approach to treat synucleinopathies, including PD. At the time of publication this was unexpected as the α-syn pathology was thought to be intracellular and the cell-to-cell prion-like spread component in the pathobiology of the disease was not yet discovered.

Direct translation of this active immunization approach to patients was not possible for at least two reasons. One was the adjuvant used, Freund's adjuvant, which is not registered for human use. More importantly, the size of α-syn imposes a significant risk for cellular autoimmunity [66, 67]. Subsequent research (Table 2) provided different solutions to tackle this topic: the activation of regulatory T cells controlling α-syn-specific, potentially

Table 2
α-syn active vaccination in experimental animal models

Animal model	Transgene	Treatment	Adjuvant	Effect	Reference
Mouse PDGF-α-syn, D-Line	h-wt-α-syn	Active IT using full length human α-syn	CFA/IFA	• Induction of α-syn-specific IgG Abs • Reduction of misfolded α-syn in neuronal cell bodies and synapses • Neuropathological improvement correlation with the strength of the immune response	[63]
1-methyl-4-phenyl-1,2,3,6-tetrahydropyridine (MPTP) C57BL/6 mouse	na	Full length human nitrotyrosine (NT)-modified and unmodified α-syn	CFA/IFA	• Immune responses exacerbate neuroinflammation and nigrostriatal degeneration • Activation of peripheral leukocytes • Exacerbations are mostly mediated by α-syn induced/specific T cells • Treg cells attenuated microglial inflammatory responses and led to robust nigrostriatal protection	[68, 71]
Rat: rAAV2/5-α-syn overexpression	h-wt-α-syn	Full length human α-syn	CFA/IFA	• High- anti-α-syn antibody response • Reduction in PD-typical aggregates • Accumulation of CD4-+, MHC II+ ramified microglia in SN • Infiltration of CD4+, Foxp3+ Treg cells in nigrostriatal system	[72]

(continued)

Table 2
(continued)

Animal model	Transgene	Treatment	Adjuvant	Effect	Reference
mPDGF-α-syn, D-Line	h-wt-α-syn	AFFITOPE®-KLH conjugates (PD01A, PD03A, others)	Alhydrogel	• Induction of an α-syn selective IgG Ab response (α-syn recognized, β-syn spared) • Generated Abs pass the BBB and bind to α-syn deposits • Reduction of pathological α-syn (oligomers, "aggregates") • Reduction of model-specific neuropathological alterations • Functional improvement (spatial memory and learning)	[62]
mThy1.2-α-syn, Line 61	h-wt-α-syn	AFFITOPE®-KLH conjugates (PD01A, PD03A, others)	Alhydrogel	• Immune response similar to D-Line • improvement in motoric function	[62]
Wt-C57Bl/6 mouse	na	• α-syn 85-99-TT P30 conjugate vaccine • α-syn 109-126-TT P30 conjugate vaccine • α-syn 126-140-TT P30 conjugate vaccine	QuilA	• All three conjugates induce h α-syn specific Abs • T cell responses to P30, but not to h α-syn • Generated Abs bound to LB and LN (DLB cases) and h α-syn in brain extracts	[60]
na	na	• α-syn-peptide-VLP	no	• No data disclosed	Jenner Institute
na	na	• 40–80 aa-long α-syn (declensional) peptides • Reflect complete pattern of abnormal phosphorylated and tri-nitrated α-syn aa residues	no	• No data disclosed	Declion Pharmaceuticals

Na not applicable, *CFA/IFA* complete/incomplete Freund's adjuvant, *rAAV* recombinant adeno-associated virus, *wt* wild type, *Treg* regulatory T cells, *TT P30* T-helper cell epitope of tetanus toxoid self-destructive, T lymphocytes; design of conjugate vaccines with α-syn stretches that a priori are too short for the activation of α-syn-specific T cells; use of antigens that mimic α-syn but differ in their amino acid sequence allowing for the generation of α-syn-specific Abs but not of α-syn-specific and, thus, potentially autoreactive T cells.

The danger of triggering cellular autoimmunity by vaccination with full-length α-syn has been recently illustrated in a PD model. Immunization with full-length, nitrated α-syn was found to aggravate the nigrostriatal degeneration occurring as a result of intracerebral injections of 1-methyl-4-phenyl-1,2,3,6-tetrahydropyridine (MPTP) [68]. Results obtained suggest that chemical modifications of the α-syn protein render it more immunogenic and thus capable of bypassing immunological self-tolerance. Importantly, in another study it was found that mice got an aggravated pathology upon vaccination with full-length, nitrated α-syn, by the effect of specific T cells [69]. The study further showed that the deleterious effects could be successfully prevented by the transfer of naturally occurring α-syn-specific regulatory T cells, which attenuated the microglia-driven neuroinflammatory processes and exhibited a robust neuroprotective effect.

Experimental evidence for a protective role for α-syn-specific regulatory T cells was independently reported by Sanchez Guajardo et al. [70]. These investigators used full-length α-syn to immunize rats overexpressing α-syn following intracerebral inoculation of α-syn gene-transduced adenoviral vectors. Vaccination was found to result in a high titer anti-α-syn Ab response, to reduce deposits of PD-typical α-syn aggregates and ameliorated the functional deficits associated with the inoculation of the α-syn-harboring adenoviral vector. A potential explanation for these findings was provided by an additional neuropathological analysis. Compared to controls, vaccinated animals accumulated CD4-positive, MHC class II-positive ramified microglia in the substantia nigra. In addition, the entire nigrostriatal system of these animals was infiltrated with cells co-expressing CD4 and Foxp3 classifying them as regulatory T cells. The study further suggested that the induction of regulatory T cells and distinctly activated microglia may, in addition to the α-syn-specific Abs, contribute to the neuroprotective activity of active vaccination. Critical in this regard will be the identification of conditions ensuring the activation of protective regulatory T cells that could prevent concomitantly activated self-reactive T cells from exerting their functions.

Ghochikyan and colleagues have recently presented another approach to the active α-syn immunotherapy, focused on short stretches of the α-syn molecule [60]. Three peptide-based epitope vaccines composed of different B-cell epitopes of human α-syn were generated and fused with a "non-self" T-helper epitope from the tetanus toxoid (P30). The three peptide-based epitopes were encoding α-syn amino acid residues 85–99, 109–126, and 126–140, and immunization of mice with these vaccines was applied with the saponin extract containing adjuvant QuilA. Vaccination produced high titers of anti-human α-syn Abs that bound to LBs and LNs on human brain sections from DLB cases and induced robust T helper cell responses to P30, but not to human α-syn.

Bachman and colleagues from the Jenner Institute (University of Oxford, UK) also built on short α-syn sequences as antigenic components for a vaccine. In their approach, virus-like particles (VLPs) are used as vehicles to display short α-syn peptides similar to VLP-based Aß-targeting Alzheimer vaccines previously tested in preclinical and clinical studies [55, 73]. These VLPs allow for the expression of multiple antigenic molecules/entities in an ordered manner and are additionally characterized by an inherent and strong adjuvant effect. Their administration results in the induction of robust Ab responses without activation of peptide-/target-specific T lymphocytes. No preclinical or clinical results have been disclosed so far using this strategy.

Declion, a company based in France, has recently announced plans for a preclinical development program built on their proprietary ModuloDEEP technology to develop a vaccine targeting α-syn in humans (Declion homepage; October 2014). This technology uses amino acid copolymers with claimed antigenic specificity, called Declensional peptides. These peptides are a mixture of 40–80 amino acid-long peptides incorporating more than one amino acid at a given position in the mix of peptides used. This method is meant to reflect the complete pattern of abnormally phosphorylated and tri-nitrated amino acid residues of α-syn and is not requiring the use of adjuvants as it is claiming to combine B- and T-cell determinants in the ModuloDEEP declensional peptides. No preclinical or clinical data have yet been published on this novel vaccination approach.

2.2.1 The AFFITOME® Approach

Rather than using native, full length α-syn, short α-syn fragments or posttranslationally modified α-syn, AFFiRiS uses AFFITOPEs®, short peptides mimicking a certain region of the α-syn molecule. Thus, the amino acid sequence of AFFITOPEs® differs from the one of the native protein [74, 75]. Moreover, AFFITOPEs® are also selected so that they do not exhibit sequence identity with other human proteins. As a result, AFFITOPEs® are "foreign" to the human immune system and thus immunological tolerance mechanisms established against "self" do not need to be overcome. Given their small size, these peptides cannot by themselves activate T cells and require conjugation to carriers for the elicitation of an Ab response. Good candidates are non-human carrier molecules such as Keyhole Limpet Hemocyanin (KLH) and Detoxified Diphtheria Toxin, which are both safe to use and have proven immunogenic in humans. Based on a physical link with the α-syn

**Screening of peptide libraries
(10⁹ peptides) with aSyn specific Ab**

Selection criteria:
- binding to selection Ab
- competition against native peptide

Candidates: n=52 (=AFFITOME®)

In silico analysis

**Remaining candidates (n=50):
in vivo selection filter**

Selection criteria:
- immunogenicity
- POC studies
- crossreactivity of Abs elicited with
  homologous proteins
- GLP toxicity/ safety
- formulation development

**AFFITOPEs® for PD vaccine development:
→ PD01 and PD03**

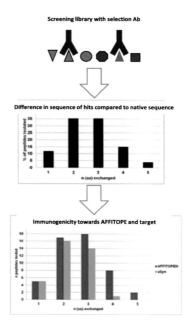

Fig. 1 The AFFITOME® technology—delineation of its principle based on the example of α-syn-targeting AFFITOPE® vaccines

mimicking peptide moieties, these carrier molecules are providing T cell help for the activation of α-syn-specific B cells and the generation of a long-lasting specific Ab response. Importantly, the T helper cells involved are specific for the carrier but not for α-syn, which adds to the safety features of AFFITOPE® vaccines as they cannot activate α-syn-specific T cells and thereby mediate a detrimental (encephalitogenic) autoimmune reaction.

For the identification of novel PD-vaccine candidates, the mechanism of molecular mimicry was exploited to select α-syn-targeting AFFITOPEs® from a pool of potential peptide candidates (Fig. 1). A monoclonal Ab recognizing the C-terminal part of α-syn (aa 110–130) was used to fish candidates from peptide phage display (7- and 12-mer) libraries, to screen for peptides binding to the selected Ab.

In a second step, identified peptides were subjected to competition experiments including aggregated forms of the α-syn molecule. Selection with the C-terminal α-syn Ab yielded a total of 52 peptides capable of (1) binding to the selection Ab and (2) competing for binding against the original peptide. As a next step, sequences of the 52 peptide hits were evaluated for homologies with all known human proteins. Peptides sharing five or more consecutive amino acids with any human molecule except α-syn were excluded at this stage.

The remaining 50 candidates were subjected to in vivo testing, which included the evaluation of their immunogenicity in different species and testing of their activity in various animal models.

An important element in these proof-of-concept (POC) studies was the exclusion of peptide candidates that would elicit Abs reacting with human proteins other than α-syn. This was done in two ways: by an open screening type approach (e.g., tissue microassays) and in addition, by focusing on molecules sharing limited sequence homology with the candidates. Key in this context was the lack of reactivity with β-syn, a highly homologous member of the synuclein family with similar expression pattern and functional redundancy, as suggested by studies on α-syn knock-out animals [76]. Moreover, β-syn cannot form/seed higher order assemblies, neither in a homologous nor in a heterologous (e.g., with α-syn) fashion [77–79]. It prevents oxidation of α-syn, regulates its expression, and inhibits its aggregation [77, 78, 80, 81]. Of note, co-expression of β-syn alleviates the pathology seen in α-syn single transgenic lines [77, 78]. Given the protective properties of β-syn, the exclusive α-syn reactivity of Abs induced is a key safety element of α-syn-targeting AFFITOPE® vaccines. The POC studies to assess α-syn AFFITOPEs® were primarily based on α-syn transgenic mouse lines. These studies encompassed the evaluation of AFFITOPE®-immunized and control animals for cerebral α-syn load, neuropathological as well as functional alterations associated with the overexpression of α-syn (see below).

This program resulted in the identification of the lead vaccine termed PD01A.

**2.2.2 PD-AFFITOPE®
Vaccines Demonstrate
Disease-Modifying Activity
in Various Transgenic
Disease Models**

During the course of their preclinical development, α-syn-targeting AFFITOPE® vaccines were evaluated in a series of transgenic animal models [62]. One of the models routinely used expresses human α-syn under the neuron-specific murine Thy1 promoter and is characterized by axonal α-syn pathology, the presence of α-syn aggregates in cortical and subcortical regions including the substantia nigra and the striatum as well as the development of behavioral motor deficits. In addition, studies are being conducted in a mouse model that overexpresses wild-type human α-syn under a PDGF-β promoter, driving expression specifically in neurons. The resulting phenotype is reminiscent of DLB based on (i) the localization of the α-syn pathology, which is found throughout the temporal cortex and the hippocampus, and (ii) altered cognitive functions.

In vivo testing of potential AFFITOPE® vaccine candidates starts with the evaluation of their immunogenicity. To this end, a set of different animal species, including α-syn-transgenic animals, is repeatedly injected at 2–4 week intervals with the vaccine candidate at different doses and relevant control agents (e.g., carrier, adjuvant). Such studies demonstrated PD01A to induce IgG-type Abs recognizing the various elements of the conjugate vaccine including the immunizing PD01A peptide but also the targeted α-syn. They did however not react with β-syn (Fig. 2) and did also not activate α-syn-specific T lymphocytes, as assessed by ELISPOT assays. Abs elicited by vaccination with PD01A were found to enter

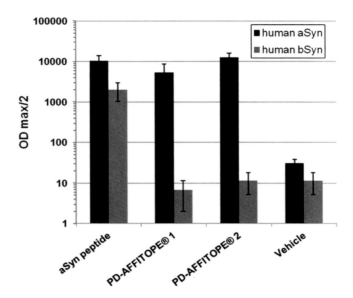

Fig. 2 Selective α-syn targeting is a key safety element of α-syn targeting AFFITOPE® vaccines. human α-syn tg animals ($n=10$/group) were vaccinated 3× with KLH conjugates containing either the original, C-terminal α-syn sequence (α-syn peptide) or 2 AFFITOPEs® mimicking this region or with vehicle (adjuvant) only. Plasma samples obtained 2 weeks after the third immunization were ana- lyzed for the presence of Abs reacting with α-syn or β-syn using an ELISA sys- tem. Results are expressed as average ± SEM

the brain based on (1) the detection of α-syn-specific Abs in the CSF of these animals following vaccination and (2) the demonstra- tion of vaccine-induced Abs binding to target structures in situ by means of immunohistochemistry [62].

AFFITOPEs® that haven proven immunogenic in wild-type animals are forwarded to POC studies in α-syn tg lines including the above described mouse models. Respective experiments are designed to cover aspects relevant to the evaluation of a causal, disease-modifying vaccine. Such studies include the determination of the cerebral load of pathological α-syn species, parameters quan- tifying the neurodegenerative process in a given animal (e.g., num- ber of neuronal dendrites and synapses, number of neurons) and the evaluation of functional deficits observed in the various lines. Typically, these experiments are done in prophylactic as well as in therapeutic settings.

The assessment of the cerebral α-syn load is based on biochem- ical and immunohistochemical methods. It is based on the assump- tion that monomeric α-syn serves physiological functions while its toxicity resides within α-syn assemblies. Vaccination with PD01A was found to reduce aggregated α-syn in both α-syn tg lines exam- ined without affecting levels of monomeric α-syn. Specifically, it reduced oligomeric α-syn in the SN and striatum of the PD/PDD model and dimeric as well as oligomeric α-syn in the neocortex and the hippocampus of the DLB model (see Figs. 3 and 4). Several features of the PD01A-induced Abs may contribute to this selective reduction of aggregated forms of α-syn including conformation-dependent reactivity and a limited affinity for α-syn monomers. PD01A also had reduced neuronal cell death, and reduced loss of their dendrites and synapses.

Importantly, the changes in the levels of α-syn are reflected in markers of neuroinflammation, which are checked as safety element of the AFFITOME® program. To this end, astrogliosis and microg-

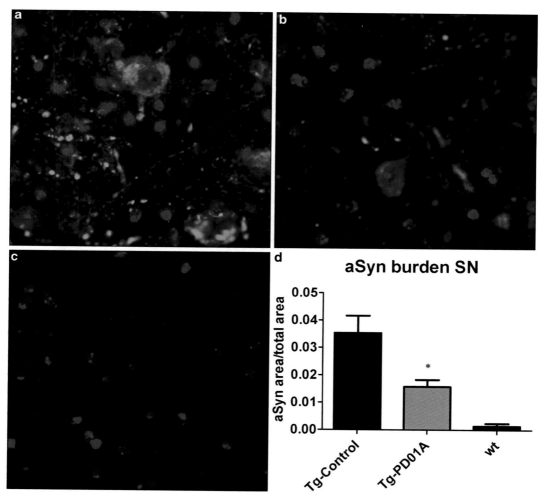

Fig. 3 Immunization with PD01A reduces α-syn load in mThy1-α-syn tg mice. α-syn levels were measured in non-tg mice and mThy1-α-syn tg mice immunized either with vehicle or PD01A ($n=10$/group) by analysis of cerebral immunofluorescence staining. (**a–c**) α-syn immunostaining of substantia nigra using the α-syn antibody LB509 (green). Cell nuclei were stained with DAPI (*blue*). (**a**) α-syn immunostaining in vehicle treated mThy1-α-syn tg mice (Tg-control); (**b**) α-syn immunostaining in PD01A treated mThy1-α-syn tg mice (Tg-PD01A); (**c**) α-syn immunostaining in vehicle treated non tg littermates (wt); (**d**) Quantification of the percentage of neuropil area positive for α-syn in substantia nigra. Results are expressed as average ± SEM. *Asterisk* (*) $p < 0.05$

liosis are quantified by means of immunohistochemistry. In addition, cytokines (e.g., IL-1Ra, IL-2, and IL-27) and chemokines (e.g., fractalkine), implicated in neuroinflammation, were assessed. PD01A-vaccinated mice showed reduced astroglial and microglial reactivity, which was associated with reduced levels of pro-inflammatory cytokines and an increase in fractalkine, known to possess anti-inflammatory properties.

The preclinical POC studies also include the functional evaluation of vaccinated α-syn tg lines, both with the Morris water maze (MWM) and by paradigms assessing their motor function and coordination, such as the body suspension test. PD01A was show to have positive functional effects in both model systems. Specifically, while vehicle-treated tg mice showed a severe deterioration of spatial memory and learning compared to non-tg animals, PD01A-vaccinated animals showed a learning curve, as well spatial memory capabilities closely resembling non-tg controls, indicating a significantly better preservation of cognitive function.

Experiments designed to unravel the mechanism by which AFFITOPE® vaccination-induced Abs lead to the clearance of pathological α-syn suggest the existence of two principal and non-exclusive pathways—the Ab-mediated augmentation of the uptake of α-syn assemblies by microglial cells [62] and the Ab-driven channeling of pathological α-syn into the lysosomal degradation pathway of neurons. Similar findings have been gained by the administration of α-syn-specific monoclonal Abs [58, 63].

2.2.3 AFFITOPE® Vaccines do not Seem to Interfere with Dopamine Reuptake, a Physiological Function of α-syn

Key to the safety evaluation of a vaccine targeting a self-protein is the assessment of side effects exerted/mediated by the effector molecules/cells. This aspect of the toxicity evaluation is termed "immunotoxicity" and summarizes negative, non-intended effects of vaccine-induced Abs in vivo. Two principle components need to be covered: (1) autoimmune reactions and (2) interference with the physiological function of the targeted molecule. The ability to test whether the specific Abs elicited by α-syn-targeting vaccines, such as PD01A, for these two criteria critically depends on model systems sharing sequence identity, at least in the respective region of the target with the native human molecule. In case of the C-terminus of α-syn, we take advantage of guinea pigs, whose α-syn protein sequence is highly homologous (90–95 %) and identical in the C-terminal region of interest.

Accordingly, repeated AFFITOPE®-immunizations were performed in guinea pigs to define potential negative effects of such vaccine-induced, α-syn specific Abs in a healthy organism. The effect on the dopamine (DA) system was studied in vivo by assessing guinea pigs vaccinated repeatedly with either a control vaccine, or the AFFITOPE® vaccine PD01A, for their striatal levels of DA, 3,4-dihydroxyphenylacetic acid (DOPAC), and homovanillic acid (HVA) using intracerebral microdialysis before and after administration of PD01A or the control vaccine. In addition, the animals

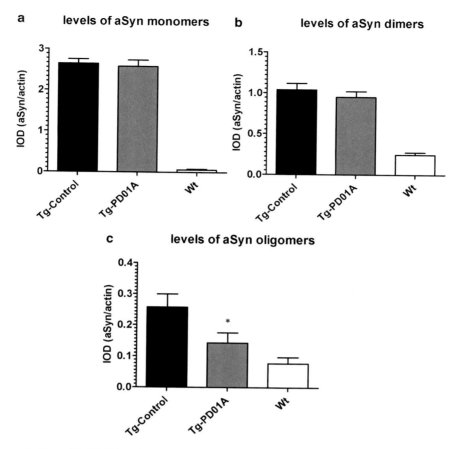

a levels of aSyn monomers

b levels of aSyn dimers

c levels of aSyn oligomers

Fig. 4 Immunization with PD01A reduces oligomeric α-syn load in mThy1-α-syn tg mice α-syn levels were measured in non-tg mice and mThy1-α-syn tg mice immunized either with vehicle (Tg-control + wt) or PD01A (Tg-PD01A; $n = 10$/group) by biochemical analysis of brain extracts. Densitometric immunoblot analysis of α-syn species ((**a**) monomers, (**b**) dimers, (**c**) oligomers). Levels of β-syn did not change with any of the treatments. β-actin was used as loading control. Results are expressed as average ± SEM. *Asterisk* (*) $p < 0.05$

received a pharmacological challenge by infusion of the DA re-uptake inhibitor nomifensine. This inhibitor was given during the post vaccination period in order to test whether AFFITOPE®-induced α-syn targeting Abs are interfering with striatal DA levels, DA metabolism or DA transport (i.e., release and reuptake) in steady state and after nomifensine challenge. Indeed, no treatment related differences in these parameters were detected (Fig. 5), suggesting that treatment with PD01A does not affect the DA system in an intact healthy brain.

2.3 Passive α-syn Immunotherapy for PD

Masliah et al. investigated the effect of treatment with the monoclonal antibody 9E4 in a PDGF α-syn transgenic model (D-line, DLB model) [64]. They found that 9E4 treatment was tolerated in animal models. Furthermore, repeated injections of the monoclonal Ab reduced the accumulation of calpain-cleaved α-syn in axons

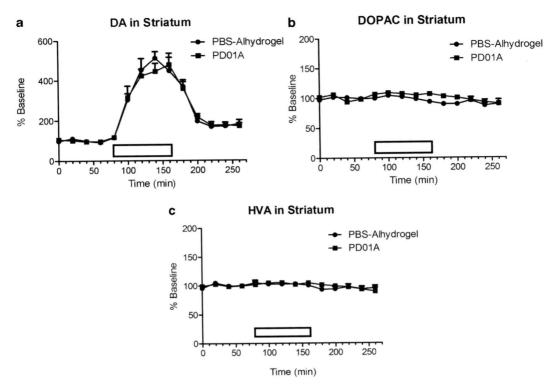

Fig. 5 Effect of repeated PD01A immunization on the DA system. To analyze the relative levels of dopamine (DA; (**a**)), 3,4-dihydroxyphenylacetic acid (DOPAC; (**b**)), and homovanillic acid (HVA; (**c**)) in guinea pig striatum after three injections of the control agent (PBS-Alhydrogel) or the PD01A vaccine tissue fluid was collected by means of microdialysis and subjected to HPLC with tandem mass spectrometry detection. *Bars* in (**a**)–(**c**) represent the time period of perfusion with the DA reuptake inhibitor nomifensine (2 μM). Nomifensine (2 μM) perfusion led to a fast and reversible block of DA reuptake and hence an increase in DA levels which was followed by reduction to baseline levels following wash out of the inhibitor as seen in (**a**). No nomifensine effects were detectable on DOPAC or HVA levels, respectively (**b** + **c**). No treatment related differences were detectable for DA, DOPAC, and HVA, suggesting that treatment with the AFFITOPE® vaccine PD01A does not affect the DA system in a healthy brain

and synapses; importantly, this reduction of α-syn was found to improve associated neurodegenerative deficits. In line with this, the Masliah team could show that the Ab crossed the blood–brain barrier and was found in neurons and microglia. Notably, the Abs were directed to the CNS, bound to cells that displayed accumulation of pathological α-syn, and promoted α-syn clearance presumably via the lysosomal pathway.

Since this discovery, the prion-like propagation mechanism of α-syn has been further elucidated.

Games and colleagues addressed if Abs directed towards the c-terminal end of the α-syn could hinder the prion-like propagation of α-syn in the brain [59]. They used Thy 1 α-syn tg mice which develop a broad α-syn pathology over time. They tested three separate antibodies (1H7, 5C1, or 5D12) directed to the C-terminus of the protein. In all cases, they found that treatment with the C-terminal directed antibodies reduced not only the accumulation of α-syn in axons, but also improved memory and motor deficits. In cell-based symptoms, Games and colleagues also observed that the cell-to-cell propagation of α-syn was reduced upon Ab treatment.

The group of Virginia Lee further explored the hypothesis that Abs to α-syn can block the prion-like propagation of pathological α-syn in an in vivo model [82]. They used non-transgenic mice that had developed LB/LN pathology through the injection of misfolded α-syn into the striatum. They found that administration of a monoclonal Ab to these mice reduced the spread of α-syn pathology in the brain of these animals and, in turn, reduced neuronal loss and improved motor skills. Lee's team was the first to demonstrate, at the example of α-syn, that prion-like propagation of misfolded proteins, a mechanism thought to be involved in various neurodegenerative diseases, can be blocked by means of passive immunotherapy.

Combined, these publications from Games et al. and Tran et al. support the potential of a passive immunotherapeutic approach to treat neurodegenerative diseases, such as Parkinson's disease. Moreover, further studies have provided insight into the importance of different forms of α-syn, which have helped to highlight that the oligomeric form and not the monomeric form is the neurotoxic species. Teams led by Ingelsson and Lannfelt [61, 65, 83, 84] found that oligomeric/fibrillar forms have particularly neurotoxic properties and suggest their use as prime therapeutic target. They generated two monoclonal Abs, mAb47 and mAb38E2, which were found to be highly selective for aggregated α-syn. They found that a passive immunotherapy approach using one of these Abs could reduce levels of α-syn in transgenic mouse models of the disease, with significantly lower levels of α-syn assemblies in the spinal cord of mice compared to placebo treated animals [61].

2.4 Clinical Progress of α-syn Immunotherapy

Two immunotherapy programs for PD have thus far made it to clinical development. The first program to modify the clinical course of the disease in PD patients was introduced by AFFiRiS in 2012 with the Phase I trial of PD01A candidate, which is an AFFITOPE® against the C-terminus of α-syn as antigen conjugated to KLH and adjuvanted with Alum [75].

The AFFiRiS PD vaccine development program focuses on AFFITOPEs® eliciting antibodies recognizing α-syn while avoiding cross reactivity with β-syn. The Phase I study (clinicaltrials.gov identifier: NCT01568099) investigated 32 subjects with early PD including 12 in each treatment group and 8 in the control group. The study completed in July 2014 and showed a strong safety profile, supporting further development of the compound for the treatment of PD (manuscript in preparation). Based on the favorable results of the study, a boost study was performed (NCT02216188) and results are anticipated within 2015.

Applying the concept of clinical maturation also to synucleinopathies, AFFiRiS moved a second candidate, PD03A, to phase I testing in two indications, PD (NCT02267434) and multiple system atrophy (NCT02270489), which are both expected to be completed in May 2016.

Hoffmann-La Roche in cooperation with Prothena (former Neotope Biosciences) is currently sponsoring two PD clinical trials. Both trials are testing the tolerability and pharmacokinetic aspects of their drug product, the monoclonal antibody, PRX002, as their primary outcome.

Their first study was a single ascending dose study of PRX002 in healthy subjects and started recruitment of approximately 40 healthy volunteers, aged 21–65, in March 2014 (clinicaltrials.gov identifier: NCT02095171). In March 2015, the company announced that all doses of PRX002 were safe and well tolerated. The study found a significant, dose dependent reduction of serum levels of free, monomeric α-syn demonstrating that this species of α-syn can be safely reduced from the blood compartment in humans by means of immunotherapy. It will be interesting to see how this connects to cerebral α-syn levels and, ultimately, to the clinical activity of the antibody. The second study is currently ongoing and is a multiple ascending dose study in patients with idiopathic PD, Hoehn and Yahr stages 1–3. Recruitment for this study started in June 2014 and is expected to be completed in April 2016 (clinicaltrials.gov identifier: NCT02157714).

Neurimmune, in cooperation with Biogen, have moved their recombinant human monoclonal antibody targeting aggregated α-syn, BIIB054, to phase I clinical trials (clinicaltrials.gov identifier: NCT02459886). BIIB054 has biophysical characteristics closely resembling those occurring in healthy centenarians. The trial's primary aim is to measure safety, tolerability, and pharmacokinetics of BIIB054 in healthy subjects. It is expected to be completed in June 2016.

A key challenge for both the current and future α-syn programs will be to find the most appropriate method to demonstrate disease modification. Four different approaches have been proposed. First, the FDA and EMA have suggested that demonstration of a clinical effect in conjunction with a biomarker effect, with the assumption that the biomarker measures something that is closer to the disease process could support a disease modification claim. The second approach, which is supported by the EMA and that has been used in other disease areas, is the demonstration that an endpoint or a clinically relevant event can be delayed for a long period of time, with a similar assumption that the endpoint could not have been delayed simply by affecting symptoms. Third, Paul Leber, Director, Division of Neuro-Pharmacological Drug Products, FDA [1981–1999] promotes an approach demonstrating a prolonged treatment response as demonstrated by a successful outcome in a randomized withdrawal or staggered start design [85]. Fourth, other modeling methods have been proposed to separate shorter-term effects, which are presumably symptomatic, from longer lasting effects, which are more likely to be disease modifying. Today, there is no consensus on the best approach to demonstrate disease modification. It will be the joint task of the scientific community, supported by data generated in these and other clinical programs, to evaluate the relevance of the above delineated approaches for the evaluation of new drugs for their disease modifying effects in PD.

References

1. Davie CA (2008) A review of Parkinson's disease. Br Med Bull 86:109–127
2. Meissner WG, Frasier M, Gasser T et al (2011) Priorities in Parkinson's disease research. Nat Rev Drug Discov 10(5):377–393
3. Parkinson J (2002) An essay on the shaking palsy. 1817. J Neuropsychiatry Clin Neurosci 14(2):223–236, discussion 222
4. Dubois B, Tolosa E, Katzenschlager R et al (2012) Donepezil in Parkinson's disease dementia: a randomized, double-blind efficacy and safety study. Mov Disord 27(10):1230–1238
5. Dauer W, Przedborski S (2003) Parkinson's disease: mechanisms and models. Neuron 39(6):889–909
6. Spillantini MG, Schmidt ML, Lee VM et al (1997) Alpha-synuclein in Lewy bodies. Nature 388(6645):839–840
7. Kosaka K (1978) Lewy bodies in cerebral cortex, report of three cases. Acta Neuropathol 42(2):127–134
8. Jellinger KA (2009) A critical evaluation of current staging of alpha-synuclein pathology in Lewy body disorders. Biochim Biophys Acta 1792(7):730–740
9. McGeer PL, McGeer EG (2008) The alpha-synuclein burden hypothesis of Parkinson disease and its relationship to Alzheimer disease. Exp Neurol 212(2):235–238
10. Iwai A, Masliah E, Yoshimoto M et al (1995) The precursor protein of non-a beta component of Alzheimer's disease amyloid is a presynaptic protein of the central nervous system. Neuron 14(2):467–475
11. Maroteaux L, Campanelli JT, Scheller RH (1988) Synuclein: a neuron-specific protein localized to the nucleus and presynaptic nerve terminal. J Neurosci 8(8):2804–2815
12. Ueda K, Fukushima H, Masliah E et al (1993) Molecular cloning of CDNA encoding an unrecognized component of amyloid in Alzheimer disease. Proc Natl Acad Sci U S A 90(23):11282–11286
13. Fortin DL, Troyer MD, Nakamura K et al (2004) Lipid rafts mediate the synaptic localization of alpha-synuclein. J Neurosci 24(30):6715–6723
14. George JM, Jin H, Woods WS et al (1995) Characterization of a novel protein regulated during the critical period for song learning in the zebra finch. Neuron 15(2):361–372
15. Murphy DD, Rueter SM, Trojanowski JQ et al (2000) Synucleins are developmentally expressed, and alpha-synuclein regulates the size of the presynaptic vesicular pool in primary hippocampal neurons. J Neurosci 20(9):3214–3220
16. Singleton AB, Farrer MJ, Bonifati V (2013) The genetics of Parkinson's disease: progress and therapeutic implications. Mov Disord 28(1):14–23
17. Edwards TL, Scott WK, Almonte C et al (2010) Genome-wide association study confirms SNPS in SNCA and the MAPT region as common risk factors for Parkinson disease. Ann Hum Genet 74(2):97–109
18. Gandhi S, Wood NW (2010) Genome-wide association studies: the key to unlocking neurodegeneration? Nat Neurosci 13(7):789–794
19. Satake W, Nakabayashi Y, Mizuta I et al (2009) Genome-wide association study identifies common variants at four loci as genetic risk factors for Parkinson's disease. Nat Genet 41(12):1303–1307
20. Simon-Sanchez J, Schulte C, Bras JM et al (2009) Genome-wide association study reveals genetic risk underlying Parkinson's disease. Nat Genet 41(12):1308–1312
21. Singleton AB, Farrer M, Johnson J et al (2003) Alpha-synuclein locus triplication causes Parkinson's disease. Science 302(5646):841
22. McNeill A, Duran R, Hughes DA et al (2012) A clinical and family history study of Parkinson's disease in heterozygous glucocerebrosidase mutation carriers. J Neurol Neurosurg Psychiatry 83(8):853–854

23. Danzer KM, Haasen D, Karow AR et al (2007) Different species of alpha-synuclein oligomers induce calcium influx and seeding. J Neurosci 27(34):9220–9232

24. Eriksen JL, Dawson TM, Dickson DW et al (2003) Caught in the act: alpha-synuclein is the culprit in Parkinson's disease. Neuron 40(3):453–456

25. Savitt JM, Dawson VL, Dawson TM (2006) Diagnosis and treatment of Parkinson disease: molecules to medicine. J Clin Invest 116(7):1744–1754

26. Winner B, Jappelli R, Maji SK et al (2011) In vivo demonstration that alpha-synuclein oligomers are toxic. Proc Natl Acad Sci U S A 108(10):4194–4199

27. Giasson BI, Duda JE, Murray IV et al (2000) Oxidative damage linked to neurodegeneration by selective alpha-synuclein nitration in synucleinopathy lesions. Science 290(5493):985–989

28. Hunot S, Boissiere F, Faucheux B et al (1996) Nitric oxide synthase and neuronal vulnerability in Parkinson's disease. Neuroscience 72(2):355–363

29. Wu DC, Teismann P, Tieu K et al (2003) Nadph oxidase mediates oxidative stress in the 1-methyl-4-phenyl-1,2,3,6-tetrahydropyridine model of Parkinson's disease. Proc Natl Acad Sci U S A 100(10):6145–6150

30. Heneka MT, Kummer MP, Latz E (2014) Innate immune activation in neurodegenerative disease. Nat Rev Immunol 14(7):463–477

31. Shavali S, Combs CK, Ebadi M (2006) Reactive macrophages increase oxidative stress and alpha-synuclein nitration during death of dopaminergic neuronal cells in co-culture: relevance to Parkinson's disease. Neurochem Res 31(1):85–94

32. Zhang W, Wang T, Pei Z et al (2005) Aggregated alpha-synuclein activates microglia: a process leading to disease progression in Parkinson's disease. FASEB J 19(6):533–542

33. Braak H, Del Tredici K, Rub U et al (2003) Staging of brain pathology related to sporadic Parkinson's disease. Neurobiol Aging 24(2):197–211

34. Dickson DW, Fujishiro H, Orr C et al (2009) Neuropathology of non-motor features of Parkinson disease. Parkinsonism Relat Disord 15(Suppl 3):S1–S5

35. Lansbury PT Jr, Brice A (2002) Genetics of Parkinson's disease and biochemical studies of implicated gene products. Curr Opin Genet Dev 12(3):299–306

36. Sacchetti B, Baldi E, Lorenzini CA et al (2002) Cerebellar role in fear-conditioning consolidation. Proc Natl Acad Sci U S A 99(12):8406–8411

37. Polymeropoulos MH, Lavedan C, Leroy E et al (1997) Mutation in the alpha-synuclein gene identified in families with Parkinson's disease. Science 276(5321):2045–2047

38. Ross OA, Braithwaite AT, Skipper LM et al (2008) Genomic investigation of alpha-synuclein multiplication and Parkinsonism. Ann Neurol 63(6):743–750

39. Fleming SM, Salcedo J, Fernagut PO et al (2004) Early and progressive sensorimotor anomalies in mice overexpressing wild-type human alpha-synuclein. J Neurosci 24(42):9434–9440

40. Fleming SM, Tetreault NA, Mulligan CK et al (2008) Olfactory deficits in mice overexpressing human wildtype alpha-synuclein. Eur J Neurosci 28(2):247–256

41. Lotharius J, Brundin P (2002) Pathogenesis of Parkinson's disease: dopamine, vesicles and alpha-synuclein. Nat Rev Neurosci 3(12):932–942

42. Masliah E, Rockenstein E, Veinbergs I et al (2000) Dopaminergic loss and inclusion body formation in alpha-synuclein mice: implications for neurodegenerative disorders. Science 287(5456):1265–1269

43. Rockenstein E, Crews L, Masliah E (2007) Transgenic animal models of neurodegenerative diseases and their application to treatment development. Adv Drug Deliv Rev 59(11):1093–1102

44. Lace G, Savva GM, Forster G et al (2009) Hippocampal tau pathology is related to neuroanatomical connections: an ageing population-based study. Brain 132(Pt 5):1324–1334

45. Jellinger KA, Kovacs GG (2011) Clinico-pathological correlations in neurodegeneration. Acta Neuropathol 122(2):115–116

46. Lim KL, Zhang CW (2013) Molecular events underlying Parkinson's disease – an interwoven tapestry. Front Neurol 4:33

47. Olanow CW, Brundin P (2013) Parkinson's disease and alpha synuclein: is Parkinson's disease a prion-like disorder? Mov Disord 28(1):31–40

48. Kordower JH, Chu Y, Hauser RA et al (2008) Lewy body-like pathology in long-term embryonic nigral transplants in Parkinson's disease. Nat Med 14(5):504–506

49. Li JY, Englund E, Holton JL et al (2008) Lewy bodies in grafted neurons in subjects with Parkinson's disease suggest host-to-graft disease propagation. Nat Med 14(5):501–503

50. Volpicelli-Daley LA, Luk KC, Patel TP et al (2011) Exogenous alpha-synuclein fibrils induce Lewy body pathology leading to synaptic dysfunction and neuron death. Neuron 72(1):57–71

51. Luk CH, Wallis JD (2009) Dynamic encoding of responses and outcomes by neurons in medial prefrontal cortex. J Neurosci 29(23):7526–7539

52. Luk KC, Kehm V, Carroll J et al (2012) Pathological alpha-synuclein transmission initi-

ates Parkinson-like neurodegeneration in non-transgenic mice. Science 338(6109):949–953

53. Watts JC, Giles K, Oehler A et al (2013) Transmission of multiple system atrophy prions to transgenic mice. Proc Natl Acad Sci U S A 110(48):19555–19560

54. Recasens A, Dehay B, Bove J et al (2014) Lewy body extracts from parkinson disease brains trigger alpha-synuclein pathology and neurodegeneration in mice and monkeys. Ann Neurol 75(3):351–362

55. Winblad B, Andreasen N, Minthon L et al (2012) Safety, tolerability, and antibody response of active abeta immunotherapy with cad106 in patients with Alzheimer's disease: randomised, double-blind, placebo-controlled, first-in-human study. Lancet Neurol 11(7):597–604

56. Doody RS, Thomas RG, Farlow M et al (2014) Phase 3 trials of solanezumab for mild-to-moderate Alzheimer's disease. N Engl J Med 370(4):311–321

57. Salloway S, Sperling R, Fox NC et al (2014) Two phase 3 trials of bapineuzumab in mild-to-moderate Alzheimer's disease. N Engl J Med 370(4):322–333

58. Bae EJ, Lee HJ, Rockenstein E et al (2012) Antibody-aided clearance of extracellular alpha-synuclein prevents cell-to-cell aggregate transmission. J Neurosci 32(39):13454–13469

59. Games D, Valera E, Spencer B et al (2014) Reducing c-terminal-truncated alpha-synuclein by immunotherapy attenuates neurodegeneration and propagation in Parkinson's disease-like models. J Neurosci 34(28):9441–9454

60. Ghochikyan A, Petrushina I, Davtyan H et al (2014) Immunogenicity of epitope vaccines targeting different b cell antigenic determinants of human alpha-synuclein: feasibility study. Neurosci Lett 560:86–91

61. Lindstrom V, Fagerqvist T, Nordstrom E et al (2014) Immunotherapy targeting alpha-synuclein protofibrils reduced pathology in (thy-1)-h[a30p] alpha-synuclein mice. Neurobiol Dis 69:134–143

62. Mandler M, Valera E, Rockenstein E et al (2014) Next-generation active immunization approach for synucleinopathies: implications for Parkinson's disease clinical trials. Acta Neuropathol 127(6):861–879

63. Masliah E, Rockenstein E, Adame A et al (2005) Effects of alpha-synuclein immunization in a mouse model of Parkinson's disease. Neuron 46(6):857–868

64. Masliah E, Rockenstein E, Mante M et al (2011) Passive immunization reduces behavioral and neuropathological deficits in an alpha-synuclein transgenic model of Lewy body disease. PLoS One 6(4):e19338

65. Nasstrom T, Goncalves S, Sahlin C et al (2011) Antibodies against alpha-synuclein reduce oligomerization in living cells. PLoS One 6(10):e27230

66. Wilcock DM, Colton CA (2008) Anti-amyloid-beta immunotherapy in Alzheimer's disease: relevance of transgenic mouse studies to clinical trials. J Alzheimers Dis 15(4):555–569

67. Menendez-Gonzalez M, Perez-Pinera P, Martinez-Rivera M et al (2011) Immunotherapy for Alzheimer's disease: rational basis in ongoing clinical trials. Curr Pharm Des 17(5):508–520

68. Benner EJ, Banerjee R, Reynolds AD et al (2008) Nitrated alpha-synuclein immunity accelerates degeneration of nigral dopaminergic neurons. PLoS One 3(1), e1376

69. Reynolds AD, Stone DK, Hutter JA et al (2010) Regulatory t cells attenuate th17 cell-mediated nigrostriatal dopaminergic neurodegeneration in a model of Parkinson's disease. J Immunol 184(5):2261–2271

70. Sanchez-Guajardo V, Barnum CJ, Tansey MG et al (2013) Neuroimmunological processes in Parkinson's disease and their relation to alpha-synuclein: microglia as the referee between neuronal processes and peripheral immunity. ASN Neuro 5(2):113–139

71. Reynolds AD, Stone DK, Mosley RL et al (2009) Nitrated {alpha}-synuclein-induced alterations in microglial immunity are regulated by cd4+ t cell subsets. J Immunol 182(7):4137–4149

72. Sanchez-Guajardo V, Annibali A, Jensen PH et al (2013) Alpha-synuclein vaccination prevents the accumulation of Parkinson disease-like pathologic inclusions in striatum in association with regulatory t cell recruitment in a rat model. J Neuropathol Exp Neurol 72(7):624–645

73. Wiessner C, Wiederhold KH, Tissot AC et al (2011) The second-generation active abeta immunotherapy cad106 reduces amyloid accumulation in app transgenic mice while minimizing potential side effects. J Neurosci 31(25):9323–9331

74. Schneeberger A, Mandler M, Mattner F et al (2010) Affitome(r) technology in neurodegenerative diseases: the doubling advantage. Hum Vaccin 6(11):948–952

75. Schneeberger A, Mandler M, Mattner F et al (2012) Vaccination for Parkinson's disease. Parkinsonism Relat Disord 18(Suppl 1):S11–S13

76. Abeliovich A, Schmitz Y, Farinas I et al (2000) Mice lacking alpha-synuclein display functional deficits in the nigrostriatal dopamine system. Neuron 25(1):239–252

77. Hashimoto M, Rockenstein E, Mante M et al (2001) Beta-synuclein inhibits alpha-synuclein aggregation: a possible role as an anti-parkinsonian factor. Neuron 32(2):213–223

78. Hashimoto M, Kawahara K, Bar-On P et al (2004) The role of alpha-synuclein assembly and metabolism in the pathogenesis of Lewy body disease. J Mol Neurosci 24(3):343–352

79. Biere AL, Wood SJ, Wypych J et al (2000) Parkinson's disease-associated alpha-synuclein is more fibrillogenic than beta- and gamma-synuclein and cannot cross-seed its homologs. J Biol Chem 275(44):34574–34579

80. Fan Y, Limprasert P, Murray IV et al (2006) Beta-synuclein modulates alpha-synuclein neurotoxicity by reducing alpha-synuclein protein expression. Hum Mol Genet 15(20):3002–3011

81. Lee HJ, Khoshaghideh F, Patel S et al (2004) Clearance of alpha-synuclein oligomeric intermediates via the lysosomal degradation pathway. J Neurosci 24(8):1888–1896

82. Tran HT, Chung CH, Iba M et al (2014) Alpha-synuclein immunotherapy blocks uptake and templated propagation of misfolded alpha-synuclein and neurodegeneration. Cell Rep 7(6):2054–2065

83. Fagerqvist T, Lindstrom V, Nordstrom E et al (2013) Monoclonal antibodies selective for alpha-synuclein oligomers/protofibrils recognize brain pathology in Lewy body disorders and alpha-synuclein transgenic mice with the disease-causing a30p mutation. J Neurochem 126(1):131–144

84. Lindstrom V, Ihse E, Fagerqvist T et al (2014) Immunotherapy targeting alpha-synuclein, with relevance for future treatment of Parkinson's disease and other Lewy body disorders. Immunotherapy 6(2):141–153

85. Leber P (1997) Slowing the progression of Alzheimer disease: methodologic issues. Alzheimer Dis Assoc Disord 11(Suppl 5):S10–S21, Discussion S37-19

Chapter 8

Tau Immunotherapy

Einar M. Sigurdsson

Abstract

Great strides have been made in recent years on the development of tau immunotherapies for Alzheimer's disease and other tauopathies. Multiple animal studies by several groups have shown efficacy of various active and passive approaches in reducing pathological tau proteins. Clinical trials are clearly warranted and a few have already been initiated. However, much remains to be clarified regarding the mechanisms of action and how efficacy can be improved and potential toxicity minimized. These are exciting times for the field and will hopefully lead to an effective therapy in the near future.

Key words Tau, Immunotherapy, Alzheimer's disease, Tauopathies, Neurofibrillary tangles, Immunization, Vaccine, Aggregates

1 Immunotherapy Against Endogenous Aggregates: From Aβ to Tau

Over the last 15 years, substantial effort has been put into the development of immunotherapies targeting various endogenous peptides and proteins. The first target was amyloid-β (Aβ) in Alzheimer's disease (AD) but more recently such therapies are being developed against other pathological aggregates in AD and several other diseases. Findings from the earliest clinical trial seemed to indicate that Aβ plaque clearance did not halt or slow the progression of dementia, emphasizing that alternative targets and prophylactic therapies should be explored [1]. Subsequently, this view has been further supported by the disappointing outcomes of Phase III Aβ antibody trials [2] and more recently of a Phase II trial of an Aβ antibody reported to have broad reactivity with various forms of Aβ [3]. Another Phase I trial of a different Aβ antibody offered renewed hope, which has dissipated to some extent with the most recent follow-up of the study subjects [4], but it warrants further evaluation in a larger trial. It is not particularly surprising that clearing Aβ may not be sufficient to halt the progression of AD after clinical symptoms because Aβ plaque burden does not correlate well with the degree of dementia. Obviously, tau pathology is another important target in AD, and the primary

Martin Ingelsson and Lars Lannfelt (eds.), *Immunotherapy and Biomarkers in Neurodegenerative Disorders*, Methods in Pharmacology and Toxicology, DOI 10.1007/978-1-4939-3560-4_8, © Springer Science+Business Media New York 2016

target in other tauopathies. Importantly, pathological tau correlates much better with memory loss than Aβ deposition [5, 6]. Hence, targeting tau may be more effective than removing Aβ once cognitive impairments are evident. Aβ targeting therapies remain attractive as a prophylactic measure and are currently being evaluated in clinical trials with such a design in familial cases of AD [7], as well as in earlier stages of its sporadic form [4]. Eventually, combination therapies targeting Aβ, tau, and other hallmarks of the disease will likely be used concurrently to prevent or slow down its progression.

2   Tau Immunotherapy: Efficacy and Mechanism of Action

Our initial pioneering approach and findings indicated that active immunization with an AD related phosphorylated tau epitope, Tau379-408[P-Ser396, 404] in JNPL3 P301L tangle model mice, reduces brain levels of aggregated tau and slows progression of the tangle-related behavioral phenotype [8, 9]. We subsequently showed that this vaccine reduces tau aggregates and prevents cognitive decline in three different tests in another animal model of NFT formation [10], and that passive tau immunotherapy targeting the same epitope is effective as well [11]. Our findings [9, 12], and several reports of neuronal uptake of antibodies suggest that intracellular tau aggregates are being cleared, directly and/or indirectly [13] (Fig. 1). Specifically, we have shown that a portion of these antibodies can enter the brain and bind to pathological tau within the endosomal/lysosomal system of neurons [9, 12]. Furthermore, inhibition of antibody uptake into neurons prevents acute antibody-mediated clearance of total and phospho-tau in primary cultures from transgenic tauopathy mice [14]. This finding indicates that, at least for acute clearance, the antibody needs to get into the neurons. Antibody-mediated clearance of extracellular tau/tangles is likely to take place concurrently and may reduce associated damage, and prevent the spread of tau pathology [15–21]. Others have reported that various different intracellular aggregates, α-synuclein, Aβ, and superoxide dismutase can be targeted with immunotherapy [22–25]. These studies support our findings and interpretations.

Over the years, since our first report [9], the promise of tau immunotherapy has been confirmed and extended by us and several other groups [10–12, 14, 19, 26–47]. These publications have shown active and passive immunizations to be effective in multiple models. Various epitopes can be targeted, namely P-Ser396 and/or P-Ser404 [9–11, 14, 27, 28, 31, 33, 41, 42, 47], P-Ser422 [29, 37], certain conformations [27, 30, 33–35, 43], total tau [19, 30, 32, 33, 38–41, 44, 45], PSer202 [46], P-Ser202, Thr205 [36], P-Ser413 [41], P-Thr231 [42], and a combination of P-Ser202,

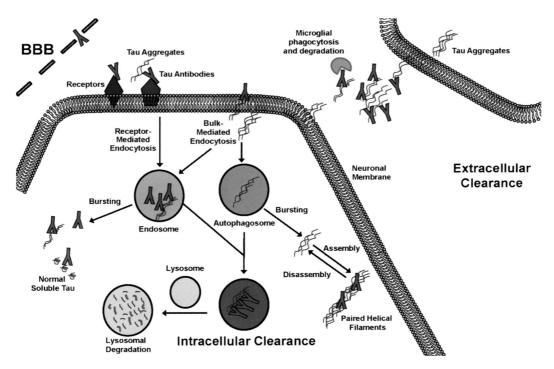

Fig. 1 Potential mechanisms for clearance and prevention of spread of pathological tau proteins. Both extra- and intracellular clearance pathways are likely to be involved, with the extent of each one depending primarily on various antibody properties and the stage of the disease. Uptake is predominantly determined by the charge of the antibody. Within the cell, the antibodies are mainly found within the endosomal/lysosomal system but some can be detected more diffusely in the cytosol after access through damaged membranes and/or bursting of endosomes. The extent of cytosolic distribution of the antibody likely depends on the abundance of its particular tau epitope within that cellular region. Some antibodies may promote lysosomal clearance by disassembling the tau aggregates and thereby facilitate access of lysosomal enzymes. Others may promote intracellular and/or extracellular tau aggregation via complex formation of antibodies and tau aggregates. Formation of such larger aggregates may prevent spreading of the pathology between neurons

Thr205, P-Thr212, Ser214, and P-Thr231 [26]. Many of these reports did not examine if the tau antibodies were taken up into neurons but some report neuronal uptake [9, 12, 14, 33, 37, 43], whereas others cannot demonstrate such detection [30, 32, 35]. The most likely explanation for these differences is that antibodies are taken up to a varying degree depending on their physicochemical properties, in particular their charge [48]. Future studies will hopefully compare the efficacy of otherwise identical antibodies that have been mutated to change their charge to increase/decrease their neuronal uptake. Such a study should provide valuable information on the potential contribution of intracellular vs. extracellular pathways for antibody-mediated clearance of tau aggregates.

Multiple scenarios can be envisioned for how each pathway can influence clearance, which may in part depend on the epitope being targeted. For example, some antibodies may disassemble tau aggregates within the endosomal/lysosomal system, and thereby facilitate access of lysosomal enzymes to promote degradation of the aggregates. Others, binding to different epitopes, may enhance aggregation via formation of antibody–tau complexes. This alternative scenario may also depend on where the interaction takes place: within intracellular vesicles; in the cytosol; within the cell membrane; and/or extracellularly. We have noticed differences in antibody location within neurons. One phospho-selective antibody, 4E6G7, bound mainly to larger aggregates within the endosomal/lysosomal system, whereas conformational antibody 6B2G12 with higher affinity for unphosphorylated tau, was also detected more diffusely in the cytosol. It is well known that endosomes routinely burst and antibodies that recognize normal tau protein to some extent may therefore be detected in the cytosol, where normal tau is abundant in soluble form. Intracellular aggregation is most likely detrimental, certainly as it builds up, but may be beneficial to some extent to reduce the pool of smaller potentially more toxic aggregates. The larger aggregates may eventually cause cell death when their bulk interferes too much with cellular function. However, such a buildup within the cell may also lead to less tau excretion, and thereby may attenuate the spread of tau pathology. It has been widely speculated that NFTs, Aβ plaques and other amyloids may be generated as a way to sequester more toxic smaller aggregates but at some point this is likely to become detrimental to the well-being of the neuron.

With regard to interaction of tau–antibody complex within the cell membrane, we have previously suggested that tau antibodies may enter the cell through damaged membranes [49]. This pathway has now been shown by others [37], reporting that tau antibody against pSer422 binds to membrane-associated tau which leads to intracellular clearance of the antibody–antigen complex.

In the matter of the extracellular scenario, some antibodies may be more efficacious than others depending on the isotype of the antibody and the epitope being targeted. Isotypes that better promote microglial phagocytosis of the antibody–antigen complex may be more effective but also more associated with inflammatory side effects although this is likely to be less of an issue for tau than Aβ. A recent report showed efficacy of an IgG2a/κ antibody but not of an IgG1/κ of similar affinity against the p-Ser404 epitope, or an IgG1/κ antibody recognizing total tau protein [47]. As discussed by the authors, IgG2a should activate more effector pathways than IgG1, which possibly may explain the different efficacies although this needs to be verified with antibodies that only differ in their isotype (Fc portion). In the case of Aβ, microglial phagocytosis of antibody–Aβ complex resulting in reduced parenchymal Aβ plaques is associated with buildup of vascular Aβ amyloid and microhemorrhages [50, 51]. Such side effects have not been reported for tau immunotherapy. The composition of extracellular tau and how it may differ from intracellular tau is also not well known. With reports of tau being released from neurons under non-pathological conditions [52–59], extracellular tau may have some normal function(s) which may need to be taken into consideration when targeting this pool (reviewed in [60]).

3   Epitope Selection

As detailed above, multiple epitopes have been targeted successfully in animals and cell culture studies. Most of these are AD associated phospho-epitopes which is a logical first choice because the relative specificity of the target minimizes potential toxicity of targeting the normal tau protein. An analogous focus is to target disease specific conformations. Such antibodies are generally of a lower affinity which may minimize efficacy but they may also recognize similar conformations in other disease-related protein aggregates and could, therefore, have broader efficacy. In AD and related disorders, these typically target β-pleated sheets, but analogous to most of the phospho-epitopes, those are found in small quantities in various normal proteins. Hence, these approaches are not entirely devoid of potential toxicity associated with targeting and clearance of normal proteins. With regard to the ability of the conformational antibodies to target similar conformations in different proteins, the profile of such binding is likely to vary depending on the antibody, the protein and the patient but this may be advantageous if the presence of such co-aggregates is not known. If known, such proteins may be more efficaciously cleared with antibodies that were specifically designed to target those particular proteins. If more than one needs to be targeted, co-administration of different antibodies can easily be performed, assuming that those exist. Pertaining to targeting all or most forms of individual proteins, both pathological and normal, such as with a total tau antibody, the key advantage is the broad selectivity which may enhance efficacy. The main disadvantage is greater risk of side effects as normal proteins may be targeted, which may reduce efficacy as well since less of the antibody is available to bind to pathological tau. However, this may not be of a major concern as the antibodies may mainly come in contact with pathological proteins, aggregates found intracellularly in the endosomal/lysosomal system or extracellularly after neuronal degradation or release from pathological neurons.

4   Potential Toxicity

While the active approach has certain advantages, it may have autoimmune side effects that may be avoided with narrower/single epitope vaccines or with passive immunization, which also allows more specific targeting of disease-related epitopes. The objective of the first reported study on tau immunization was to test the feasibility of active induction of neuroimmune disorder in mice [61]. A combination of very strong adjuvants was used with full length recombinant tau, resulting in neurological deficits. Similar effects were later reported by the same investigators after multiple injections of these adjuvants with phospho-tau peptides [62]. More recently, treatment of Aβ plaque mice with a total tau antibody has increased mortality, which raises some concerns about targeting normal tau epitopes [63]. We have observed enhanced mortality in some mixed mouse strain backgrounds after more than five injections of p-tau immunogen in alum adjuvant (unpublished results). This appears to be related to enhanced immune response in certain genetic backgrounds, even with such a mild adjuvant. These animals are fine with 4–5 immunizations and maintain relatively high antibody titers for over a year after the last immunization. These findings indicate that immune response needs to be carefully monitored during active tau immunizations. Eventually, the choice of adjuvant, immunogen, and number of injections should be tailor-made for individual patients.

Besides immune system related side effects, clearance of normal tau may also be detrimental as referred to earlier. In our long-term in vivo tau immunotherapy studies, we have not observed reductions in total tau levels but have detected such decrease acutely in cell culture [9–11, 14]. However, tau knockout mice are relatively normal [64–67], although they do show some deficits with age [68, 69], suggesting that some lowering of tau levels is likely not detrimental as related proteins may at least partially take over their function (see also [70] for review). In the context of AD, lowering tau levels reduces Aβ associated toxicity in in vitro and in vivo models [71–73], further alleviating major concerns with possible therapy-associated clearance of total cellular tau protein.

5   Antibody Engineering

Within the passive approach, antibody engineering may lead to further improvements. It is well known from other fields that antibody properties such as charge (isoelectric point), size, valency, affinity and avidity for the target, affinity for FcRn, and glycosylation influence its pharmacodynamics and pharmacokinetics, including cellular uptake [48]. These important aspects are only beginning to be studied in the tau immunotherapy field. All the tau antibodies that we have generated and studied to date are taken up into neurons, and all have isoelectric point in the neutral to basic range (unpublished observations). Size matters as well. Fab fragments of two of these antibodies are taken up to a greater extent in brain slices than intact antibodies [33]. However, the intact antibodies are predominantly associated with tau aggregates within the endosomal/lysosomal system, whereas the Fab fragments spread more diffusely throughout the neuronal cytosol. Furthermore, the intact tau antibodies are prominently taken up into neurons in tauopathy slices but not in wild-type slices, whereas the Fabs are taken up to a similar degree in both pathological and normal slices [33]. Regarding other properties, to the best of our knowledge, the influence of target affinity/avidity, valency, FcRn affinity, and glycosylation on efficacy, distribution, and clearance has not been studied for tau antibodies. We, however, have shown that neuronal uptake of whole antibodies in primary and brain slice culture is predominantly through low affinity FcγII/III receptors, which has been confirmed by others [43], and to a lesser extent via fluid-phase (bulk) endocytosis [14]. Tau Fabs which lack the Fc antibody portion are primarily taken up by the latter pathway [33]. The therapeutic utility of such tau antibody fragments has not been well studied but such smaller entities as well as diabodies, and single chain variable fragments (scFv's) may be particularly promising as imaging agents for in vivo detection of tau aggregates within the brain. The main focus of development of tau imaging agents has been on β-sheet binding dye derivatives [74], but antibody-based probes should be more specific, assuming sufficient target engagement can be obtained. We have reported that tau antibody derived scFv allows in vivo detection of tau aggregates in transgenic mice using the In Vivo Imaging System (IVIS) and that the IVIS signal correlates well with the degree of tau pathology [75]. This finding has major implications for experimental and clinical use of this approach to monitor tau pathology and assess the efficacy of various tau targeting therapies.

6   Clinical Trials

There are currently six Phase I clinical trials on tau immunotherapy in progress. One is being performed by Axon Neuroscience SE which is testing AADvac1, an active vaccine consisting of a KLH-conjugate of a tau peptide 294–305 in patients with mild-to-moderate AD [38, 76]. Another one is being conducted by AC Immune and Janssen, which according to their press release is testing ACI-35, a liposome-based phospho-tau peptide active vaccine in mild-to-moderate AD. Further information on the trial has yet to be deposited in clinical trial databases. A mouse study on ACI-35 indicates that the tau epitope is Tau393-408[P-Ser396, 404] [31]. In addition to these two active trials, four passive trials have been recently initiated. Two include healthy subjects and two individuals with Progressive Supranuclear Palsy (PSP). Bristol-Meyers Squibb is conducting two trials in these two groups on one of the tau antibodies they obtained with the purchase of iPerian [77, 78]. It binds to a postulated pathological tau fragment (tau1-224) but should recognize normal tau as well [40]. Roche is studying their P-Ser422 antibody in healthy subjects who presumably do not have this epitope [29, 37, 79], and C2N Diagnostics/Abbvie are treating PSP patients with tau antibody C2N-8E12 [80]. It is not clear if it is the humanized version of the apparent lead antibody of C2N Diagnostics which binds to tau25-30 [32]. Clinical trials by several other companies will likely be initiated in the near future [81].

7   Future Studies

It is now important to clarify if and how efficacy versus toxicity of the tau antibodies or immunogen depend on: (1) which epitope(s) are being targeted; (2) affinity/avidity towards the target; (3) targeting single versus multiple epitopes; (4) the isotype of the antibody; (5) whole antibody versus antibody fragments; (6) the adjuvant used for active immunization; (7) whether tau is targeted intracellularly and/or extracellularly; (8) disease stage; (9) the route of administration; (10) dose and frequency of injection, and; (11) development of anti-ideotypic antibodies. Many of these issues have been addressed to some extent and will continue to be clarified in animals and culture models but will eventually have to be evaluated in clinical trials. Immunotherapies such as these targeting self-antigens are best suited to be personalized, taking into account the disease epitope and immune response profiles of each patient for individually suited therapies. Ongoing and future advances in imaging and other biomarkers as well as haplotype mapping and other immune system profiling should greatly facilitate such tailored approaches.

Acknowledgements

E.M.S. is supported by NIH grants NS077239, AG032611, and AG020197. He is an inventor on patents on tau immunotherapy and related diagnostics that are assigned to New York University. This technology is licensed to and is being co-developed with H. Lundbeck A/S.

References

1. Holmes C, Boche D, Wilkinson D et al (2008) Long-term effects of A beta(42) immunisation in Alzheimer's disease: follow-up of a randomised, placebo-controlled phase I trial. Lancet 372(9634):216–223

2. Aisen PS, Vellas B (2013) Passive immunotherapy for Alzheimer's disease: what have we learned, and where are we headed? J Nutr Health Aging 17(1):49–50

3. Fagan T (2014) Crenezumab disappoints - Phase 2 - Researchers remain hopeful. http://www.alzforum. org/news/conference-coverage/crenezumab-disappoints-phase-2-researchers-remain-hopeful. Accessed 13 Aug 2014

4. Strobel G (2015) Aducanumab, solanezumab, gantenerumab data lift crenezumab, as well. http://www.alzforum.org/news/conference-coverage/aducanumab-solanezumab-gantenerumab-data-lift-crenezumab-well. Accessed 21 Aug 2015

5. Wilcock GK, Esiri MM (1982) Plaques, tangles and dementia: a quantitative study. J Neurol Sci 56(2-3):343–356

6. Arriagada PV, Growdon JH, Hedley-Whyte ET, Hyman BT (1992) Neurofibrillary tangles but not senile plaques parallel duration and severity of Alzheimer's disease. Neurology 42(3 Pt 1):631–639

7. Strobel G (2014) NIH director announces $100M prevention trial of Genentech antibody. http://www. alzforum.org/news/conference-coverage/nih-director-announces-100m-prevention-trial-genentech-antibody. Accessed 13 Aug 2014

8. Sigurdsson EM. Immune therapy for AD plaques and tangles. [Project period begin date 09/30/2001]. NIH, 1R01AG020197

9. Asuni AA, Boutajangout A, Quartermain D, Sigurdsson EM (2007) Immunotherapy targeting pathological tau conformers in a tangle mouse model reduces brain pathology with associated functional improvements. J Neurosci 27(34):9115–9129

10. Boutajangout A, Quartermain D, Sigurdsson EM (2010) Immunotherapy targeting pathological tau prevents cognitive decline in a new tangle mouse model. J Neurosci 30(49):16559–16566

11. Boutajangout A, Ingadottir J, Davies P, Sigurdsson EM (2011) Passive immunization targeting pathological phospho-tau protein in a mouse model reduces functional decline and clears tau aggregates from the brain. J Neurochem 118(4):658–667

12. Krishnamurthy PK, Deng Y, Sigurdsson EM (2011) Mechanistic studies of antibody-mediated clearance of tau aggregates using an ex vivo brain slice model. Front Psychiatry 2:59

13. Sigurdsson EM (2009) Tau-focused immunotherapy for Alzheimer's disease and related tauopathies. Curr Alzheimer Res 6(5):446–450

14. Congdon EE, Gu J, Sait HB, Sigurdsson EM (2013) Antibody uptake into neurons occurs primarily via clathrin-dependent Fcgamma receptor endocytosis and is a prerequisite for acute tau protein clearance. J Biol Chem 288(49):35452–35465

15. Frost B, Jacks RL, Diamond MI (2009) Propagation of tau misfolding from the outside to the inside of a cell. J Biol Chem 284(19):12845–12852

16. Clavaguera F, Bolmont T, Crowther RA et al (2009) Transmission and spreading of tauopathy in transgenic mouse brain. Nat Cell Biol 11(7):909–913

17. Kim W, Lee S, Jung C, Ahmed A, Lee G, Hall GF (2010) Interneuronal transfer of human tau between Lamprey central neurons in situ. J Alzheimers Dis 19(2):647–664

18. Liu L, Drouet V, Wu JW et al (2012) Trans-synaptic spread of tau pathology in vivo. PLoS ONE 7(2):e31302

19. Kfoury N, Holmes BB, Jiang H, Holtzman DM, Diamond MI (2012) Trans-cellular propagation of tau aggregation by fibrillar species. J Biol Chem 287(23):19440–19451

20. Santa-Maria I, Varghese M, Ksiezak-Reding H, Dzhun A, Wang J, Pasinetti GM (2012) Paired helical filaments from Alzheimer disease brain induce intracellular accumulation of tau protein in aggresomes. J Biol Chem 287(24):20522–20533

21. Wu JW, Herman M, Liu L et al (2013) Small misfolded tau species are internalized via bulk endocytosis and anterogradely and retrogradely transported in neurons. J Biol Chem 288(3):1856–1870

22. Masliah E, Rockenstein E, Adame A et al (2005) Effects of alpha-synuclein immunization in a mouse model of Parkinson's disease. Neuron 46(6):857–868

23. Tampellini D, Magrane J, Takahashi RH et al (2007) Internalized antibodies to the A beta

domain of APP reduce neuronal A beta and protect against synaptic alterations. J Biol Chem 282(26):18895–18906

24. Masliah E, Rockenstein E, Mante M et al (2011) Passive immunization reduces behavioral and neuropathological deficits in an alpha-synuclein transgenic model of Lewy body disease. PLoS ONE 6(4), e19338

25. Urushitani M, Ezzi SA, Julien JP (2007) Therapeutic effects of immunization with mutant superoxide dismutase in mice models of amyotrophic lateral sclerosis. Proc Natl Acad Sci U S A 104(7):2495–2500

26. Boimel M, Grigoriadis N, Lourbopoulos A, Haber E, Abramsky O, Rosenmann H (2010) Efficacy and safety of immunization with phosphorylated tau against neurofibrillary tangles in mice. Exp Neurol 224(2):472–485

27. Chai X, Wu S, Murray TK et al (2011) Passive immunization with anti-tau antibodies in two transgenic models: reduction of tau pathology and delay of disease progression. J Biol Chem 286(39):34457–34467

28. Bi M, Ittner A, Ke YD, Gotz J, Ittner LM (2011) Tau-targeted immunization impedes progression of neurofibrillary histopathology in aged P301L tau transgenic mice. PLoS One 6(12):e26860

29. Troquier L, Caillierez M, Burnouf S et al (2012) Targeting phospho-Ser422 by active tau immunotherapy in the THY-Tau22 mouse model: a suitable therapeutic approach. Curr Alzheimer Res 9(4):397–405

30. d'Abramo C, Acker CM, Jimenez HT, Davies P (2013) Tau passive immunotherapy in mutant P301L mice: antibody affinity versus specificity. PLoS ONE 8(4):e62402

31. Theunis C, Crespo-Biel N, Gafner V et al (2013) Efficacy and safety of a liposome-based vaccine against protein tau, assessed in Tau. P301L mice that model tauopathy. PLoS One 8(8):e72301

32. Yanamandra K, Kfoury N, Jiang H et al (2013) Anti-tau antibodies that block tau aggregate seeding in vitro markedly decrease pathology and improve cognition in vivo. Neuron 80(2):402–414

33. Gu J, Congdon EE, Sigurdsson EM (2013) Two novel tau antibodies targeting the 396/404 region are primarily taken up by neurons and reduce tau protein pathology. J Biol Chem 288(46):33081–33095

34. Castillo-Carranza DL, Gerson JE, Sengupta U, Guerrero-Munoz MJ, Lasagna-Reeves CA, Kayed R (2014) Specific targeting of tau oligomers in hTau mice prevents cognitive impairment and tau toxicity following injection with brain-derived tau oligomeric seeds. J Alzheimers Dis 40:S97–S111

35. Castillo-Carranza DL, Sengupta U, Guerrero-Munoz MJ et al (2014) Passive immunization with tau oligomer monoclonal antibody reverses tauopathy phenotypes without affecting hyperphosphorylated neurofibrillary tangles. J Neurosci 34(12):4260–4272

36. Walls KC, Ager RR, Vasilevko V, Cheng D, Medeiros R, LaFerla FM (2014) p-Tau immunotherapy reduces soluble and insoluble tau in aged 3xTg-AD mice. Neurosci Lett 575:96–100

37. Collin L, Bohrmann B, Gopfert U, Oroszlan-Szovik K, Ozmen L, Gruninger F (2014) Neuronal uptake of tau/pS422 antibody and reduced progression of tau pathology in a mouse model of Alzheimer's disease. Brain 137(Pt 10):2834–2846

38. Kontsekova E, Zilka N, Kovacech B, Novak P, Novak M (2014) First-in-man tau vaccine targeting structural determinants essential for pathological tau-tau interaction reduces tau oligomerisation and neurofibrillary degeneration in an Alzheimer's disease model. Alzheimers Res Ther 6(4):44

39. Selenica ML, Davtyan H, Housley SB et al (2014) Epitope analysis following active immunization with tau proteins reveals immunogens implicated in tau pathogenesis. J Neuroinflammation 11:152

40. Bright J, Hussain S, Dang V et al (2015) Human secreted tau increases amyloid-beta production. Neurobiol Aging 36(2):693–709

41. Umeda T, Eguchi H, Kunori Y et al (2015) Passive immunotherapy of tauopathy targeting pSer413-tau: a pilot study in mice. Ann Clin Transl Neurol 2(3):241–255

42. Sankaranarayanan S, Barten DM, Vana L et al (2015) Passive immunization with phospho-tau antibodies reduces tau pathology and functional deficits in two distinct mouse tauopathy models. PLoS One 10(5):e0125614

43. Kondo A, Shahpasand K, Mannix R et al (2015) Antibody against early driver of neurodegeneration cis P-tau blocks brain injury and tauopathy. Nature 523(7561):431–436

44. Yanamandra K, Jiang H, Mahan TE et al (2015) Anti-tau antibody reduces insoluble tau and decreases brain atrophy. Ann Clin Transl Neurol 2(3):278–288

45. Funk KE, Mirbaha H, Jiang H, Holtzman DM, Diamond MI (2015) Distinct therapeutic mechanisms of tau antibodies: promoting microglial clearance vs. blocking neuronal uptake. J Biol Chem 290(35):21652–62

46. d'Abramo C, Acker CM, Jimenez H, Davies P (2015) Passive immunization in JNPL3 trans-

genic mice using an array of phospho-tau specific antibodies. PLoS One 10(8):e0135774

47. Ittner A, Bertz J, Suh LS, Stevens CH, Gotz J, Ittner LM (2015) Tau-targeting passive immunization modulates aspects of pathology in tau transgenic mice. J Neurochem 132(1): 135–145

48. Bumbaca D, Boswell CA, Fielder PJ, Khawli LA (2012) Physiochemical and biochemical factors influencing the pharmacokinetics of antibody therapeutics. AAPS J 14(3):554–558

49. Sigurdsson EM (2008) Immunotherapy targeting pathological tau protein in Alzheimer's disease and related tauopathies. J Alzheimers Dis 15:157–168

50. Pfeifer M, Boncristiano S, Bondolfi L et al (2002) Cerebral hemorrhage after passive anti-Abeta immunotherapy. Science 298(5597):1379

51. Morgan D (2009) The role of microglia in antibody-mediated clearance of amyloid-beta from the brain. CNS Neurol Disord Drug Targets 8(1):7–15

52. Chai X, Dage JL, Citron M (2012) Constitutive secretion of tau protein by an unconventional mechanism. Neurobiol Dis 48(3):356–366

53. Shi Y, Kirwan P, Smith J, MacLean G, Orkin SH, Livesey FJ (2012) A human stem cell model of early Alzheimer's disease pathology in Down syndrome. Sci Transl Med 4(124):124ra29

54. Saman S, Kim W, Raya M et al (2012) Exosome-associated tau is secreted in tauopathy models and is selectively phosphorylated in cerebrospinal fluid in early Alzheimer disease. J Biol Chem 287(6):3842–3849

55. Simon D, Garcia-Garcia E, Royo F, Falcon-Perez JM, Avila J (2012) Proteostasis of tau. Tau overexpression results in its secretion via membrane vesicles. FEBS Lett 586(1):47–54

56. Yamada K, Cirrito JR, Stewart FR et al (2011) In vivo microdialysis reveals age-dependent decrease of brain interstitial fluid tau levels in P301S human tau transgenic mice. J Neurosci 31(37):13110–13117

57. Plouffe V, Mohamed NV, Rivest-McGraw J, Bertrand J, Lauzon M, Leclerc N (2012) Hyperphosphorylation and cleavage at D421 enhance tau secretion. PLoS One 7(5):e36873

58. Karch CM, Jeng AT, Goate AM (2012) Extracellular tau levels are influenced by variability in tau that is associated with tauopathies. J Biol Chem 287(51):42751–42762

59. Pooler AM, Phillips EC, Lau DH, Noble W, Hanger DP (2013) Physiological release of endogenous tau is stimulated by neuronal activity. EMBO Rep 14(4):389–394

60. Medina M, Avila J (2014) The role of extracellular tau in the spreading of neurofibrillary pathology. Front Cell Neurosci 8:113

61. Rosenmann H, Grigoriadis N, Karussis D et al (2006) Tauopathy-like abnormalities and neurologic deficits in mice immunized with neuronal tau protein. Arch Neurol 63(10):1459–1467

62. Rozenstein-Tsalkovich L, Grigoriadis N, Lourbopoulos A et al (2013) Repeated immunization of mice with phosphorylated-tau peptides causes neuroinflammation. Exp Neurol 248:451–456

63. Mably AJ, Kanmert D, Mc Donald JM et al (2015) Tau immunization: a cautionary tale? Neurobiol Aging 36(3):1316–1332

64. Harada A, Oguchi K, Okabe S et al (1994) Altered microtubule organization in small-caliber axons of mice lacking tau-protein. Nature 369(6480):488–491

65. Dawson HN, Ferreira A, Eyster MV, Ghoshal N, Binder LI, Vitek MP (2001) Inhibition of neuronal maturation in primary hippocampal neurons from tau deficient mice. J Cell Sci 114(6):1179–1187

66. Tucker KL, Meyer M, Barde YA (2001) Neurotrophins are required for nerve growth during development. Nat Neurosci 4(1):29–37

67. Fujio K, Sato M, Uemura T, Sato T, Sato-Harada R, Harada A (2007) 14-3-3 proteins and protein phosphatases are not reduced in tau-deficient mice. Neuroreport 18(10):1049–1052

68. Ikegami S, Harada A, Hirokawa N (2000) Muscle weakness, hyperactivity, and impairment in fear conditioning in tau-deficient mice. Neurosci Lett 279(3):129–132

69. Lei P, Ayton S, Finkelstein DI et al (2012) Tau deficiency induces parkinsonism with dementia by impairing APP-mediated iron export. Nat Med 18(2):291–295

70. Ke YD, Suchowerska AK, van der Hoven J et al (2012) Lessons from tau-deficient mice. Int J Alzheimers Dis 2012:873270

71. Rapoport M, Dawson HN, Binder LI, Vitek MP, Ferreira A (2002) Tau is essential to beta-amyloid-induced neurotoxicity. Proc Natl Acad Sci U S A 99(9):6364–6369

72. Roberson ED, Scearce-Levie K, Palop JJ et al (2007) Reducing endogenous tau ameliorates amyloid beta-induced deficits in an Alzheimer's disease mouse model. Science 316(5825): 750–754

73. Ittner LM, Ke YD, Delerue F et al (2010) Dendritic function of tau mediates amyloid-beta toxicity in Alzheimer's disease mouse models. Cell 142(3):387–397

74. Congdon EE, Krishnaswamy S, Sigurdsson EM (2014) Harnessing the immune system for treatment and detection of tau pathology. J Alzheimers Dis 40:S113–S121

75. Krishnaswamy S, Lin Y, Rajamohamedsait WJ, Rajamohamedsait HB, Krishnamurthy P, Sigurdsson EM (2014) Antibody-derived in vivo imaging of tau pathology. J Neurosci 34(50):16835–16850

76. Axon Neuroscience SE (2015) NCT01850238: safety study of AADvac1, a tau peptide-KLH-conjugate active vaccine to treat Alzheimer's disease. ClinicalTrials. gov

77. Bristol-Meyers Squibb (2015) NCT02294851: a randomized, double-blind, placebo-controlled, single ascending dose study of intrave-nously administered BMS-986168 in healthy subjects. ClinicalTrials.gov

78. Bristol-Meyers Squibb (2015) NCT02460094: Multiple ascending dose study of intravenously administered BMS-986168 in patients with progressive supranuclear palsy (CN002-003). ClinicalTrials.gov

79. Hoffmann-La-Roche (2015) NCT02281786: a study of RO6926496 in healthy volunteers. ClinicalTrials.gov

80. C2N Diagnostics - Abbvie (2015) NCT02494024: safety, tolerability and pharma-cokinetics of C2N-8E12 in subjects with progressive supranuclear palsy. ClinicalTrials.gov

81. Pedersen JT, Sigurdsson EM (2015) Tau immunotherapy for Alzheimer's disease. Trends Mol Med 21(6):394–402

Chapter 9

Active and Passive Immunotherapy Against Tau: Effects and Potential Mechanisms

Kiran Yanamandra, Marc I. Diamond, and David M. Holtzman

Abstract

The aggregation, hyperphosphorylation, and accumulation of the microtubule-associated protein tau is a hallmark for several neurodegenerative diseases, including Alzheimer's disease. These diseases are known as tauopathies. In tauopathies, the tau protein becomes hyperphosphorylated and forms intracellular neurofibrillary tangles visualized within dystrophic neurites and cell bodies. Evidence suggests that some tau aggregates can become extracellular where they potentially propagate between cells and induce tau pathology in previously unaffected cells. The amount of tau pathology correlates well with the load of neurofibrillary tangles, synaptic loss, and functional decline in humans as well as in transgenic mouse models of tauopathy. Several active and passive immunization studies targeting tau in transgenic mouse models have shown reduced tau pathology, although the mechanism(s) underlying these effects is not clear. In this chapter, we review the recent active and passive immunization strategies targeting tau in mouse models and our understanding of potential mechanisms underlying the effects seen.

Key words Tau, Immunotherapy, Alzheimer's disease, Neurodegeneration, Antibody

1 Tau Protein and Neurodegenerative Disease

The microtubule-associated protein tau stabilizes microtubules and promotes axonal transport. In neurons, it is found mainly in axons, but it is also expressed in astrocytes and oligodendrocytes. In the adult human brain, tau is encoded by the gene *MAPT* (microtubule-associated protein tau) on chromosome 17q21. It has six splice isoforms. The presence or absence of exons 2 and 3, encode a region in the N-terminus, creating 0, 1, or 2N regions. Exon 10 encodes one of four microtubule binding repeat sequences, and its presence or absence creates 4 repeat (4R) or 3 repeat (3R) tau [1, 2]. Tau is thus referred to by the number of N and R sequences, e.g., 1N3R.

Aggregation and accumulation of amyloid-β (Aβ) and tau are pathological hallmarks of Alzheimer's disease (AD). In the disease, specific posttranslational modifications of tau occur. Hyper-phosphorylation and hyperacetylation are described in aggregated

Martin Ingelsson and Lars Lannfelt (eds.), *Immunotherapy and Biomarkers in Neurodegenerative Disorders*, Methods in Pharmacology and Toxicology, DOI 10.1007/978-1-4939-3560-4_9, © Springer Science+Business Media New York 2016

forms of tau, such as neurofibrillary tangles (NFTs), although it is not clear if these are primary or secondary events in the process of tau aggregation. In normal aging, NFTs containing tau occur in virtually all brains in certain regions, including CA1 of the hippocampus and entorhinal cortex. However, after Aβ deposition begins to occur in the neocortex, the process is associated with progression of tauopathy to the neocortex in AD [3]. Strong data supports the idea that Aβ aggregation somehow drives progression of tau aggregation and its associated neurodegeneration that occurs in AD, but the mechanism is unknown. In certain forms of frontotemporal dementia (FTD), progressive supranuclear palsy (PSP), corticobasal degeneration (CBD), and Pick's disease, tau aggregates and forms NFTs and is hyperphosphorylated even in the absence of Aβ aggregation [4]. In some inherited cases of FTD, mutations in the *MAPT* gene also cause tau aggregation, NFTs, and tau hyperphosphorylation. These diseases are collectively termed tauopathies [4].

2   Active Immunization with Tau Peptides

Analogous to targeting of Aβ [5], multiple active and passive immunization strategies against tau have been tested in mouse models of tauopathy. The data from these studies are summarized in Tables 1 and 2. In initial active immunization studies on tau, investigators immunized wild-type female C57Bl/6 mice expressing only murine tau with recombinant human tau protein administered intraperitoneally. This caused encephalomyelitis accompanied by the formation of apparent NFTs in wild-type mice [6]. True NFTs have typically not been found in wild-type mice in the absence of human tau expression. The same group then used a human transgenic tau model expressing double mutant K257T/P301S tau alone in which one-half of the animals had induced inflammation at 6–7 weeks of age by administration of myelin oligodendrocyte glycoprotein. These two groups were subcutaneously injected at 4 months of age with three tau peptides mixed together—(Tau195-213 [P202/205], Tau207-220 [P212/214], and Tau224-238 [P231])—that contained phosphorylation sites recognized by the AT8, AT100, and AT180 monoclonal antibodies that stain pathological tau. Immunized mice showed decreased tau pathology and neurofibrillary tangle burden by Gallyas staining, and decreased phosphorylated forms of tau as recognized by immunostaining with the AT8 and AT180 antibodies. In addition, immunized mice showed increased lectin positive microglial staining compared to controls. The astrocytic burden was unaffected [7].

In another study, phospho-tau peptide (Amino acids 379–408, with pSer 396 and 404) containing the PHF1 phospho-tau epitope antibody), was subcutaneously injected in the JNPL3

Table 1

Active immunization with tau peptides

	Target peptide	Mouse model	Adjuvant	Onset of pathology	Type of inj.	Start of treatment	IHC	Biochemistry	Microglial/astrocytes activation	Antibody in neuron	Behavior tests
Boimel et al. 2010 [7]	Tau195-213 [P202/205], Tau207-220 [P212/214] and Tau224-238 [P231]	K257T/P301S tau double tg mice	Complete Freund	6 months	SC	4 months	Tau pathology reduced in cortex, hippocampus and brain stem	–	Increased microglia	–	–
Asuni et al. 2007 [8]	Tau379-408 [P396/404]	JNPL3	Aluminum	~3 months	SC	2 months	Tau pathology reduced in dentate gyrus, motor cortex and brain stem	Soluble ptau increased and no change in insoluble p-tau	–	Yes	Improvement in rotarod, transverse beam and maximum velocity tests
Boutajangout et al. 2010 [9]	Tau 379-408 [P396/404]	htau/PS1 mice (htau model cross withPS1 M146L model)	Aluminum	2 months	IP	3–4 months	Tau pathology reduced in piriform cortex	Soluble ptau decreased and no change in insoluble p-tau	No difference	–	Improvement in radial arm maze and closed field symmetrical maze testes
Bi et al. 2011 [12]	Tau 395-406 [P396/404]	pR5 mice (P301L)	KLH with complete or incomplete freund	6 months	IP	4, 8 and 18 months	Tau pathology reduced in amygdala and CA1 region	–	Increased astrogliosis in old mice	No	–
Troquier et al. 2012 [13]	Tau417-427 (P422); Tau420-426 (P422)	THY-Tau22	Complete or incomplete freund	3 months	IP	3.5 months	Decrease trend of tau pathology at CA1 region	Insoluble ptau was decreased	–	–	Improvement in Y-maze test

IHC immunohistochemistry, KLH keyhole limpet hemocyanin, IP intraperitoneal injection, SC subcutaneous injection

Table 2
Passive Immunization by using tau antibodies

	Abs for immunization	Mouse model	Treatment	Onset of pathology	Type of inj.	Dose	IHC	Biochemistry	Microglial/ astrocytes activation	Antibody in neurons	Behavior tests
Chia et al. 2011 [16]	PHF-1, MC1 and IgG (control antibody)	JNPL3 & P301S (Thy1 promoter)	2–6 months	4.5–5 months	IP	15 mg/kg 3 inj/week	Tau pathology reduced in brain stem and spinal cord	Insoluble tau level was reduced	No difference	No	Improvement in rotarod
Boutajangout et al. 2011 [17]	PHF-1, IgG	JNPL3	2–5 months	~3 months	IP	250 μg/ 125 μl	Tau pathology reduced in dentate gyrus	Insoluble tau level was reduced	No difference	Yes	Improvement in traverse beam test
d'Abramo et al. 2013 [18]	MC1,PHF1, DA31 (pan antibody), Saline (control)	JNPL3	3–7 months; 7–10 months	4.5–5 months	IP	10 mg/kg	Tau pathology reduced in CA1 region	Total tau and Insol. phospho-tau reduced	No difference	No	–
Yanamandra et al. 2013 [20]	Anti-tau antibodies (HJ8.5, HJ9.3, HJ9.4) and HJ3.4 (control antibody)	P301S (prp promoter)	6–9 months	6 months	ICV	605 μg/ 3months	Tau pathology reduced at piriform, entorhinal cortex and amygdala	Insoluble tau and seeding activity reduced	Decreased microglial activity	–	Improvement in contextual fear conditioning test
Castillo-Carranza et al. 2014 [19]	Tau oligomer antibody (TOMA), IgG (control)	JNPL3	8 months	4.5–5 months	ICV, IV	Single inj. 1 μg for ICV, 30 μg/ IV	Tau pathology reduced in CA1 region	Tau oligomers were reduced	No difference	No	Improvement in rotarod and Y-maze test
Yanamandra et al. 2015 [21]	Anti-tau antibody HJ8.5	P301S (prp promoter)	6–9 months	6 months	IP	50 mg/kg, 10 mg/kg	Tau pathology reduced in CA1 celllayer, decreased brain atrophy	Insoluble tau reduced	–	–	Improvement in Inverted and Ledge test

IHC immunohistochemistry, *IP* intraperitoneal injection, *ICV* intracerebroventricular injection, *IV* intravenous injection

(P301L tau transgenic mouse) model. Control mice received aluminum adjuvant alone. One group of mice was treated from 2 until 5 months of age and another group from 2 until 8 months of age. At the end of the treatment, both 5 and 8 month old mice went through a battery of sensorimotor tests before sacrifice. Quantitative immunostaining with the anti-tau antibodies MC1 and PHF1 showed reduced tau pathology in the dentate gyrus, motor cortex, and brainstem regions. Western blotting showed increased soluble phospho-tau and no difference in insoluble phospho-tau. Treated mice showed improvement in rotarod, transverse beam, and maximum velocity tests. This treatment was more effective at the earlier time point of 5 months of age as compared to the later 8 month time point [8]. The same group also immunized mice expressing human tau under the control of the normal tau promoter that were crossed with PS1 transgenic mice (htau/PS1) mice [9]. Mice were immunized with the tau peptide 379–408 containing the PHF1 tau antibody epitope pSer 396 and 404. The htau/PS1 mice were obtained by crossing htau mice expressing all 6 isoforms of tau on a mouse tau knockout background [10] with a model carrying the M146L presenilin mutation that causes a form of dominantly inherited AD [11]. The mice received intraperitoneal injections, with three injections every 2 weeks beginning at 3–4 months of age with subsequent administration at monthly intervals. Control groups received aluminum adjuvant alone. Immunotherapy reduced PHF1 reactive tau pathology compared to controls as assessed by immunostaining in the piriform cortex. Soluble PHF1 reactive tau levels were decreased by Western blot, but there was no difference in insoluble phospho-tau levels compared to controls. No difference in microgliosis or astrogliosis was noted. However immunized mice showed improvement in the radial arm maze and closed field symmetrical maze tests compared to control groups [9].

In another study, pR5 mice that express human P301L tau under the control of Thy 1.2 promoter were immunized with a 12 amino acid peptide of Tau 395–406 containing the PHF1 epitope pS396 and pS404. Three different age groups of 4, 8 and 18 months of age were immunized intraperitoneally with tau peptide linked to keyhole limpet hemocyanin (KLH). Tau-KLH was dissolved in PBS and emulsified with complete or incomplete Freund's adjacent at 1:1 ratio. Control mice received KLH with complete Freund's adjacent. Immunostaining showed reduced phosphorylated tau in the amygdala and CA1 regions. In addition, increased astrogliosis was observed in older age group mice. No anti-tau antibodies were found inside neurons of treated pR5 mice [12].

Troquier et al. used THY-Tau22 transgenic mice, which develop hippocampal neurofibrillary tangle-like inclusions at 3–6 months of age. Tau peptide vaccine containing phospho-Ser422 was injected peritoneally at 3 months of age. Control mice received adjuvant alone. The first two injections were administered every 2 weeks, followed by injections given monthly. There was no effect on phosphorylated tau species stained by the anti-tau antibodies AT100 and pS422 in the hippocampal CA1 region. In the biochemical analysis, insoluble tau was decreased by AT100 and pS422 detection. Following active immunization, an increase in tau levels was observed in the blood. Cognitive improvement was also observed in immunized mice in the Y-maze test [13]. Taken together, active immunization with different tau peptides has reduced tau pathology and improved behavior in human tau transgenic mice. However, compared to results with Aβ vaccination, the effects on pathology and behavior do not appear to be as strong, and the underlying mechanism(s) remains unknown.

3 Passive Immunization by Using Anti-Tau Antibodies

In an initial passive immunization study, JNPL3 and P301S tau transgenic mice (at age 2–3 months, prior to the onset of tau pathology) were administered the PHF1 anti-tau monoclonal antibody [14] or the conformation specific antibody MC1 [15] intraperitoneally at 15 mg/kg three times a week for 2 months followed by 10 mg/kg twice a week for the next 2 months. P301S mice were given 15 mg/kg of antibody twice weekly. PHF1 recognizes phospho tau at pSer396/404 on both normal tau and disease-associated tau. MC1 recognizes tau only in a pathological conformation. Both treatments reduced insoluble tau levels [16]. Phospho-tau was reduced in both the brainstem and spinal cord. Treated mice showed improvement in the rotarod test. No alteration in activation of microglia or astrocytes was observed in treated vs. control mice [16]. In another passive immunization study with JNPL3 tau transgenic mice, the PHF1 antibody was intraperitoneally administered for 13 weeks from 2 to 3 months of age, i.e., prior to the onset of pathology in this model. As compared to IgG control treated mice, the tau antibody treated mice showed decreased PHF1 tau pathology in the dentate gyrus. While a decrease in insoluble phospho-tau was observed, there was no change in total insoluble tau levels as measured by Western blot. Treated mice also performed better in the transverse beam task, and similar degrees of micro- and astrogliosis was observed in treated vs. control mice [17].

In another study, d'Abramo et al. treated female JNPL3 mice animals with intraperitoneal injections of either the MC1 or DA31 anti-tau antibodies of 10 mg/kg weekly from 3 to 7 months of age and compared these with saline treated mice. Another group of mice received MC1 weekly from 7 to 10 months of age. P301L mice sacrificed at 7 months of age or treated with saline from 7 months until 10 months were used as control groups. The MC1 antibody reduced soluble and insoluble tau in the forebrain of

P301L Tau mice compared to the DA31 treated mice. Mice treated with the MC1 antibody from 7 to 10 months showed decreased phospho-tau immunostaining as assessed by the anti-tau antibodies CP13 and RZ3 in the hippocampal CA1 region. In addition, decreased phosphorylated, insoluble tau was noted in the forebrain of treated mice [18].

A recent study assessed the effects of that administration of a single dose of 1 or 30 μg of an anti-tau oligomeric monoclonal antibody (TOMA) by intracerebroventricular or intravenous injection in 8 month old JNPL3 mice. A control group received nonspecific IgG–rhodamine and wild type mice received saline injections. Four days after intracerebroventricular injection with TOMA, mice showed improved performance on the rotarod [19]. Tau oligomers were reduced as assessed by Western blot and immunofluorescence assays, with no change in monomeric tau. Four to six days after intravenous injection of the TOMA antibody there was improved performance of mice on both the rotarod and Y-maze task. The investigators also noted an increase in tau oligomers in the periphery following peripheral administration of TOMA [19].

Our group [20] hypothesized that anti-tau antibodies might function by blocking cell to cell spread of a pathological form of tau. We first screened antibodies that blocked the ability of extracellular tau aggregates to seed intracellular tau. We then chose antibodies with various efficacies in blocking tau seeding and tested them in vivo. P301S Tau transgenic mice were treated with one of three different anti-tau antibodies (HJ8.5, HJ9.3, and HJ9.4), a control antibody, or phosphate-buffered saline with infusion into the lateral ventricles for 3 months, beginning at 6 months of age. Each anti-tau antibody targets a different, non-phosphorylated tau epitope. Quantitative immunostaining showed that all three monoclonal anti-tau antibodies strongly reduced the abnormally phosphorylated tau stained by the AT8 phospho-tau antibody in different brain regions. Two of three anti-tau antibodies reduced insoluble tau levels from cortical brain tissues as assessed by biochemical analysis. This treatment also significantly reduced pathological seeding activity in the treated soluble brain lysates of P301S mice compared to control groups. Of the three antibodies tested, HJ8.5 and HJ9.4 significantly improved memory deficits in a conditioned fear test [20]. These experiments were consistent with a mechanism of action based on binding extracellular tau aggregates.

In a follow-up study, the most potent antibody, HJ8.5 in the prior study, was further studied assessed with peripheral administration (intraperitoneal). Two different doses of HJ8.5, 10 mg/kg or 50 mg/kg, were administered weekly to 6 month old male P301S mice for three months. HJ8.5 at 50 mg/kg strongly reduced insoluble tau levels compared to controls. Interestingly, both doses of antibody resulted in decreased cortical and hippocampal brain atrophy compared to the control treated P301S mice. Both doses of HJ8.5 treatment reduced hippocampal CA1 cell layer stained with the p-tau antibody AT8 as well as Thio-S positive tau aggregates in piriform cortex and amygdala. Mice treated with HJ8.5 at 50 mg/kg showed a decrease in motor/sensorimotor deficits compared to control group. Moreover, HJ8.5 treatment resulted in a dose-dependent increase of tau in plasma [21]. All the above studies support the idea that anti-tau antibodies should considered as a potential treatment for tauopathies.

4   Propagation of Tau

In AD and other tauopathies, tau pathology starts in a particular brain region and then progresses or spreads to other regions that are anatomically connected. Normally, monomeric tau is closely associated with microtubules. Yet monomeric tau under physiological conditions is released into both the interstitial fluid (ISF) and CSF, and tau aggregates may also be present in the ISF [22]. Tau antibodies that enter the CNS could thus be targeting extracellular tau aggregates as well as monomeric tau. What is the evidence that extracellular tau aggregates are important in disease pathogenesis? In cultured cells, tau aggregates can be released into the extracellular space, and these aggregates have been shown to be transferred to neighboring cells [23, 24]. In vivo injection of the brain extracts from human mutant P301S tau mice into the hippocampus and cerebral cortex of ALZ17 mice, which express the longest form of the wild type human four repeat isoform and never develop tau deposits, induced tau pathology, with spread of the pathology from sites of injection to neighboring brain regions [25]. Isolation of tau oligomers from Alzheimer's disease brains by immunoprecipitation followed by injection into the wild type C57BL/6 mice was found to induce tau aggregation by seeding endogenous murine tau, and to induce tau pathology at distant sites after prolonged incubation [26]. Two independent research groups showed in similar animal models that by restricting the expression of P301L tau in the entorhinal cortex, tau aggregates spread to neighboring cells and also synaptically connected regions in the hippocampus [27, 28]. In young mice, tau pathology was limited to the entorhinal cortex. However, in aged mice, tau aggregates spread to the synaptically connected granular layer of the dentate gyrus, CA region of the hippocampus, and the cingulate cortex. Infusion of synthetic fibrils of recombinant full length human tau with P301S mutation into the hippocampus of the young P301S tau transgenic mice induced rapid formation of neurofibrillary tangle-like inclusions at the injection sites. The pathology spread to synaptically connected regions in a time and dose-dependent manner [29], although it is difficult to exclude spreading of the inoculum itself.

Following injection of brain extract from tauopathies such as AD into the hippocampus and cerebral cortex of ALZ17 mice, there was induction of tau inclusions. Human tauopathy brain extracts injected into non-transgenic 3 month old C57BL/6 mice also resulted in the formation of tau inclusions. Furthermore, induced pathology in mouse brain could induce more pathology upon reinjection into a next generation of mice [30]. Finally, a recent study found that stably expressed tau repeat domain will propagate distinct amyloid conformations in a clonal fashion in culture [31]. Reintroduction of tau from these lines into naive cells reestablished identical clones. Further, the two "artificial" tau strains produced in vitro induced distinct pathologies in vivo as determined by successive inoculations into three generations of transgenic mice. Immunopurified tau from these mice created the original strains in culture. Finally, the cell culture system enabled isolation of multiple disease-associated strains from tauopathy patients. Together with other studies, this demonstrates that some form(s) of tau has essential characteristics of a prion. The studies above clearly indicate that tau aggregates formed in one region propagate a specific tau conformation to neighboring neuronal cells. It may be that certain anti-tau antibodies are able to block or decrease this process.

Tau seeding and spreading appears to be mediated by specific conformations of tau protein. For proteins that aggregate in neurodegenerative diseases, including tau, specific conformations may determine patterns of both spreading pathology and toxicity. Small aggregates of pathogenic proteins, termed oligomers, are generally more neurotoxic than the insoluble mature fibrils [32]. Therefore, it may be very important to target such species to create the most effective immunotherapy. As mentioned earlier, passive immunization studies targeting different phosphorylation or pathological forms of the tau have been shown to reduce tau pathology. However, most effects do not appear overly robust in animal models using this strategy, indicating that we need to better understand antibody mechanisms, particularly those of antibodies that have strong effects. The best treatment results to date appear to have been accomplished with anti-tau antibodies that do not specifically target a phosphorylated or acetylated form of tau but can recognize a host of different forms [20, 21]. To best design anti-tau immunotherapy approaches, understanding these effects will be critical.

5   Tau Species to Be Targeted

Tau is hyperphosphorylated in neurodegenerative conditions, and phosphorylated tau is present in paired helical filaments and NFTs. In a Drosophila model, it was shown that neurodegeneration occurs even in the absence of NFTs [33] and that the presence of

NFTs in mouse neurons does not always mark dying or sick cells [34, 35]. It may be that particular aggregated forms of tau are key in eliciting neurodegeneration, but this is not known.

It has recently been shown that tau can misfold into specific conformational states and epigenetically propagate multiple amyloid conformations in clonal cell lines and in vivo [31]. Therefore, tau conformers can be in distinct tau aggregated forms or "strains" may predominate in patients with different types of tauopathies. Different tau antibodies are likely to differentially bind to these different strains or tau conformations. Therefore, in immunotherapy, a key may be to choose antibodies that can either target multiple conformations or to target very specific conformations associated with a particular disease. In both active and passive immunization, by selecting pathological forms of tau peptides in active immunization or utilizing antibodies targeting pathological tau or tau oligomers, there was reduction of tau pathology and also improvement in behavioral deficits in tau transgenic mouse models (Tables 1 and 2). Of the studies published to date, infusion of anti-tau antibodies directly into the lateral ventricle of the brain appear to have had the greatest effect in decreasing tau pathology versus other treatments in transgenic mice [20]. Interestingly, all the 3 anti-tau antibodies used in this study appeared to immunoprecipitate unique forms of tau species from brain lysates of transgenic mice as assessed by atomic force microscopy [20]. This indicates that different anti-tau antibodies may differentially recognize unique tau conformations. Depending on the location within the brain that such antibodies can access, the antibodies may sequester soluble or aggregated forms of tau in the extracellular or intracellular space and might also prevent monomeric tau from forming oligomeric or fibrillar species. While some studies suggest that anti-tau antibodies access the cytoplasm [17, 36, 37], this has not been observed in other studies [16, 18–20].

6   Potential Mechanism in Blocking Extracellular Tau Spread/Toxicity

In contrast to Aβ that is secreted and forms extracellular plaques, tau forms primarily intracellular amyloids. However, in vivo microdialysis indicates that tau is released from cells under physiological conditions. Moreover, tau is present in relatively high levels in the ISF of wild-type mice at concentrations of ~50 ng/ml—even in the absence of neurodegeneration or injury [22]. Studies from cultured cells have shown that certain forms of tau can escape cells and spread in a prion like manner to neighboring cells. Such secretion of tau into the extracellular space from neurons is independent of cell death [38, 39]. In addition, recent studies showed that tau release by neurons is regulated by excitatory neuronal activity [40, 41]. It is not yet clear whether under either normal or pathological conditions tau aggregates are also secreted into the brain extracellular space along with monomers via similar mechanisms. Once the tau aggregates are released from the cells into the extracellular space, they may sequester monomeric tau [22]. These extracellular aggregates could be taken up by adjacent cells or connected cells or may be taken up by the same cells and increase the intracellular burden of aggregated tau.

Blocking of tau aggregates that are more prone to initiate seeding activity in adjacent cells or promote the clearance of extracellular tau conformers by microglia, neurons, or other cells may be important mechanisms in tau immunotherapy. While the study by Yanamandra et al. (2013) suggests that anti-tau antibodies may block spreading of extracellular tau seeds from one cell to another, this has not yet been definitively proven. If an antibody is able to target forms of extracellular tau seeds or conformers, there can be several possible fates of the tau protein, as discussed in the following section. In addition, it is possible that extracellular forms of tau are toxic. Targeting these forms, independent of blocking spreading per se, could potentially lead to beneficial effects on synaptic/neuronal function.

7   Clearance of Tau and Tau Aggregates

7.1   Neurons

If an anti-tau antibody binds extracellular tau, the anti-tau antibody/tau complex might still be taken up by neurons. There are two main protein degradation systems present in cells (including neurons), namely the proteasomal and lysosomal systems. The proteasome mainly degrades soluble and short lived ubiquitinated proteins. Lysosome-mediated degradation mediates multiple mechanisms including macroautophagy [42]. Non-functional misfolded proteins can be cleared for the purpose of detoxification by either of these systems.

Certain neurons express high affinity FcγR1 receptors on their membrane [43, 44]. The low affinity Fc receptors FcγII and FcγIII are not expressed in neurons and are exclusively expressed in microglia in brain [44–46]. High affinity FcγRI receptors recognize the Fc domain of IgG and can initiate antibody uptake [47]. If the antibody enters the cytoplasm via this mechanism, it could then bind cytosolic tau aggregates and initiate its clearance by lysosomal pathways. In such a location, it could also theoretically bind to cytosolic antibody receptor TRIM21 and trigger antibody/tau degradation by the proteasome and initiate signaling pathways of the innate immune system [48, 49]. With the knowledge that tau can be present in the extracellular space, one study suggests that antibody bound to extracellular tau aggregates can be taken up by the neurons in a clathrin-dependent Fcγ receptor mediated endocytosis and further degraded by proteolytic enzymes in lysosomes [36, 37]. In contrast, recent studies using tau antibodies targeting extracellular tau species showed no detectable amount of uptake of anti-tau antibodies into neurons [18, 19] or non-neuronal cells in vitro [20]. Further in vitro and in vivo work will be required to sort out the role of neurons in uptake, degradation, and seeding of tau in the presence and absence of different anti-tau antibodies.

7.2 Microglia and Astrocytes

In neurodegenerative disease and other tauopathies, tau aggregation is linked to the activation of microglia and astrocytes in transgenic mouse models [50–54]. Microglia and astrocytes are phagocytic in nature. Once anti-tau antibodies in vivo sequester extracellular tau aggregates, their metabolic fate is not yet clear. Passive immunization with anti-Aβ antibodies has been noted to reduce microgliosis chronically [55] though acute application of anti-Aβ antibodies can lead to rapid microglial activation if the antibodies bind aggregated Aβ and have an intact Fc domain [56]. Microglia express low affinity FcγII and FcγIII receptors in the cytoplasm and on the surface of the cells. These receptors are not present on astrocytes. These receptors have the potential to recognize antibody/tau aggregate complexes and initiate the multiple immune effector pathways including antibody mediated cellular uptake, phagocytosis, and release of inflammatory mediators [57]. Antibody mediated clearance of extracellular α-synuclein was showed to occur mainly in microglia through Fcγ receptors and not in neuronal cells or astrocytes [46]. Certain antibodies against amyloid-β were shown to trigger microglial cells to clear plaques through Fc receptor-mediated phagocytosis and subsequent peptide degradation [58]. In temporal neocortex of Alzheimer's patients, the size distribution of dense-core plaques was proportional to the microglial response but not to the astrocyte response. However, plaque-associated reactive astrocytes may be protecting neurons form surrounding plaques [59]. The role of astrocytes in tau pathology in the presence or absence of anti-tau antibodies is not yet clear. Astrocytes may be activated indirectly by antibody/tau complexes and activate microglial release of some inflammatory signals or cytokines.

In some anti-tau immunotherapies that have been tested by using anti-pathological tau antibodies, no change in activation of microglia or astrocytes was found [16, 17]. After 3 months of anti-tau antibody administration into tau transgenic mice, activated microglia were reduced in proportion to the reduction of tau pathology in treated mice [20]. This is also consistent with a study in which several months of passive immunization with anti-Aβ antibodies showed reduced Aβ plaques and reduced microgliosis [60]. In cases in which there is reduction of microgliosis upon passive administration of anti-tau antibodies, this could simply reflect lower levels of tau aggregation due to the anti-tau antibody therapy. In BV2-murine cultured immortalized microglial-like cells, anti-tau antibody increased the uptake of tau aggregates compared to control conditions. However, no difference in uptake of tau aggregates in presence or absence of anti-tau antibody was noted using primary neurons [21]. Using in vivo models, whether and how microglia and astrocytes play a role in anti-tau antibody mediated tau clearance still remains an open question.

7.3 Peripheral Sink and Cerebrospinal Fluid

Peripheral administration of anti-Aβ antibodies in PDAPP transgenic mice reduces Aβ burden. One mechanism that may account for part of this effect is by facilitating Aβ efflux or clearance from the brain to the periphery in a "peripheral sink" type of mechanism [61–63]. Anti-Aβ antibodies were also shown to sequester extracellular soluble Aβ in the central nervous system to potentially further block its aggregation [61, 64]. It is thought that antibodies cannot effectively penetrate cells and directly access cytoplasmic proteins under normal circumstances. In tau immunotherapy, it is also possible that anti-tau antibodies can sequester extracellular tau species effectively in the brain, not allowing prion-like spreading of tau to seed tau in adjacent cells. Antibodies to tau could thus promote tau monomer and aggregate clearance via binding to tau in the extracellular space and promoting efflux of tau antibody/tau complexes via the brain ISF and CSF into the periphery [65, 66]. It is also possible that anti-tau antibody in the periphery could accelerate CNS to plasma efflux of tau via bulk flow or blood–brain barrier mediated mechanisms as proposed with the peripheral sink Aβ hypothesis. As the mechanism(s) by which tau can exit the CNS to the periphery have not yet been worked out, future experiments will need to address these issues.

8 Summary

Active and passive immunization of tau has shown promising results in reducing tau pathology and improving brain dysfunction, indicating that these approaches should be further considered as therapeutic strategies for tauopathies. In immunotherapy studies, tau antibodies may be targeting tau species in either the extracellular or intracellular space and promoting tau clearance by multiple pathways. Extracellular tau clearance may be mediated by microglial, astrocytic, or neuronal mediated uptake followed by lysosomal degradation. It is also interesting to consider the possibility of antibody mediated clearance of tau monomer and aggregate via CSF and ISF flow into the periphery, as well as tau clearance via a "peripheral sink" mechanism. In this scenario, antibodies could promote tau efflux into the peripheral blood stream without requiring antibody entry into the CNS. We have summarized several possible mechanisms of anti-tau antibody-mediated clearance of tau in Fig. 1. While studies suggest that some of these mechanisms may be operative, it is not yet clear which of these is the most

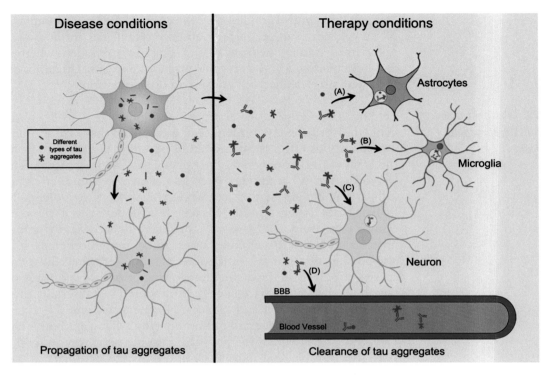

Fig. 1 Possible clearance mechanisms of tau aggregates by antibodies: In disease conditions, different forms of tau aggregates can be released into the extracellular space and propagate into neighboring cells to induce the aggregation of intracellular tau (Shown in *left panel*). Under therapeutic conditions (*right panel*), anti-tau antibodies trap tau aggregates in the extracellular space and induce clearance by different mechanisms, possibly via astrocytes (*A*), microglia (*B*) or neuronal mediated clearance mechanisms (*C*). (*D*) Anti-tau antibodies could also promote efflux of tau from central nervous system by crossing the blood–brain barrier and binding tau in the CNS, promoting clearance via ISF/CSF flow ultimately into the plasma. It is also possible that anti-tau antibodies present in the blood can somehow increase the normal efflux of tau from CNS to plasma

important. We suggest that the choice of antibody is likely critical to see the best possible efficacy. Our own data suggests that targeting all forms of tau species and blocking the prion-like propagation of pathological forms of tau into adjacent cells may be most important. However, much more work needs to be done in this area to better understand the underlying mechanism(s) of these potentially very promising effects.

Acknowledgements

This work was supported by research grants from the Tau consortium and C2N Diagnostics (M.I.D. and D.M.H.).

References

1. Goode BL, Feinstein SC (1994) Identification of a novel microtubule binding and assembly domain in the developmentally regulated inter-repeat region of tau. J Cell Biol 124(5):769–782

2. Gustke N, Trinczek B, Biernat J, Mandelkow EM, Mandelkow E (1994) Domains of tau protein and interactions with microtubules. Biochemistry 33(32):9511–9522

3. Musiek ES, Holtzman DM (2012) Origins of Alzheimer's disease: reconciling cerebrospinal fluid biomarker and neuropathology data regarding the temporal sequence of amyloid-beta and tau involvement. Curr Opin Neurol 25(6):715–720. doi:10.1097/WCO.0b013e32835a30f4

4. Mandelkow EM, Mandelkow E (2012) Biochemistry and cell biology of tau protein in neurofibrillary degeneration. Cold Spring Harb Perspect Med 2(7):a006247. doi:10.1101/cshperspect.a006247, Pii: a006247

5. Brody DL, Holtzman DM (2008) Active and passive immunotherapy for neurodegenerative disorders. Annu Rev Neurosci 31:175–193. doi:10.1146/annurev.neuro.31.060407.125529

6. Rosenmann H, Grigoriadis N, Karussis D, Boimel M, Touloumi O, Ovadia H, Abramsky O (2006) Tauopathy-like abnormalities and neurologic deficits in mice immunized with neuronal tau protein. Arch Neurol 63(10):1459–1467. doi:10.1001/archneur.63.10.1459, Pii: 63/10/145

7. Boimel M, Grigoriadis N, Lourbopoulos A, Haber E, Abramsky O, Rosenmann H (2010) Efficacy and safety of immunization with phosphorylated tau against neurofibrillary tangles in mice. Exp Neurol 224(2):472–485. doi:10.1016/j.expneurol.2010.05.010, Pii: S0014-4886(10)00168-8

8. Asuni AA, Boutajangout A, Quartermain D, Sigurdsson EM (2007) Immunotherapy targeting pathological tau conformers in a tangle mouse model reduces brain pathology with associated functional improvements. J Neurosci 27(34):9115–9129. doi:10.1523/JNEUROSCI.2361-07.2007, pii:27/34/9115

9. Boutajangout A, Quartermain D, Sigurdsson EM (2010) Immunotherapy targeting pathological tau prevents cognitive decline in a new tangle mouse model. J Neurosci 30(49):16559–16566. doi:10.1523/JNEUROSCI.4363-10.2010, pii: 30/49/16559

10. Andorfer C, Acker CM, Kress Y, Hof PR, Duff K, Davies P (2005) Cell-cycle reentry and cell death in transgenic mice expressing nonmutant human tau isoforms. J Neurosci 25(22):5446–5454. doi:10.1523/JNEUROSCI.4637-04.2005, pii: 25/22/5446

11. Duff K, Eckman C, Zehr C, Yu X, Prada CM, Perez-tur J, Hutton M, Buee L, Harigaya Y, Yager D, Morgan D, Gordon MN, Holcomb L, Refolo L, Zenk B, Hardy J, Younkin S (1996) Increased amyloid-beta42(43) in brains of mice expressing mutant presenilin 1. Nature 383(6602):710–713. doi:10.1038/383710a0

12. Bi M, Ittner A, Ke YD, Gotz J, Ittner LM (2011) Tau-targeted immunization impedes progression of neurofibrillary histopathology in aged P301L tau transgenic mice. PLoS One 6(12), e26860. doi:10.1371/journal.pone.0026860, pii: PONE-D-11-15839

13. Troquier L, Caillierez R, Burnouf S, Fernandez-Gomez FJ, Grosjean ME, Zommer N, Sergeant N, Schraen-Maschke S, Blum D, Buee L (2012) Targeting phospho-Ser422 by active Tau immunotherapy in the THYTau22 mouse model: a suitable therapeutic approach. Curr Alzheimer Res 9(4):397–405, doi:CAR-EPUB-20120123-019 [pii]

14. Otvos L Jr, Feiner L, Lang E, Szendrei GI, Goedert M, Lee VM (1994) Monoclonal antibody PHF-1 recognizes tau protein phosphorylated at serine residues 396 and 404. J Neurosci Res 39(6):669–673. doi:10.1002/jnr.490390607

15. Jicha GA, Weaver C, Lane E, Vianna C, Kress Y, Rockwood J, Davies P (1999) cAMP-dependent protein kinase phosphorylations on tau in Alzheimer's disease. J Neurosci 19(17):7486–7494

16. Chai X, Wu S, Murray TK, Kinley R, Cella CV, Sims H, Buckner N, Hanmer J, Davies P, O'Neill MJ, Hutton ML, Citron M (2011) Passive immunization with anti-Tau antibodies in two transgenic models: reduction of Tau pathology and delay of disease progression. J Biol Chem 286(39):34457–34467. doi:10.1074/jbc.M111.229633, pii: M111.229633

17. Boutajangout A, Ingadottir J, Davies P, Sigurdsson EM (2011) Passive immunization targeting pathological phospho-tau protein in a mouse model reduces functional decline and clears tau aggregates from the brain. J Neurochem 118(4):658–667. doi:10.1111/j.1471-4159.2011.07337.x

18. d'Abramo C, Acker CM, Jimenez HT, Davies P (2013) Tau passive immunotherapy in mutant P301L mice: antibody affinity versus specificity. PLoS One 8(4):e62402. doi:10.1371/journal.pone.0062402, pii: PONE-D-13-01397

19. Castillo-Carranza DL, Sengupta U, Guerrero-Munoz MJ, Lasagna-Reeves CA, Gerson JE, Singh G, Estes DM, Barrett AD, Dineley KT, Jackson GR, Kayed R (2014)

Passive immunization with Tau oligomer monoclonal antibody reverses tauopathy phenotypes without affecting hyperphosphorylated neurofibrillary tangles. J Neurosci 34(12):4260–4272. doi:10.1523/JNEUROSCI.3192-13.2014, pii: 34/12/4260

20. Yanamandra K, Kfoury N, Jiang H, Mahan TE, Ma S, Maloney SE, Wozniak DF, Diamond MI, Holtzman DM (2013) Anti-tau antibodies that block tau aggregate seeding in vitro markedly decrease pathology and improve cognition in vivo. Neuron 80(2):402–414. doi:10.1016/j.neuron.2013.07.046,pii:S0896-6273(13)00670-3

21. Yanamandra K, Jiang H, Mahan TE, Maloney SE, Wozniak DF, Diamond MI, Holtzman DM (2015) Anti-tau antibody reduces insoluble tau and decreases brain atrophy. Ann Clin Transl Neurol 2(3):278–288. doi:10.1002/acn3.176

22. Yamada K, Cirrito JR, Stewart FR, Jiang H, Finn MB, Holmes BB, Binder LI, Mandelkow EM, Diamond MI, Lee VM, Holtzman DM (2011) In vivo microdialysis reveals age-dependent decrease of brain interstitial fluid tau levels in P301S human tau transgenic mice. J Neurosci 31(37):13110–13117. doi:10.1523/JNEUROSCI.2569-11.2011, pii: 31/37/13110

23. Guo JL, Lee VM (2011) Seeding of normal Tau by pathological Tau conformers drives pathogenesis of Alzheimer-like tangles. J Biol Chem 286(17):15317–15331. doi:10.1074/jbc.M110.209296, pii: M110.209296

24. Frost B, Jacks RL, Diamond MI (2009) Propagation of tau misfolding from the outside to the inside of a cell. J Biol Chem 284(19):12845–12852. doi:10.1074/jbc.M808759200, pii: M808759200

25. Clavaguera F, Bolmont T, Crowther RA, Abramowski D, Frank S, Probst A, Fraser G, Stalder AK, Beibel M, Staufenbiel M, Jucker M, Goedert M, Tolnay M (2009) Transmission and spreading of tauopathy in transgenic mouse brain. Nat Cell Biol 11(7):909–913. doi:10.1038/ncb1901, pii: ncb1901

26. Lasagna-Reeves CA, Castillo-Carranza DL, Sengupta U, Guerrero-Munoz MJ, Kiritoshi T, Neugebauer V, Jackson GR, Kayed R (2012) Alzheimer brain-derived tau oligomers propagate pathology from endogenous tau. Sci Rep 2:700. doi:10.1038/srep00700

27. Liu L, Drouet V, Wu JW, Witter MP, Small SA, Clelland C, Duff K (2012) Trans-synaptic spread of tau pathology in vivo. PLoS One 7(2), e31302. doi:10.1371/journal.pone.0031302, pii: PONE-D-11-23353

28. de Calignon A, Polydoro M, Suarez-Calvet M, William C, Adamowicz DH, Kopeikina KJ, Pitstick R, Sahara N, Ashe KH, Carlson GA, Spires-Jones TL, Hyman BT (2012) Propagation of tau pathology in a model of early Alzheimer's disease. Neuron 73(4):685–697. doi:10.1016/j.neuron.2011.11.033, pii: S0896-6273(12)00038-4

29. Iba M, Guo JL, McBride JD, Zhang B, Trojanowski JQ, Lee VM (2013) Synthetic Tau fibrils mediate transmission of neurofibrillary tangles in a transgenic mouse model of Alzheimer's-like tauopathy. J Neurosci 33(3):1024–1037. doi:10.1523/JNEUROSCI.2642-12.2013, pii: 33/3/1024

30. Clavaguera F, Akatsu H, Fraser G, Crowther RA, Frank S, Hench J, Probst A, Winkler DT, Reichwald J, Staufenbiel M, Ghetti B, Goedert M, Tolnay M (2013) Brain homogenates from human tauopathies induce tau inclusions in mouse brain. Proc Natl Acad Sci U S A 110(23):9535–9540. doi:10.1073/pnas.1301175110, pii: 1301175110

31. Sanders DW, Kaufman SK, DeVos SL, Sharma AM, Mirbaha H, Li A, Barker SJ, Foley AC, Thorpe JR, Serpell LC, Miller TM, Grinberg LT, Seeley WW, Diamond MI (2014) Distinct Tau prion strains propagate in cells and mice and define different tauopathies.. doi:10.1016/j.neuron.2014.04.047, pii: Neuron, doi:S0896-6273(14)00362-6

32. Haass C, Selkoe DJ (2007) Soluble protein oligomers in neurodegeneration: lessons from the Alzheimer's amyloid beta-peptide. Nat Rev Mol Cell Biol 8(2):101–112. doi:10.1038/nrm2101, pii: doi:nrm2101

33. Wittmann CW, Wszolek MF, Shulman JM, Salvaterra PM, Lewis J, Hutton M, Feany MB (2001) Tauopathy in Drosophila: neurodegeneration without neurofibrillary tangles. Science 293(5530):711–714. doi:10.1126/science.1062382, pii: 1062382

34. Kuchibhotla KV, Wegmann S, Kopeikina KJ, Hawkes J, Rudinskiy N, Andermann ML, Spires-Jones TL, Bacskai BJ, Hyman BT (2014) Neurofibrillary tangle-bearing neurons are functionally integrated in cortical circuits in vivo. Proc Natl Acad Sci U S A 111(1):510–514. doi:10.1073/pnas.1318807111, pii: 1318807111

35. de Calignon A, Fox LM, Pitstick R, Carlson GA, Bacskai BJ, Spires-Jones TL, Hyman BT (2010) Caspase activation precedes and leads to tangles. Nature 464(7292):1201–1204. doi:10.1038/nature08890, pii: nature08890

36. Congdon EE, Gu J, Sait HB, Sigurdsson EM (2013) Antibody uptake into neurons occurs

primarily via clathrin-dependent Fcgamma receptor endocytosis and is a prerequisite for acute tau protein clearance. J Biol Chem 288(49):35452–35465. doi:10.1074/jbc. M113.491001, pii: M113.491001

37. Sigurdsson EM (2009) Tau-focused immunotherapy for Alzheimer's disease and related tauopathies. Curr Alzheimer Res 6(5):446–450, pii: CAR-7

38. Karch CM, Jeng AT, Goate AM (2012) Extracellular Tau levels are influenced by variability in Tau that is associated with tauopathies. J Biol Chem 287(51):42751–42762. doi:10.1074/jbc.M112.380642, pii: M112.380642

39. Chai X, Dage JL, Citron M (2012) Constitutive secretion of tau protein by an unconventional mechanism. Neurobiol Dis 48(3):356–366. doi:10.1016/j.nbd.2012.05.021, pii: S0969-9961(12)00207-0

40. Yamada K, Holth JK, Liao F, Stewart FR, Mahan TE, Jiang H, Cirrito JR, Patel TK, Hochgrafe K, Mandelkow EM, Holtzman DM (2014) Neuronal activity regulates extracellular tau in vivo. J Exp Med 211(3):387–393. doi:10.1084/jem.20131685, pii: jem.20131685

41. Pooler AM, Phillips EC, Lau DH, Noble W, Hanger DP (2013) Physiological release of endogenous tau is stimulated by neuronal activity. EMBO Rep 14(4):389–394. doi:10.1038/embor.2013.15, pii: embor201315

42. Ding WX, Yin XM (2008) Sorting, recognition and activation of the misfolded protein degradation pathways through macroautophagy and the proteasome. Autophagy 4(2):141–150, pii: doi:5190

43. Mohamed HA, Mosier DR, Zou LL, Siklos L, Alexianu ME, Engelhardt JI, Beers DR, Le WD, Appel SH (2002) Immunoglobulin Fc gamma receptor promotes immunoglobulin uptake, immunoglobulin-mediated calcium increase, and neurotransmitter release in motor neurons. J Neurosci Res 69(1):110–116. doi:10.1002/jnr.10271

44. Andoh T, Kuraishi Y (2004) Direct action of immunoglobulin G on primary sensory neurons through Fc gamma receptor I. FASEB J 18(1):182–184. doi:10.1096/fj.02-1169fje, pii: 02-1169fje

45. Niu N, Zhang J, Guo Y, Zhao Y, Korteweg C, Gu J (2011) Expression and distribution of immunoglobulin G and its receptors in the human nervous system. Int J Biochem Cell Biol 43(4):556–563. doi:10.1016/j.biocel.2010.12.012, pii: S1357-2725(10)00424-3

46. Bae EJ, Lee HJ, Rockenstein E, Ho DH, Park EB, Yang NY, Desplats P, Masliah E, Lee SJ (2012) Antibody-aided clearance of extracellular alpha-synuclein prevents cell-to-cell aggregate transmission. J Neurosci 32(39):13454–13469. doi:10.1523/JNEUROSCI.1292-12.2012, pii: 32/39/13454

47. Ravetch JV, Bolland S (2001) IgG Fc receptors. Annu Rev Immunol 19:275–290. doi:10.1146/annurev.immunol.19.1.275, pii: 19/1/275

48. McEwan WA, Tam JC, Watkinson RE, Bidgood SR, Mallery DL, James LC (2013) Intracellular antibody-bound pathogens stimulate immune signaling via the Fc receptor TRIM21. Nat Immunol 14(4):327–336. doi:10.1038/ni.2548, pii: ni.2548

49. Mallery DL, McEwan WA, Bidgood SR, Towers GJ, Johnson CM, James LC (2010) Antibodies mediate intracellular immunity through tripartite motif-containing 21 (TRIM21). Proc Natl Acad Sci U S A 107(46):19985–19990. doi:10.1073/pnas.1014074107, pii: 1014074107

50. Bellucci A, Westwood AJ, Ingram E, Casamenti F, Goedert M, Spillantini MG (2004) Induction of inflammatory mediators and microglial activation in mice transgenic for mutant human P301S tau protein. Am J Pathol 165(5):1643–1652. doi:10.1016/S0002-9440(10)63421-9, pii: S0002-9440(10)63421-9

51. Ikeda M, Shoji M, Kawarai T, Kawarabayashi T, Matsubara E, Murakami T, Sasaki A, Tomidokoro Y, Ikarashi Y, Kuribara H, Ishiguro K, Hasegawa M, Yen SH, Chishti MA, Harigaya Y, Abe K, Okamoto K, St George-Hyslop P, Westaway D (2005) Accumulation of filamentous tau in the cerebral cortex of human tau R406W transgenic mice. Am J Pathol 166(2):521–531. doi:10.1016/S0002-9440(10)62274-2, pii: S0002-9440(10)62274-2

52. Sasaki A, Kawarabayashi T, Murakami T, Matsubara E, Ikeda M, Hagiwara H, Westaway D, George-Hyslop PS, Shoji M, Nakazato Y (2008) Microglial activation in brain lesions with tau deposits: comparison of human tauopathies and tau transgenic mice TgTauP301L. Brain Res 1214:159–168. doi:10.1016/j.brainres.2008.02.084, pii: S0006-8993(08)00554-4

53. Zilka N, Stozicka Z, Kovac A, Pilipcinec E, Bugos O, Novak M (2009) Human misfolded truncated tau protein promotes activation of microglia and leukocyte infiltration in the transgenic rat model of tauopathy. J Neuroimmunol 209(1-2):16–25. doi:10.1016/j.jneuroim.2009.01.013, pii: S0165-5728(09)00020-4

54. Yoshiyama Y, Higuchi M, Zhang B, Huang SM, Iwata N, Saido TC, Maeda J, Suhara T, Trojanowski JQ, Lee VM (2007) Synapse loss and microglial activation precede tangles in a P301S tauopathy mouse model. Neuron 53(3):337–351. doi:10.1016/j.neuron.2007.01.010, pii: S0896-6273(07)00030-X

55. Wilcock DM, DiCarlo G, Henderson D, Jackson J, Clarke K, Ugen KE, Gordon MN, Morgan D (2003) Intracranially administered anti-Abeta antibodies reduce beta-amyloid deposition by mechanisms both independent of and associated with microglial activation. J Neurosci 23(9): 3745–3751, doi:23/9/3745 [pii]

56. Bacskai BJ, Kajdasz ST, Christie RH, Carter C, Games D, Seubert P, Schenk D, Hyman BT (2001) Imaging of amyloid-beta deposits in brains of living mice permits direct observation of clearance of plaques with immunotherapy. Nat Med 7(3):369–372. doi:10.1038/85525, pii: 85525

57. Gessner JE, Heiken H, Tamm A, Schmidt RE (1998) The IgG Fc receptor family. Ann Hematol 76(6):231–248

58. Bard F, Cannon C, Barbour R, Burke RL, Games D, Grajeda H, Guido T, Hu K, Huang J, Johnson-Wood K, Khan K, Kholodenko D, Lee M, Lieburg I, Motter R, Nguyen M, Soriano F, Vasquez N, Weiss K, Welch B, Seubert P, Schenk D, Yednock T (2000) Peripherally administered antibodies against amyloid beta-peptide enter the central nervous system and reduce pathology in a mouse model of Alzheimer disease. Nat Med 6(8):916–919. doi:10.1038/78682

59. Serrano-Pozo A, Muzikansky A, Gomez-Isla T, Growdon JH, Betensky RA, Frosch MP, Hyman BT (2013) Differential relationships of reactive astrocytes and microglia to fibrillar amyloid deposits in Alzheimer disease. J Neuropathol Exp Neurol 72(6):462–471. doi:10.1097/NEN.0b013e3182933788

60. Wilcock DM, Munireddy SK, Rosenthal A, Ugen KE, Gordon MN, Morgan D (2004) Microglial activation facilitates Abeta plaque removal following intracranial anti-Abeta antibody administration. Neurobiol Dis 15(1):11–20, doi:S0969996103001955 [pii]

61. Dodart JC, Bales KR, Gannon KS, Greene SJ, DeMattos RB, Mathis C, DeLong CA, Wu S, Wu X, Holtzman DM, Paul SM (2002) Immunization reverses memory deficits without reducing brain Abeta burden in Alzheimer's disease model. Nat Neurosci 5(5):452–457. doi:10.1038/nn842, pii: nn842

62. DeMattos RB, Bales KR, Cummins DJ, Dodart JC, Paul SM, Holtzman DM (2001) Peripheral anti-A beta antibody alters CNS and plasma A beta clearance and decreases brain A beta burden in a mouse model of Alzheimer's disease. Proc Natl Acad Sci U S A 98(15):8850–8855. doi:10.1073/pnas.151261398, pii: 151261398

63. DeMattos RB, Bales KR, Cummins DJ, Paul SM, Holtzman DM (2002) Brain to plasma amyloid-beta efflux: a measure of brain amyloid burden in a mouse model of Alzheimer's disease. Science 295(5563):2264–2267. doi:10.1126/science.1067568, pii: 295/5563/2264

64. Yamada K, Yabuki C, Seubert P, Schenk D, Hori Y, Ohtsuki S, Terasaki T, Hashimoto T, Iwatsubo T (2009) Abeta immunotherapy: intracerebral sequestration of Abeta by an anti-Abeta monoclonal antibody 266 with high affinity to soluble Abeta. J Neurosci 29(36):11393–11398. doi:10.1523/JNEUROSCI.2021-09.2009, pii: 29/36/11393

65. Abbott NJ (2004) Evidence for bulk flow of brain interstitial fluid: significance for physiology and pathology. Neurochem Int 45(4):545–552. doi:10.1016/j.neuint.2003.11.006, pii: S0197018603002675

66. Iliff JJ, Wang M, Liao Y, Plogg BA, Peng W, Gundersen GA, Benveniste H, Vates GE, Deane R, Goldman SA, Nagelhus EA, Nedergaard M (2012) A paravascular pathway facilitates CSF flow through the brain parenchyma and the clearance of interstitial solutes, including amyloid beta. Sci Transl Med 4(147):147ra111. doi:10.1126/scitranslmed.3003748, pii: 4/147/147ra111

Chapter 10

Immunotherapy on Experimental Models for Huntington's Disease

Anne Messer

Abstract

The misfolding mutant Huntingtin protein (HTT) has been identified as the primary trigger of dysregulation and degeneration in Huntington's disease (HD). In order to counteract the abnormal protein–protein interactions and aggregation that characterize this and related protein misfolding diseases, antibody fragments that bind near the pathogenic region have been identified and characterized, and then engineered for improved affinity, intracellular solubility, and bispecific function. HD is a paradigm disease for misfolding proteins, since the readouts are exceptionally robust in cell and animal models. Candidate antibody fragments include single-chain Fv (scFv) and single domain antibodies (dAb, VL, VH). They have been selected from phage display libraries, or cloned from monoclonal antibodies of known specificity for the HTT Exon1 targets.

Preclinical immunotherapies have been tested with gene delivery via transgenes, or delivered using AAV or lentiviral gene therapy vectors. These intrabodies can strongly affect the HD phenotype across a range of epitopes and model systems. Given that individuals with HD can be identified genetically in a premanifest stage of disease, the potential for immunotherapeutic interventions is very promising.

Key words Trinucleotide repeats, Polyglutamine expansion, Fibrillar aggregates, Single-chain Fv (scFv)

1 Introduction

Huntington's disease (HD) is an autosomal dominant neuropsychiatric disorder, caused by expansion of a trinucleotide CAG repeat in the DNA, encoding polyglutamine (polyQ.) This results in a mutant protein, huntingtin (HTT), with abnormally long polyQ tracts that misfold and interact abnormally. Age of onset is inversely related to repeat size, with polyQ > 36 generally leading to adult onset between ages 35–55, while polyQ > 60 can show juvenile onset. The adult onset disease is characterized clinically by a movement disorder that is largely chorea, with personality changes that can mimic schizophrenia or psychosis manifesting either before or after the onset of motor problems. The juvenile motor disorder tends to be more rigid-akinetic, and the psychiatric

Martin Ingelsson and Lars Lannfelt (eds.), *Immunotherapy and Biomarkers in Neurodegenerative Disorders*, Methods in Pharmacology and Toxicology, DOI 10.1007/978-1-4939-3560-4_10, © Springer Science+Business Media New York 2016

component shows a higher incidence of dementia and loss of executive function. Neuropathologically, the symptoms are mirrored in the brain regions that can be identified as abnormal on MRI, and later *postmortem*. The adult onset form shows severe cell loss in the basal ganglia with additional cortical pathology, while juvenile HD affects cortex more widely, and can also involve the cerebellum. The HTT protein is extremely large (>3000 amino acids); however, the pathogenic species appears to primarily involve an N-terminal fragment, which facilitates modeling.

HD is a paradigm disease, having been among the first genes mapped by the Human Genome Project, and the second of what are now 14 known genetic diseases caused by expansion of CAG repeats in the coding region [1]. Given that severity is inversely related to repeat size, and that the truncated HTT Exon1 can trigger pathogenesis, it has been possible to model the disorder on a compressed timescale by utilizing constructs in which the CAG repeat size is >70. The most prevalent models have included cultured cells, yeast, *C. elegans*, *Drosophila*, and transgenic mice. More recently, rats, sheep, and non-human primates have also been reported. The robust readouts that are possible in these models allow for efficient testing of immunotherapies. A combination of human studies and these models has clarified that the triggering primary defect in HD is an intracellular misfolding protein that can lead to transcriptional dysregulation in the nucleus, mitochondrial and transport defects in the cytoplasm, and increases in a range of cellular stress pathways [2].

Immunotherapy could include both active vaccination, and passive delivery of systemic antibodies or antibody fragments delivered as proteins or genes. Systemic approaches have the appeal that the HTT mutant gene is expressed ubiquitously, and it may be necessary to correct peripheral as well as CNS sites. However, the greatest sites of damage are within the brain, which has been the strongest initial target. Approaches utilizing intracellular antibody fragments, known as intrabodies, have the potential to target a very early step in intracellular pathogenesis. Intrabodies can alter the kinetics of misfolding and turnover of both mutant and partnered complexes; reduce access of the misfolded HTT species to partner proteins; and, independently or via molecular fusions, alter the subcellular localization of pathogenic protein (Fig. 1). Intrabodies can also be used for target validation and rational drug design. This chapter first describes the models that are available for HD preclinical testing, followed by a review of the current status of intrabody studies that target the CNS using delivery of antibody fragments as genes. Active vaccination and future protein delivery strategies are also noted briefly.

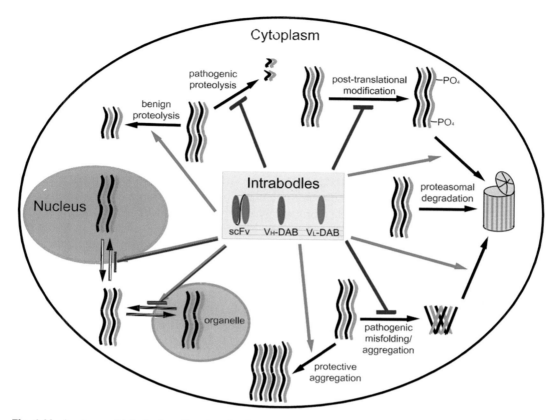

Fig. 1 Mechanisms of intrabody action. Intrabodies may alter target proteins through one or a combination of a variety of actions. Depicted here are several of the more likely possible mechanisms, and steps at which intervention with intrabodies could block a pathogenic cascade. *Black arrows* indicate transitions and modifications of a protein, including misfolding, proteolytic processing, proteasomal degradation, posttranslational modification, and transport between organelles and subcellular compartments. *Green arrows* indicate pathways where stimulation by intrabodies could be therapeutic. *Red perpendicular lines* indicate stages where inhibitory intrabodies could be useful. Intrabodies may be beneficial by stimulating or inhibiting protein transport between subcellular compartments depending on the compartment involved, as depicted by the *dual green/red arrows*. Additionally, several of the protein modifications such as proteasomal degradation, here depicted in the cytoplasm, may occur within organelles such as the nucleus, so intrabody targeting to subcellular compartments to alter protein modifications could also be favorable. Figure reprinted with permission from: Miller TW, Messer A (2006) Gene therapy for CNS diseases using intrabodies. In: Michael G. Kaplitt and Matthew During (eds) *Gene therapy in the brain*. Elsevier, pp 133–149

2   HD Models for Testing

The identification of the gene and its truncated pathogenic product has allowed the creation of cellular and animal models of the disease, which are critical for therapeutic testing. Since severity tracks with repeat number, it is also possible to accelerate the process tremendously by using very large numbers of repeats, and including only HTTExon1. Very early and severe HD does exist clinically; therefore, models using long repeats are not simply evaluating artifactual processes. Longer repeats also appear to be generated somatically during aging [3].

In situ HD models have been created by transfecting cultured cell lines (neuronal and non-neuronal) with HTTExon1-polyQ-GFP. Over 48–72 h, these models show length-dependent formation of intensely fluorescent SDS-insoluble aggregates that can be assessed semi-quantitatively [4]. A temperature-sensitive, conditionally immortalized rat embryonic striatal cell line, ST14A, developed by the Cattaneo group, has proved most valuable due to high transfection efficiency and some neuronal phenotypes [5]. Transfectability is particularly important when co-transfecting with HTTExon1, along with one or more antibody-based test reagents. Readouts are robust [6, 7]. Organotypic slice cultures can also be used, with delivery of particles containing multiple genes, although their consistency tends to be lower, due to the difficulty of perfectly replicating gene delivery and conditions [8].

Candidate intrabodies can be efficiently delivered as transgenes into invertebrate models of HD. Disease progression is rapid, and testing for combinatorial therapies with small molecule drugs is facilitated in these models. *Drosophila* lack an endogenous gene containing HTTExon1, allowing an HTTExon1 transgene to be presented on a null background, with either specific or pan-neuronal promoter systems. The UAS-HTT-exon-1-Q93 model develops through the larval stages, but exhibits reduced eclosion rates, an adult life span shortened to ~6–9 days in the flies that do hatch, and neurodegeneration observed by progressive loss of the photoreceptor cells of the eye in the HD fly [9]. This model allowed the first in vivo demonstration of anti-HTT intrabody correction of phenotype.

Transgenic mice have been used very extensively, and available mouse models, phenotypes, advantage and disadvantages have been recently reviewed [2]. Transgenic fragment models, including the R6 transgenic lines [10], are the most common for intrabody testing, since there is onset of symptoms in 6–12 weeks, and morbidity in 12–30 weeks for three of them. However, studies of delivery to full-length models based on the human MHTT expressed from yeast or bacterial artificial chromosomes, such as YAC128 and BAC97 [11–13] or knock-in, e.g., [14, 15], are also very valuable, despite a lengthy time course.

3 Anti-HD Intrabodies

In order to counteract the primary effects of the misfolding mutant protein fragment, the most promising approaches to date have utilized single-chain Fvs (scFvs) and single-domain (Dabs or nanobodies). Peptide antigens on both the N-terminal and C-terminal regions in close proximity to the misfolding polyQ have been used in selections from phage and yeast display libraries, or the relevant binding sites have been cloned from mouse monoclonal antibodies. The diagram below shows the selection targets for constructs that have been tested in situ and in vivo as immunotherapeutics.

C4		Happ 1&3	EM48

MATLEKLMKAFESLKSFQQQQQQQ(n)PPPPPPPPPPPQLPQPPPQAQPLLPQPQPPPPPPPPPPPGPAVAEEPLHRPK

VL12.3	MW1&2	MW7		MW7

3.1 Anti-N17 Intrabodies and Their Effects

3.1.1 C4 scFv

The first anti-HTT intrabody, C4 scFv, was selected from a naïve human spleen scFv phage-display library by panning in solution with a peptide of the N-terminal amino acid residues 1–17 of HTT [4]. Although many scFv fragments fold poorly in the reducing environment of the cytoplasm, this construct displayed excellent intracellular folding properties, which in retrospect is likely due to its negative charge at neutral pH [16]. In vitro affinity is high (ca. 8 nM), and this construct can counteract in situ length-dependent mHTT Exon1 aggregation and toxicity in several cell lines, as well as organotypic slice cultures [4, 6, 8, 17]. Critically, this intrabody preferentially binds soluble mHTT Exon1 fragments, with much weaker affinity for endogenous full length HTT [17, 18]. This should enhance its long-term safety profile, given that conditional deletion of wild-type HTT in forebrain neurons of transgenic mice elicited a progressive neurodegeneration [19]. C4 scFv has been tested in vivo in both *Drosophila* and mouse models of HD.

C4 scFv Correction of the HD *Drosophila* Phenotypes

The C4 scFv gene was expressed in flies using the UAS-GAL4 system, so that crossing the *elav*-GAL4 flies to those harboring both the UAS- C4 scFv and UAS-*HTT* exon 1 gave pan-neuronal co-expression. Intrabody expression corrected eclosion rates from 23 % up to 100 %, extended adult life span by 30 %, and slowed both neurodegeneration and aggregation [18]. However, flies still died prematurely, with adults building up aggregates and evidence of neurodegeneration. We therefore tested several combinatorial approaches to improve the phenotype. Small molecules that show mild systemic correction have the potential to complement and enhance the effects of intrabodies. The transgenic *Drosophhila* model has the potential for rapid screening of this process. Complex combinatorial effects were elicited by treating intrabody-expressing HD flies with cystamine at different stages of the life cycle [20]. An additional compound which showed promising preliminary results in flies was nicotinamide. This was moved directly into mice for small molecule testing, where it improved motor deficits and upregulated PGC-1alpha and BDNF gene expression in HDR6/1 mice [21]. The doses used did not, however, appear to confer long-term neuroprotection. Further studies will be required to establish the extent to which potential enhancements are in the direct intrabody functional pathways vs. parallel, complementary pathways.

Drospohila intrabody experiments have provided insight into the protective effects of anti-HTT Exon1 constructs, with a differentiation of neuroprotection vs. longevity. Even with pan-neuronal expression of mHTT and intrabody driven by the same promoters, rescue of life span can diverge from effects on individual neurons. The small molecule complementation of the intrabody effects provides additional information on classes of therapies that may be worthwhile to use in combination in the clinic.

C4 scFv in Mouse Models

An assessment of mammalian brain efficacy and safety of C4 scFv was tested, using adeno-associated viral vectors (AAV2/1) for intrastriatal delivery of C4 scFv intrabody genes into inbred B6. HDR6/1 mice. Quantitatively, both the size and number of HTT aggregates were significantly reduced at early to middle stages of disease [22]. Confocal imaging with an anti-HA antibody, used to identify the presence of intrabody, confirmed that most transduced cells lack HTT aggregates initially. However, with time, aggregates built up again. We hypothesize that the kinetics of aggregation are such that a small fraction of the mutant protein can misfold during the time that the intrabody is dissociated from its target, and that over a period of months this "escaped" fibrillar species becomes insoluble and resistant to further intrabody correction. A bifunctional fusion construct that can immediately increase the turnover of bound protein is one approach to solving this problem, as described below. Vector spread in these initial experiments was also suboptimal. Newer delivery vectors, and combinatorial therapies based on the fly data, are being used to follow up on these partial corrections. Nanobodies with extremely high affinity are also being considered.

3.1.2   VL12.3

A second intrabody to the region N-terminal to the polyQ was selected from a non-immune human yeast surface display library, using HTT AA1-20 rather than AA1-17 as a target. An scFv intrabody was selected, shown to have full binding activity with only the light chain, and further engineered as a variable light chain only single-domain intrabody (V_L). To enhance biological functionality in the cytoplasm, the V_L intrabody was then engineered to fold in the reducing environment of the cell via a series of substitutions of cysteine with hydrophobic residues, followed by additional rounds of affinity maturation. This intrabody could correct HD phenotype in cell culture models at a lower dose than C4 scFv [23, 24]. Although initial testing in an HD *Drosophila* model was disappointing, the powerful in situ data justified testing in vivo in mouse models.

Southwell et al. delivered VL12.3 using AAV in both the R6/2 transgenic mice, and a model made by injecting mHTT Exon 1 into striatum using a lentivirus. In the latter model, with very high expression of mHTTExon 1, and co-administration of the toxic protein and its binder, VL12.3 improved behavior and neuropathology [25]. However, VL12.3 binding appears to block cytoplasmic retention of HTT resulting in higher levels of antigen-antibody complex in the nucleus of transduced cells [26], This may explain the modest increase in toxicity in the HDR6/2 mouse model [25]. Because VL12.3 causes nuclear retention of mHTT, it may need to be delivered prior to the onset of aggregation of mHTT exon 1 fragments to have a therapeutic effect.

3.1.3 Comparing the Two Anti-N1-17 Intrabodies

The difference in the in vivo efficacy of the two anti-N-term antibody fragments offers an opportunity to fine-tune our concept of epitope dominance, antigen choice, subcellular localization of antigen-antibody complex, and target validation. C4 scFv was selected in solution against the highly-conserved AA1-17, and increases cytoplasmic retention of HTTExon1, reducing toxicity [27]. This differs from the in vivo nuclear localization of VL12.3, which can be detrimental. Re-targeting fusion constructs may be necessary to improve efficacy in this case.

3.2 Intrabodies that Target HTT Exon 1 Regions C-Terminal to the PolyQ

3.2.1 Happ

The proline-rich region immediately C-terminal to the polyQ domain of HTT Exon 1 contains two pure polyproline (polyP) series, interrupted by a unique proline-rich stretch. If this domain is not included in Exon 1 fragments, aggregation is accelerated [28, 29]. The Patterson lab has investigated a series of intrabodies against this region C-terminal to the polyQ. The first generation was an scFv cloned from the variable domains of the monoclonal antibody MW7, which binds to the two polyP stretches [30]. scFv-MW7 has been shown to reduce mHTT-induced aggregation and enhance survival in an HEK293 culture model of HD [31]. Intracellular solubility may have been limiting, and this intrabody has the potential to bind other proteins containing a polyP stretch. Additional anti-proline-rich domain intrabodies (Happ 1 and Happ 3) were selected from a non-immune human recombinant scFv phage library [26]. Similar to VL12.3, these Happ intrabodies bound via a single light-chain domain. Doses to prevent aggregation and toxicity were effective at a 2:1 ratio of intrabody to mHTT Exon 1-103Q for Happ1 vs. a 4:1 ratio for scFv-MW7 [26]. All three intrabodies accelerated the clearance of this very rapidly-aggregating mHTTExon1 in HEK293 cells, presumably by allowing the bound target to remain soluble and therefore subject to normal turnover mechanisms [26]. It appears that the mechanism of Happ1- induced clearance of mHTT is due to enhanced calpain cleavage of the first 15AA of mHTT followed by lysosomal degradation [32].

Intrastriatal AAV delivery of Happ1 was found to be beneficial in a variety of in vivo assays in diverse mouse models, including an acute unilateral lentiviral model; and R6/2, N171-82Q, YAC128, and BACHD transgenic HD mouse lines [25]. In all five mouse models, intrastriatal AAV delivery of Happ1 showed improvement of the neuropathology, as well as correction of a variety of motor and cognitive phenotypes [25, 32]. The N171-82Q model also showed increased body weight and a 30 % increased life span. It would be extremely interesting to combine these treatments with intrabodies targeting the N-terminal region of HTTExon1, and/or combinatorial therapies with small molecules.

3.2.2   EM48 scFv

mEM48, a mouse monoclonal antibody that recognizes a human-specific epitope in the C-terminus of HTT Exon 1, is a valuable immunocytochemical reagent for following aggregated protein in mice expressing human HTT [33]. When cloned as an scFv and expressed as an intrabody, scFvEM48 suppressed the cytoplasmic, but not nuclear, toxicity of mHTTExon1 in HEK293 cells, possibly via increased ubiquitination and degradation of cytoplasmic mutant HTT [34]. Delivery into the striatum of transgenic N171-82Q HD using adenovirus, which primarily transduces glia, led to reduced neuropil aggregate formation, and motor deficits of N171-82Q during an 8- week test [34]. Longer testing periods, and delivery to other cell types, should be very interesting.

4   Multifunctional Engineered Constructs

4.1   Targeting for Degradation

A major problem that became evident from the fly and mouse in vivo data is that the protein is only prevented from misfolding during the time that it is actually bound to the intrabody. Aggregates therefore begin build up over weeks or months, even in the presence of high levels of the intrabody. To enhance the function of the bound C4 scFv intrabodies, we added a targeting signal to induce rapid turnover of bound HTTExon1. Proteins containing a PEST motif, an enriched region of amino acids Proline (P), Glutamic Acid (E), Serine (S), and Threonine (T), typically have a short half life, and are degraded by the proteasome [35]. Recently, our lab fused Mouse Ornithine Decarboxylase PEST motif to anti-N1-17 C4 scFv, leading to significant turnover of antigen, while not changing solubility of the intrabody [36]. It is important to note that C4 scFv maintains mHTT in a monomeric soluble conformation, which allows mHTT Exon 1 to enter the proteasome and undergo degradation. Aggregated mHTT fragments have been reported to be resistant to degradation by the proteasome [37], and fusion of the PEST motif to an *anti-fibrillar* scFv, 6E failed to enhance clearance of the already misfolded conformer of the mHTT protein. This underlines the role of the target antigen conformation for potential use of the intrabody-PEST approach. Levels of aggregated mHTT can also be reduced by induction of autophagic/lysosomal pathway of intracellular protein degradation [38–40]. Therefore, it may be possible to use a fusion construct similar to that employed by Bauer et al. to target intrabody-mHTT Exon1 complexes to the lysosome for degradation by chaperone-mediated autophagy [41]. However, if the charge of the protein becomes too positive, the intrabody fusion construct will become unstable in the cytoplasm [16]

4.2 Targeting for Protein and Systemic Delivery

All of the in vivo preclinical studies cited above utilized delivery of the antibody fragments as transgenes, either by direct intercrossing (*Drosophila*) or using gene therapy vectors and injecting intracranially (mice). A novel multifunctional construct that fused a conformation-specific anti-alpha-synuclein scFv with a carrier peptide derived from ApoB demonstrated correction of several phenotypic markers in a Parkinson's mouse model [42]. Given that these conformation-specific nanobodies can cross-react with HTT, and that there is evidence for extracellular aggregated HTT in human and mouse brains, this approach may have promise for HD as well [43].

5 Active Vaccination

The mutant HTT protein is expressed ubiquitously, and effects of the mutation are observed in many peripheral tissues, in addition to the brain. This includes immune dysfunction [44, 45], muscle changes [46], and diabetes [47], among others.

An active vaccination protocol has the potential to target these diverse effects, directly ameliorating non-neuronal components of the clinical syndrome, as well as possibly providing a beneficial feedback effect on the CNS phenotype. In an early proof of concept, DNA vaccination with HTTExon1-72Q-GFP was able to correct the glucose intolerance in aging HDR6/1 mice [13]. Recently, safety and immunogenicity for a broad series of peptide, protein, and DNA plasmid immunization protocols, have been tested using fragment (R6/1), and knock-in (zQ175) mouse models of HD. Critically, all tested protocols were safe, with no acute or long-term disease exacerbation. A combination of three non-overlapping KLH-conjugated *HTT* Exon1 coded peptides, conjugated to KLH gave the most robust responses, although an N586-82Q plasmid, delivered via gene gun, also showed significant ELISA responses (Ramsingh et al., Human Mol Gen, in press). Full efficacy trials should be conducted.

6   Conclusions and Future Directions

Harnessing the power of the immune system has great potential to rescue cellular function in HD. With the primary source of pathogenesis both within the brain and within neurons, the challenges are substantial, and the animal models are essential. There are several antibody Fv fragments that show significant correction when delivered as genes directly into the affected brain regions. Multifunctional fusions, similar to those already in use for cancer and toxin clearance, have shown efficacy in further enhancing intracellular clearance via the proteasome, and in systemic delivery in a related PD model. Further combinatorial therapies that utilize multiple antigenic targets, in addition of small molecules that counteract downstream pathogenic processes, and possible systemic active immunization, should greatly enhance the power of these immunotherapies.

Acknowledgments

We thank members of the Messer lab group, especially Drs. David Butler and Abigail Snyder-Keller, and Kevin Manley for helpful discussions of the manuscript. Work in the Messer lab was supported in part by grants from NIH/NINDS NS053912 and NS061257, and NSF REU #DBI1062963; Hereditary Disease Foundation, High Q Foundation/CHDI, Huntington's Disease Society of America, and the Michael J. Fox Foundation.

References

1. Wexler NS, Rose EA, Housman DE (1991) Molecular approaches to hereditary diseases of the nervous system: Huntington's disease as a paradigm. Annu Rev Neurosci 14:503–529

2. Crook ZR, Housman D (2011) Huntington's disease: can mice lead the way to treatment? Neuron 69(3):423–435

3. Gonitel R, Moffitt H, Sathasivam K, Woodman B, Detloff PJ, Faull RL et al (2008) DNA instability in postmitotic neurons. Proc Natl Acad Sci U S A 105(9):3467–3472

4. Lecerf JM, Shirley TL, Zhu Q, Kazantsev A, Amersdorfer P, Housman DE et al (2001) Human single-chain Fv intrabodies counteract in situ huntingtin aggregation in cellular models of Huntington's disease. Proc Natl Acad Sci U S A 98(8):4764–4769

5. Ehrlich ME, Conti L, Toselli M, Taglietti L, Fiorillo E, Taglietti V et al (2001) ST14A cells have properties of a medium-size spiny neuron. Exp Neurol 167(2):215–226

6. Kvam E, Nannenga BL, Wang MS, Jia Z, Sierks MR, Messer A (2009) Conformational targeting of fibrillar polyglutamine proteins in live cells escalates aggregation and cytotoxicity. PLoS One 4(5):e5727

7. Miller TW, Messer A (2005) Intrabody applications in neurological disorders: progress and future prospects. Mol Ther 12(3):394–401

8. Murphy RC, Messer A (2004) A single-chain Fv intrabody provides functional protection against the effects of mutant protein in an organotypic slice culture model of Huntington's disease. Brain Res Mol Brain Res 121(1-2):141–145

9. Steffan JS, Agrawal N, Pallos J, Rockabrand E, Trotman LC, Slepko N et al (2004) SUMO modification of Huntingtin and Huntington's disease pathology. Science 304(5667):100–104

10. Mangiarini L, Sathasivam K, Seller M, Cozens B, Harper A, Hetherington C et al (1996) Exon 1 of the HD gene with an expanded CAG repeat is sufficient to cause a progressive

neurological phenotype in transgenic mice. Cell 87(3):493–506

11. Gray M, Shirasaki DI, Cepeda C, Andre VM, Wilburn B, Lu XH et al (2008) Full-length human mutant huntingtin with a stable polyglutamine repeat can elicit progressive and selective neuropathogenesis in BACHD mice. J Neurosci 28(24):6182–6195

12. Slow EJ, van Raamsdonk J, Rogers D, Coleman SH, Graham RK, Deng Y et al (2003) Selective striatal neuronal loss in a YAC128 mouse model of Huntington disease. Hum Mol Genet 12(13):1555–1567

13. Miller TW, Shirley TL, Wolfgang WJ, Kang X, Messer A (2003) DNA vaccination against mutant huntingtin ameliorates the HDR6/2 diabetic phenotype. Mol Ther 7(5 Pt 1):572–579

14. Wheeler VC, Gutekunst CA, Vrbanac V, Lebel LA, Schilling G, Hersch S et al (2002) Early phenotypes that presage late-onset neurodegenerative disease allow testing of modifiers in Hdh CAG knock-in mice. Hum Mol Genet 11(6):633–640

15. Menalled LB, Sison JD, Dragatsis I, Zeitlin S, Chesselet MF (2003) Time course of early motor and neuropathological anomalies in a knock-in mouse model of Huntington's disease with 140 CAG repeats. J Comp Neurol 465(1):11–26

16. Kvam E, Sierks MR, Shoemaker CB, Messer A (2010) Physico-chemical determinants of soluble intrabody expression in mammalian cell cytoplasm. Protein Eng Des Sel 23(6):489–498

17. Miller TW, Zhou C, Gines S, MacDonald ME, Mazarakis ND, Bates GP et al (2005) A human single-chain Fv intrabody preferentially targets amino-terminal Huntingtin's fragments in striatal models of Huntington's disease. Neurobiol Dis 19(1-2):47–56

18. Wolfgang WJ, Miller TW, Webster JM, Huston JS, Thompson LM, Marsh JL et al (2005) Suppression of Huntington's disease pathology in Drosophila by human single-chain Fv antibodies. Proc Natl Acad Sci U S A 102(32):11563–11568

19. Dragatsis I, Levine MS, Zeitlin S (2000) Inactivation of Hdh in the brain and testis results in progressive neurodegeneration and sterility in mice. Nat Genet 26(3):300–306

20. Bortvedt SF, McLear JA, Messer A, Ahern-Rindell AJ, Wolfgang WJ (2010) Cystamine and intrabody co-treatment confers additional benefits in a fly model of Huntington's disease. Neurobiol Dis 40(1):130–134

21. Hathorn T, Snyder-Keller A, Messer A (2011) Nicotinamide improves motor deficits and upregulates PGC-1alpha and BDNF gene expression in a mouse model of Huntington's disease. Neurobiol Dis 41(1):43–50

22. Snyder-Keller A, McLear JA, Hathorn T, Messer A (2010) Early or late-stage anti-N-terminal Huntingtin intrabody gene therapy reduces pathological features in B6.HDR6/1 mice. J Neuropathol Exp Neurol 69(10):1078–1085

23. Colby DW, Garg P, Holden T, Chao G, Webster JM, Messer A et al (2004) Development of a human light chain variable domain (V(L)) intracellular antibody specific for the amino terminus of huntingtin via yeast surface display. J Mol Biol 342(3):901–912

24. Colby DW, Chu Y, Cassady JP, Duennwald M, Zazulak H, Webster JM et al (2004) Potent inhibition of huntingtin aggregation and cytotoxicity by a disulfide bond-free single-domain intracellular antibody. Proc Natl Acad Sci U S A 101(51):17616–17621

25. Southwell AL, Ko J, Patterson PH (2009) Intrabody gene therapy ameliorates motor, cognitive, and neuropathological symptoms in multiple mouse models of Huntington's disease. J Neurosci 29(43):13589–13602

26. Southwell AL, Khoshnan A, Dunn DE, Bugg CW, Lo DC, Patterson PH (2008) Intrabodies binding the proline-rich domains of mutant huntingtin increase its turnover and reduce neurotoxicity. J Neurosci 28(36):9013–9020

27. Butler DC, Snyder-Keller A, De Genst E, Messer A (2014) Differential nuclear localization of complexes may underlie in vivo intrabody efficacy in Huntington's disease. Protein Eng Des Sel 27(10):359–363

28. Rockabrand E, Slepko N, Pantalone A, Nukala VN, Kazantsev A, Marsh JL et al (2007) The first 17 amino acids of Huntingtin modulate its sub-cellular localization, aggregation and effects on calcium homeostasis. Hum Mol Genet 16(1):61–77

29. Qin ZH, Wang Y, Sapp E, Cuiffo B, Wanker E, Hayden MR et al (2004) Huntingtin bodies sequester vesicle-associated proteins by a polyproline-dependent interaction. J Neurosci 24(1):269–281

30. Ko J, Ou S, Patterson PH (2001) New anti-huntingtin monoclonal antibodies: implications for huntingtin conformation and its binding proteins. Brain Res Bull 56(3-4):319–329

31. Khoshnan A, Ko J, Patterson PH (2002) Effects of intracellular expression of anti-huntingtin antibodies of various specificities on mutant huntingtin aggregation and toxicity. Proc Natl Acad Sci U S A 99(2):1002–1007

32. Southwell AL, Bugg CW, Kaltenbach LS, Dunn D, Butland S, Weiss A et al (2011) Perturbation with intrabodies reveals that calpain cleavage is required for degradation of huntingtin exon 1. PLoS One 6(1):e16676

33. Smith DL, Portier R, Woodman B, Hockly E, Mahal A, Klunk WE et al (2001) Inhibition of polyglutamine aggregation in R6/2 HD brain slices-complex dose-response profiles. Neurobiol Dis 8(6):1017–1026

34. Wang CE, Zhou H, McGuire JR, Cerullo V, Lee B, Li SH et al (2008) Suppression of neuropil aggregates and neurological symptoms by an intracellular antibody implicates the cytoplasmic toxicity of mutant huntingtin. J Cell Biol 181(5):803–816

35. Rechsteiner M, Rogers SW (1996) PEST sequences and regulation by proteolysis. Trends Biochem Sci 21(7):267–271

36. Butler DC, Messer A (2011) Bifunctional anti-huntingtin proteasome-directed intrabodies mediate efficient degradation of mutant huntingtin exon 1 protein fragments. PLoS One 6(12):e29199

37. Verhoef LG, Lindsten K, Masucci MG, Dantuma NP (2002) Aggregate formation inhibits proteasomal degradation of polyglutamine proteins. Hum Mol Genet 11(22):2689–2700

38. Ravikumar B, Duden R, Rubinsztein DC (2002) Aggregate-prone proteins with polyglutamine and polyalanine expansions are degraded by autophagy. Hum Mol Genet 11(9):1107–1117

39. Rose C, Menzies FM, Renna M, Acevedo-Arozena A, Corrochano S, Sadiq O et al (2010) Rilmenidine attenuates toxicity of polyglutamine expansions in a mouse model of Huntington's disease. Hum Mol Genet 19(11):2144–2153

40. Sarkar S, Rubinsztein DC (2008) Huntington's disease: degradation of mutant huntingtin by autophagy. FEBS J 275(17):4263–4270

41. Bauer PO, Goswami A, Wong HK, Okuno M, Kurosawa M, Yamada M et al (2010) Harnessing chaperone-mediated autophagy for the selective degradation of mutant huntingtin protein. Nat Biotechnol 28(3):256–263

42. Spencer B, Emadi S, Desplats P, Eleuteri S, Michael S, Kosberg K et al (2014) ESCRT mediated uptake and degradation of brain targeted alpha-synuclein-single chain antibody attenuates neuronal degeneration in vivo. Mol Ther 22(10):1753–1767

43. Messer A (2014) Engineered antibody therapies coming of age for aging brains. Mol Ther 22(10):1725–1727

44. Kwan W, Trager U, Davalos D, Chou A, Bouchard J, Andre R et al (2012) Mutant huntingtin impairs immune cell migration in Huntington disease. J Clin Invest 122(12):4737–4747

45. Wild E, Magnusson A, Lahiri N, Krus U, Orth M, Tabrizi SJ et al (2011) Abnormal peripheral chemokine profile in Huntington's disease. PLoS Curr 3:RRN1231

46. Strand AD, Aragaki AK, Shaw D, Bird T, Holton J, Turner C et al (2005) Gene expression in Huntington's disease skeletal muscle: a potential biomarker. Hum Mol Genet 14(13):1863–1876

47. Wood NI, Goodman AO, van der Burg JM, Gazeau V, Brundin P, Bjorkqvist M et al (2008) Increased thirst and drinking in Huntington's disease and the R6/2 mouse. Brain Res Bull 76(1-2):70–79

Part III

Biomarkers for Neurodegenerative Disorders

Chapter 11

Cerebrospinal Fluid Biomarkers in Alzheimer's Disease

Henrik Zetterberg and Jonathan M. Schott

Abstract

Alzheimer's disease (AD) is a progressive neurodegenerative disease, which typically shows an initial predilection for brain regions involved in episodic memory consolidation before progressing to affect also other cognitive functions. Neuropathologically, the disease is characterised by accumulation of a 42-amino acid-long protein called amyloid β (Aβ42), as well as N-terminally truncated fragments thereof in extracellular senile plaques. In addition to senile plaques, there are intraneuronal inclusions of hyperphosphorylated tau protein in neurofibrillary tangles and neuroaxonal degeneration and loss. Clinical chemistry tests for these pathologies have been developed and applied to cerebrospinal fluid samples. Here, we review what these markers have taught us about the disease process in AD and how they can be used as diagnostic tests in clinical practice as well as inclusion criteria and outcome measures for clinical trials. We describe both how such analyses are currently performed in clinical chemistry laboratories and the ongoing efforts to standardise analysis between different sites. Finally, we are also providing an overview of new markers in various stages of development and implementation.

Key words Alzheimer's disease, Biomarkers, Cerebrospinal fluid, Plasma, Tau, Amyloid, Clinical trials, Clinical diagnosis

Abbreviations

AD	Alzheimer's disease
fAD	Familial AD
CJD	Creutzfeldt-Jakob disease
APP	Amyloid precursor protein
sAPPα	Soluble APP alpha
sAPPβ	Soluble APP beta
BACE1	Beta-site APP-cleaving enzyme
CNS	Central nervous system
CSF	Cerebrospinal fluid
T-tau	Total-tau
P-tau	Phospho-tau
Aβ42	Amyloid β-42
MCI	Mild cognitive impairment

Martin Ingelsson and Lars Lannfelt (eds.), *Immunotherapy and Biomarkers in Neurodegenerative Disorders*, Methods in Pharmacology and Toxicology, DOI 10.1007/978-1-4939-3560-4_11, © Springer Science+Business Media New York 2016

NFL   Neurofilament light
TGF-β   Transforming growth factor-β
TNF-α   Tumour necrosis factor α
IL-1β   Interleukin 1β
CCL2   C-C chemokine ligand 2
CV   Coefficient of variation
HIV   Human immunodeficiency virus
QC   Quality control
GCBS   Global Consortium for Biomarker Standardization
IFCC   International Federation of Clinical Chemistry and Laboratory Medicine
ELISA   Enzyme-linked immunosorbent assay

1   Introduction

In 1906, Alois Alzheimer described the clinical characteristics of a female patient in her 50s with a progressive memory disorder that eventually, and prematurely, ended her life [1]. The neuropathology was striking with three main features: (1) gross atrophy due to neuronal degeneration and loss, (2) extracellular argyrophilic accumulations called senile plaques, and (3) intraneuronal inclusions called neurofibrillary tangles [2]. In 1911, Emil Kraepelin named this condition Alzheimer's disease (AD) in his influential textbook on psychiatry. For many decades, AD was considered a rare brain disorder found in patients who developed dementia in middle age. However, during the 1960s, it was noted that many elderly who died demented actually displayed neuropathological changes similar to those of AD [3], and the term senile dementia of Alzheimer type was coined. Over time, the distinction between early-onset AD and senile dementia of the Alzheimer type faded out and AD was introduced as the common term for both entities [4].

In 1966, Roth and colleagues found a positive correlation between plaque counts and how demented the patient had been prior to death [5], which stimulated research on the molecular composition of the plaque. In 1984, Glenner and Wong managed to purify and partially sequence a protein derived from twisted β-pleated sheet fibrils in cerebrovascular amyloidosis of AD brains that reacted to antisera made against plaque-containing brain extracts [6]. They called the protein amyloid fibril protein β. The year after, Masters and Beyreuther established the presence of an approximately 40-amino acid-long protein, with a sequence similar to that Glenner and Wong had reported, in plaques from brains of patients with AD and Down's syndrome [7]. The protein, or peptide, was originally called the A4 protein because of its 4 kDa molecular weight. This term has now virtually disappeared in favour of amyloid β (Aβ).

It is now known that the predominant Aβ forms in senile plaques are Aβ4–42 (Aβ starting at amino acid 4 in the Aβ domain and ending at amino acid 42 after a stretch of hydrophobic amino acids making the protein self-adhesive), Aβ1–42, Aβ1–40 and pyro-glutamate-modified Aβ3–42 [8].

In 1986, data were published showing that an abnormally hyperphosphorylated form of tau protein is the main component of neurofibrillary tangles [9, 10]. Tau is a microtubule-binding axonal protein that promotes microtubule assembly and stability. Abnormal phosphorylation and truncation of tau may lead to disassembly of microtubules and impaired axonal transport with compromised neuronal function, which is believed to cause tau aggregation into paired helical filaments and neurofibrillary tangles [11].

2   Alzheimer's Disease: Key Molecules Involved

The identification of Aβ as the main component of plaques initiated a search for the gene from which it is coded. In 1987, 2 years after Aβ had been sequenced, the gene of its precursor protein (amyloid precursor protein, APP) was cloned, sequenced and localised to chromosome 21 [12, 13]. A gene-dose effect of the triplication of the *APP* gene in Down's syndrome (trisomy 21) is thought to explain the plaque pathology and cognitive deficits which typically occurs in Down's syndrome patients already in early adulthood. However, some studies have reported a similar frequency of pathology in mental retardation of other causes, for which there is not an extra *APP* gene [14].

APP is a type I transmembrane protein with one membrane-spanning domain and is expressed not only in the brain but also in other tissues. The secreted form of APP was soon found to be identical to an already known plasma antichymotrypsin protease involved in coagulation, nexin-2 [15]. The exact function of APP in the brain remains elusive, but the protein appears to be involved in several biological processes, such as brain development, synaptic plasticity and neuroprotection [16]. Mutations in the *APP* gene have been identified in some cases of familial AD (fAD) cases [17–19], all of which influence Aβ and promote a pro-amyloidogenic state. The enzymes responsible for amyloidogenic APP-processing (β- and γ-secretase) were subsequently identified and causative fAD mutations were found in the presenilin genes that encode the proteins that build up the active site of γ-secretase [20]. There is now convincing data suggesting that most fAD-causing presenilin mutations (of which there are at least 170) lead to γ-secretase dysfunction, so that relatively more Aβ42 is produced when dysfunctional γ-secretase fails to process amyloidogenic Aβ42 to less aggregation-prone Aβ37/38/39 variants [21], thus promoting brain amyloidosis. That mutations in both the substrate (APP) and one of the key enzymes (γ-secretase) can cause AD by promoting brain amyloidosis and that different preparations of Aβ are neurotoxic in in vitro and in vivo models [22] have fuelled the notion that Aβ accumulation actually drives the disease process in AD, and that tangle formation (tau pathology) and neurodegeneration are downstream events. This view was formalised in the amyloid cascade hypothesis of AD [23], which (with some minor modifications) remains the predominant hypothesis of AD pathogenesis [24]. More recent evidence for a central role of Aβ in the aetiology of AD was the identification that a rare *APP* mutation substituting amino acid 673 in APP from alanine to threonine (position 2 in the Aβ domain) and resulting in decreased β-secretase-mediated Aβ production decreases the risk of AD in an Icelandic cohort [25].

One common criticism against the hypothesis is that it is based primarily on mechanisms operating in fAD and it is not clear how relevant these are for sporadic AD, which (by definition) does not have autosomal dominant heritability, and includes the vast majority of patients diagnosed with AD. Specifically, it has been proposed that the cognitive decline may have more heterogeneous causes in late-onset AD compared to early-onset AD [26]. However, recent evidence has demonstrated that, unlike familial AD which occurs due to relative or absolute overproduction of pathological forms of Aβ, sporadic AD may be caused by a relative failure of clearance leading to accumulation of short forms of Aβ [27].

Genetic factors are important not only in fAD but also in sporadic AD. Twin studies suggest that 40–70 % of the risk of sporadic AD could be explained by genetic factors [28, 29]. The most important susceptibility gene for sporadic AD is the *APOE* ε4 gene variant, which accounts for about 50 % of the risk [30], but many more low-risk loci exist [31]. Genome-wide association studies have identified susceptibility genes linked to at least three molecular pathways that may be involved in AD pathogenesis: (1) endosomal vesicle recycling, (2) cholesterol metabolism and (3) the innate immune system [32]. Further, exome sequencing has identified a rare, heterozygous loss-of-function mutation in a microglia-regulating gene (*TREM2*) that renders microglia overactive to brain amyloidosis and increases the risk of clinical AD at least fourfold [33, 34]. It is not yet possible to relate these pathways to each other or to APP definitively, but some suggestions emerge from the literature, and they may all be targets for therapy.

As described above, and as supported by genetic and neuropathological data, the definitions of AD and old-age dementia have changed dramatically during the last century, with AD no longer considered a rare cause of early-onset dementia but a broad diagnosis including most patients with age-related dementia. However, despite this development there is a debate regarding the relationship between AD and normal aging, and the relative roles of the different pathological hallmarks of AD to clinical presentation of the disease. At the core of this debate are some facts that are difficult to reconcile, including that (1) a degree of brain atrophy is common in normal elderly subjects and is also seen in brain regions primarily associated with AD, including the hippocampus, albeit to a lesser extent than in AD [35]; (2) autopsy and biomarker studies suggest that around one-third of non-demented elderly have plaque pathology [36, 37]; (3) autopsy studies indicate that Aβ plaque pathology appears first in neocortical association areas and only later in the hippocampus [38]; (4) tau pathology may appear decades before plaque pathology in AD [39]; (5) the location and spread of tau pathology are more closely related to the cognitive loss in AD than the location and spread of Aβ pathology [40]; and (6) mutations in the *MAPT* gene, which encodes the tau protein, most often cause frontotemporal lobar degeneration and not AD (with some exceptions [41, 42]), while mutations in *APP* and *presenilin* genes cause AD rather than frontotemporal lobar degeneration.

3 CSF in Alzheimer's Disease

Cerebrospinal fluid (CSF) is located in the cerebral ventricles and also surrounds the brain and the spinal cord. It communicates freely with the brain interstitial fluid, and may thereby serve as a biochemical window into the brain. CSF investigations in AD were pioneered by Gottfries and colleagues in the late 1960s and early 1970s, who reported reduced CSF monoamine metabolite concentrations, suggesting a breakdown of these neurotransmitter systems in the deteriorating brain [43, 44], and elevated CSF lactate concentration as a sign of tissue hypoxia [45]. During the 1990s tests for proteins thought to reflect the core neuropathology of AD were developed. Established and candidate biomarkers are discussed below and a summary is given in Fig. 1.

3.1   CSF Aβ42

Initially, just after the identification of aggregation-prone Aβ proteins ending at amino acids 40 and 42 in senile plaques [6, 7, 46], the protein was thought to be an abnormal side product of APP metabolism invariably associated with AD. The natural secretion of Aβ from untransfected primary cells therefore came as a surprise [47]. Since then, it has been established that APP can enter at least three proteolytic clearance pathways: (1) amyloidogenic processing that primarily leads to production of Aβ42 and Aβ40 (but also some shorter, less aggregation-prone fragments) by successive β- and γ-secretase cleavages; (2) non-amyloidogenic processing that leads to production of sAPPα and possibly also a C-terminal fragment called p3 (this fragment should consist of Aβ17–40/42, but has been difficult to verify using modern techniques; it is possible that it is quickly degraded into shorter fragments); and (3) another non-amyloidogenic processing pathway involving concerted cleavages of APP by β- and α-secretase resulting in production of Aβ1–14/15/16 fragments at the expense of longer Aβ fragments [48].

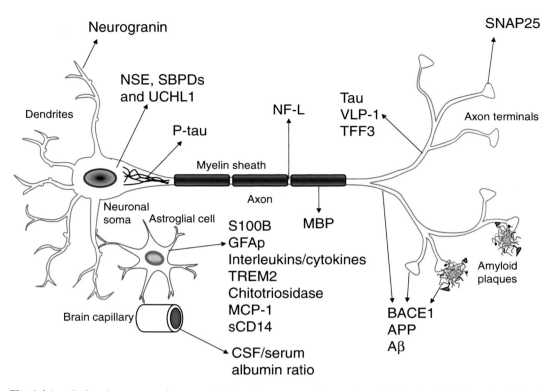

Fig. 1 A tangle-bearing neuronal soma with dendrites, axon and axon terminals is depicted. An astroglial cell, a blood vessel and senile plaques are also represented. Key biomarkers for different pathologies and cell compartments, discussed in detail in the text, are indicated

The first assay for CSF Aβ42 was published in 1995 [49]. Using this enzyme-linked immunosorbent assay (ELISA), AD patients were shown to have reduced levels of CSF Aβ42, a finding which has since been replicated and verified in hundreds of papers [50]. This reduction is thought to reflect Aβ42 sequestration in senile plaques in the brain, as evidenced by both autopsy and *in vivo* imaging studies [51–54]. In 1999, the first paper showing a reduction in CSF Aβ42 in patients with mild cognitive impairment (MCI) who later developed AD dementia was published [55]. Since then, numerous studies have verified that low CSF Aβ42 levels are highly predictive of future AD, both in MCI [56–59] and cognitively normal cohorts [60–62]. Causal mutations aside, CSF Aβ42 remains the earliest biomarker currently available in AD, and as a result CSF Aβ42 is now incorporated into new criteria for the diagnosis of AD, also in pre-dementia stages [63]. Low CSF Aβ42 concentrations in the absence of senile plaques have also been reported in neuroinflammatory conditions, e.g. bacterial meningitis [64], multiple sclerosis [65], human immunodeficiency virus (HIV)-associated dementia [66] and Lyme neuroborreliosis [67], and are often accompanied by biomarker evidence of a general reduction in APP metabolites, e.g. secreted forms of APP, which is not typical of AD [50].

Besides Aβ42, several other Aβ isoforms are present in CSF. The most abundant variant in CSF is Aβ40, which is relatively unchanged in AD. The ratio of CSF Aβ42 to Aβ40 has been suggested to have stronger diagnostic accuracy for AD compared to CSF Aβ42 alone [68]. There are also several other C- or N-terminally truncated Aβ isoforms in CSF, which may be altered in AD [69], also in the earliest clinical stages [70].

3.2 CSF T-tau

The first CSF total tau (T-tau) assay was published in 1993 [71]. This was a sandwich ELISA in which a monoclonal antibody against the mid-domain of tau was combined with a polyclonal anti-tau antiserum. Two years later, the first assay based on three mid-region monoclonal antibodies, which recognises all tau isoforms irrespective of phosphorylation state, was published [72]. This assay is today known as the "Innogenetics assay". Using this assay, AD patients were shown to have clearly elevated T-tau levels [71, 72], a finding that has been replicated in hundreds of papers, using several different assays, in many different clinical contexts [50]. It has been shown that CSF T-tau levels correlate with imaging measures of hippocampal atrophy [73] and grey matter degeneration [74], findings in keeping with the known high expression of tau in thin unmyelinated axons of the cortex [75]. In response to acute brain injury, CSF T-tau levels are dynamic; they increase during the first few days following injury and stay elevated for a few weeks until they normalise [76, 77]. This has led to the view that elevated CSF T-tau levels reflect ongoing axonal degeneration, which in turn may indicate disease activity. Indeed, CSF T-tau predicts the rapidity of the clinical course in AD; the higher the levels, the more rapid the clinical disease progression [78]. Accordingly, in severe and rapid neurodegeneration, e.g. as in Creutzfeldt-Jakob disease (CJD), CSF T-tau elevations orders of magnitude higher than in typical AD are seen [79].

Two recent discoveries have made the tau biomarker field more complex. These include (1) the finding that tau secretion from cultured cells [80] and mouse neurons [81] may be stimulated by Aβ in the absence of neuronal death [81]; and (2) that most of the tau in CSF seems to be fragmented [82].

Tau secretion in the absence of neurodegeneration is not unexpected as it has been known for decades that tau is present in CSF also of healthy individuals [83]. Nonetheless this raises some important issues from a practical perspective as it confirms that tau elevation cannot simply be considered a surrogate marker of neurodegeneration. Moreover, the mechanism of tau elevation in AD may well be at least partially independent of neuronal death. The latter would be consistent with tau changes seen in other forms of brain injury and the observation of intraneuronal increase in tau expression following acute experimental brain injury in animals [84].

The finding that most CSF tau seems to be in fragmented forms is consistent with well-established evidence that endogenous tau fragments are found in tangles [85]. It may also explain why it has been important to have capture and detection antibodies located closely to each other in T-tau assays, and why combinations of distally located N- and C-terminal antibodies do not work [82]. The clinical significance of these fragments is not known and it remains challenging to accomplish a reliable quantification, including determination of reference samples.

3.3 CSF P-tau

The first CSF assay for phosphorylated tau (P-tau), the form of tau that is believed to show the closest association with neurofibrillary tangle load, was published in 1995 [72]. Since then, a variety of P-tau assays measuring different forms of phosphorylated tau proteins have been developed [86]. Broadly speaking, these assays correlate well with one another, and show similar findings in AD [86]. CSF P-tau levels correlate with neurofibrillary tangle pathology in AD [54, 87], but a major outstanding research question is why other tauopathies, including some forms of frontotemporal lobar degeneration and progressive supranuclear palsy, do not show P-tau elevation, at least not as systematically as seen in AD. It is possible that these disorders show disease-specific tau phosphorylation, or that tau is processed or truncated in a way that is not recognised by available assays. However, determining the relative specificity of P-tau elevation and AD has considerable advantages in differentiating different neurodegenerative diseases. For example, the ratio of T-tau to P-tau is a quite specific test for CJD [88, 89]. There are at present only three conditions in addition to AD in which elevated CSF P-tau levels have been reported: (1) term and preterm newborns, possibly reflecting physiological tau phosphorylation in brain development [90], (2) herpes encephalitis [91] and (3) superficial CNS siderosis [92, 93]. For obvious reasons, these conditions are not often considered as differential diagnoses for AD. Nevertheless, they may shed light on mechanisms behind CSF P-tau increase, as may emerging data on tau phosphorylation in hibernating squirrels [94] and hamsters [95], as well as in anaesthesia [96], by pointing to physiological and pathological conditions in which tau phosphorylation occurs, potentially as a consequence of reduced neuronal activity.

3.4 Diagnostic Performance of Combined CSF T-tau, P-tau and Aβ42 Tests

Multiple studies have investigated the diagnostic accuracy of combined CSF tests for T-tau, P-tau and Aβ42 [83]. These studies collectively show a diagnostic accuracy of 80–90% in cross-sectional studies aiming to distinguish AD from controls and in longitudinal studies aiming to determine which MCI patients that will develop AD [83]. Higher diagnostic performance is typically seen in single-centre studies [56, 97], whereas large multicentre studies tend to report slightly lower sensitivities and specificities [58, 98].

The association of elevated T-tau and P-tau and reduced Aβ42 with AD neuropathology has been validated in autopsy [57] and brain biopsy [54] studies. To date, the CSF Aβ42, T-tau and P-tau do not seem to markedly differ between patients with typical, amnestic AD and posterior cortical atrophy, a rarer variant of AD (where visuospatial dysfunction dominates [99, 100]. In addition, the influence of AD phenotype on CSF biomarkers has been less thoroughly explored in other clinical variants of AD, including AD presenting with logopenic primary progressive aphasia [101] or corticobasal degeneration [102].

3.5 Longitudinal Changes in CSF AD Biomarkers

Recent data show that it is possible to identify longitudinal changes in CSF Aβ42, T-tau and P-tau in cognitively healthy controls followed over several years [103–105], although most studies (with exceptions [103]) show that CSF AD biomarkers are essentially stable once patients have converted to AD [70, 106, 107]. This biomarker stability (at least during short-term follow-up) may be useful in clinical trials to help identify effects of interventions on the intended biological target, such as altered Aβ metabolism in response to an anti-Aβ treatment. One of the relatively few longitudinal studies of cognitively normal individuals where repeated lumbar punctures were made suggests that Aβ42 and tau changes occur in parallel and predict incident cognitive symptoms better than absolute baseline levels [105]. CSF measurements may track trajectories of specific Aβ and APP metabolites [108–111], as well as downstream effects, such as reduced axonal degeneration in response to a disease-modifying drug [112, 113].

4 Candidate AD Biomarkers and Markers of Other Pathologies

As explained above, despite sharing the same core pathology, AD does show heterogeneity both in terms of phenotype and pathological co-morbidities. Thus, aetiologically, phenotypically and pathologically, AD in an 85-year-old person with type II diabetes, hypertension and sleep apnoea is likely to show considerable differences compared to a patient with AD in an otherwise healthy 60-year-old with a positive family history. There are also several other conditions that may contribute to AD-like cerebral dysfunction [114]. A recent clinicopathologic study reported that dementia with Lewy bodies, cerebrovascular disease, frontotemporal lobar degeneration and hippocampal sclerosis is the most prevalent AD mimics [115]. Interestingly, the clinical phenotype can vary considerably although the same brain plaque and tangle pathology can be seen, as demonstrated for the non-amnestic disease AD variants including posterior cortical atrophy, and logopenic or progressive non-fluent aphasia [114]. A vision in the biomarker research field is to develop biomarkers that can not only determine the core underlying pathologies in AD, but could also be used as adjuncts to neuroimaging and neuropsychology measures in order to understand and predict the molecular basis of the phenotypic diversity seen for individual cases.

4.1 CSF BACE1

As described above, in the amyloidogenic pathway, Aβ is produced through proteolytic processing of APP by β- and γ-secretases. The major β-secretase in the brain is the β-site APP-cleaving enzyme 1 (BACE1) [116]. Increased BACE1 activity has been measured in postmortem samples from patients with AD [117]. The activity and concentration of BACE1 can also be measured in CSF, but the results have been conflicting. Holsinger et al. found an increase in the activity of CSF BACE1 in AD patients as well as in patients with other dementias [118, 119] compared to non-neurological controls. The activity of CSF BACE1 was also found to be elevated in patients with MCI who progressed to AD compared to subjects with MCI who remained stable or developed other forms of dementia [120]. Many studies, however, have failed to show any significant difference in BACE1 activity between MCI and AD patients compared to controls [121, 122], and one study suggested that CSF BACE1 activity may drop in advanced disease stages [123]. Altogether, the discrepant results of these studies suggest that the diagnostic value of BACE1 in AD is limited. However, the marker may still be valuable in certain circumstances, e.g. in clinical trials of putative BACE1 inhibitors.

4.2 CSF sAPPα/ sAPPβ

Theoretically, secreted forms of APP should be excellent fluid markers of amyloidogenic (sAPPβ) and non-amyloidogenic (sAPPα) APP processing. The proteins are readily measureable in CSF but several studies have failed to show any differences between AD patients and controls [97, 120, 124]. In the context of MCI, one study reported elevated CSF sAPPβ in patients with MCI compared with controls [124], and another study showed increased levels of CSF sAPPβ in MCI patients who progressed to AD compared to patients who remained stable [125]. Studies that grouped patients on the basis of CSF tau and Aβ markers into those with and without biomarker support for AD found elevated levels of CSF sAPPα and sAPPβ in the group displaying AD-like changes [126–128]. However, in the absence of a cognitively normal control group these studies did not take into account that the differences might have been driven by lower levels of sAPPα and sAPPβ among non-AD cases, and not increase in AD. Similarly to BACE1, the results of studies exploring CSF sAPPα and sAPPβ as potential biomarkers for AD have been sufficiently inconsistent and are still not useful in clinical practice. However, these biomarkers may be valuable in clinical trials to monitor the effect of novel therapies targeting APP metabolism.

4.3 Aβ Oligomers

The correlation between amyloid plaque cerebral load and disease severity is poor [129]. To reconcile this observation with the amyloid cascade hypothesis, it has been suggested that most of the presumed Aβ toxicity is exerted by soluble portions of Aβ, while the plaques *per se* are relatively inert. Walsh et al. showed that soluble oligomers of Aβ inhibit hippocampal long-term potentiation in rats [130] and others have reported that they can lead to abnormal phosphorylation of tau as well as neuritic dystrophy [131–133]. Higher levels of oligomers have been shown in the brains of AD patients compared to controls [134, 135], but results from several studies trying to replicate these findings in CSF have been inconsistent. Some studies have found elevated CSF Aβ oligomer levels in patients with AD [136–140] or in cognitively normal older adults with an AD-like biomarker profile [141], while others have not found this relationship [134, 142]. A consistent problem when developing oligomer assays is the unreliable quantification due to their low concentration in CSF. Moreover, "oligomers" include species ranging from dimers to protofibrils and most studies to date are using methods that cannot distinguish between these various forms.

4.4 Blood-Brain Barrier Biomarkers

The best established biomarker so far for the integrity of the blood-brain barrier is CSF/serum albumin ratio. Typically, this ratio is normal in patients with pure AD [143], whereas patients with cerebral small vessel disease generally have increased CSF/serum albumin ratio [144]. The same finding is often present in Lyme disease (neuroborreliosis), where there typically also is an increased number of CSF monocytes and evidence of immunoglobulin production within the CNS [145]. Other less well-established blood-brain biomarkers in CSF include secretory Ca^{2+}-dependent phospholipase A2 activity [146] and antithrombin III [147]. More research is warranted in this field, especially to develop assays to differentiate between specific forms of blood-brain barrier dysfunction.

4.5 Additional Biomarkers for Neurodegeneration

CSF biomarker candidates, other than tau proteins, that may reflect AD-like neurodegeneration are visinin-like protein 1 (VLP-1), a neuronal protein which is elevated in AD patients and correlates with T-tau concentration [148], and trefoil factor 3 (TFF3), a gastrointestinal protein with unknown function in the CNS, which just emerged as a strong predictor of brain atrophy rates in the Alzheimer's Disease Neuroimaging Initiative [149].

An established biomarker for subcortical axonal degeneration, frequently seen in potential AD mimics, such as cerebral small vessel disease [150–152], frontotemporal lobar degeneration [153, 154] and HIV-associated dementia [155], is neurofilament light protein (NFL). NFL, as well as other members of the neurofilament group of proteins, acts as an integral part of the neural cytoskeleton, providing structural support for predominantly large-calibre myelinated axons.

Elevated CSF NFL levels indicate involvement of these axons in the disease process and can help differentiating pure AD from the conditions listed above as combined T-tau and NFL increases are common in mixed forms of AD and cerebrovascular disease. These mixed CSF findings are very common in unselected patients undergoing evaluation because of suspected neurodegenerative disease [156]. NFL is also a useful biomarker for damage severity in several other conditions characterised by white matter lesions and injury to subcortical brain regions such as amyotrophic lateral sclerosis [157], various CNS infections [91] and stroke [158].

4.6 Biomarkers for Inflammation, Oxidative Stress and Microglial Activation

Inflammation, oxidative stress and microglial activation in AD may be downstream phenomena of neurodegeneration, although recent genetic data suggest that they may well contribute to pathogenesis in susceptible individuals [33, 34]. Possible triggers are the accumulation of abnormal proteins (aggregated Aβ in the case of AD) and/or mediators released from dying cells. Such triggers may lead to overshoot inflammation in some individuals, e.g. carriers of a recently described loss-of-function mutation in the microglia-controlling triggering receptor expressed on myeloid cells-2 (*TREM2*) gene [33, 34], perhaps making them more likely to develop clinical AD in response to Aβ.

Many studies have examined potential biomarkers linked to inflammatory processes. Cytokines, such as interleukin 6, transforming growth factor (TGF)-β, tumour necrosis factor α (TNF-α) and interleukin 1β (IL-1β), have been measured in CSF of AD patients, but in one meta-analysis the only consistent finding was of increased CSF levels of TGF-β in AD compared with control groups [159]. Additional candidate inflammatory biomarkers for AD include the cytokine osteopontin, which was elevated in CSF from AD patients [160] and the TNF-α-induced pro-inflammatory agent lipocalin 2, which has been found at lower concentrations in CSF from MCI and AD patients compared with controls [161]. Another study found that CSF lipocalin 2, also known as neutrophil gelatinase-associated lipocalin, occurred at lower levels in AD and stable MCI patients compared with patients who had AD and vascular risk factors [162].

It should be noted that the biomarker literature is tainted by studies reporting CSF cytokine or interleukin concentrations that are below the analytical sensitivity of the employed assays (IL-1β is just one example), and that standard clinical chemistry tests for neuroinflammation, including CSF leukocyte count and general signs of IgG or IgM production within the CNS, are generally negative in AD and other primary neurodegenerative diseases [163]. Where the CSF shows cells or unmatched oligoclonal bands non-AD pathology should be considered and should motivate further investigation of the patient to exclude infections, multiple sclerosis, neuroinflammatory and conditions that may contribute to the cognitive symptoms [164].

Isoprostanes, in particular a subclass called F2-isoprostanes, are the most examined CSF biomarkers for oxidative stress. They are prostaglandin-like compounds produced by free radical-dependent peroxidation of arachidonic acid [165]. Studies report elevated F2-isoprostane levels in AD CSF [166–170] in a manner that appears to be downstream of Aβ pathology [171]. CSF isoprostanes correlate to clinical disease progression in the MCI and dementia stages of AD, especially in *APOE* ε4-carrying patients [172], and may serve as damage response markers. Pilot studies suggest that the levels of oxidative DNA damage repair products are elevated in CSF from mixed vascular and Alzheimer's dementia patients [173], and that reduced levels of mitochondrial DNA in CSF suggest depletion of mitochondria [174], which may reflect oxidative stress, but these studies await replication.

Neuroinflammation is tightly linked to activation of the inflammatory M1 phenotype of microglia, the macrophages of the brain. Chitotriosidase is an enzyme that is secreted by activated macrophages [175] and its plasma levels are increased in patients with the lysosomal storage disorder Gaucher's disease [176]. Increased CSF chitotriosidase activity has been found in AD patients compared with non-demented controls [177]. A glycoprotein that has great homology with chitotriosidase but lacks its enzymatic activity is YKL-40 [178]. YKL-40 is expressed in both microglia and astrocytes and elevated levels have been reported in both prodromal AD and cerebrovascular disease [179, 180].

Another microglial marker, the C-C chemokine receptor 2, is expressed on monocytes and one of its ligands, C-C chemokine ligand 2 (CCL2), that can be produced by microglia is important for the recruitment of monocytes in the CNS [181]. Higher CSF CCL2 levels have been associated with a faster cognitive decline in MCI patients who developed AD [182]. CCL2 levels in CSF were increased in AD patients compared with healthy controls [183, 184], as well as in the MCI stage of the disease [185]. However, one study failed to report any significant differences between AD patients and controls [186]. Another study found elevated CSF CCL2 levels in AD patients compared with controls, but there was an age-dependent increase in the biomarker level that may have affected the result [187]. Moreover, one study reported elevated levels of a soluble form of CD14 in the CSF from AD (and Parkinson's disease) patients compared with healthy controls [188]. CD14 is a surface protein, mainly expressed by macrophages. As a cofactor for toll-like receptors, CD14 is essential for the recognition of pathogens by the innate immune system of the brain. Another microglial biomarker that has been detected in CSF of AD patients is neopterin, a degradation product deriving from the purine nucleotide guanosine triphosphate. However, no significant differences between AD and controls have been seen to date [189].

Taken together, biomarker studies support involvement of low-grade neuroinflammation, oxidative stress and microglial activation in the AD process, but to date no single biomarker has emerged as being sufficiently robust to have clinical utility. Future longitudinal studies of healthy individuals will most likely help to determine what order these markers change in relation to plaque and tangle pathology and neurodegeneration in AD. A recent study found that CSF levels of several proteins possibly associated with microglia activity predicted longitudinal reduction of CSF Aβ42 in cognitively healthy subjects, suggesting involvement of inflammatory pathways early in the AD disease process [104].

4.7 Biomarkers for Synaptic Changes

Loss of synapses is highly correlated with decrease in neurocognitive function in AD patients [190]. Therefore, a biomarker that reflects this pathology has very significant potential both for diagnosis and prognosis. Synaptic proteins such as synaptotagmin, growth-associated protein 43, synaptosomal-associated protein 25, rab3a and neurogranin are abundant in brain tissue, but present at very low concentrations in CSF [191], thus presenting analytical challenges. Nevertheless, the dendritic protein neurogranin has been detected in CSF and elevated levels in AD dementia and prodromal AD have been observed using a semi-quantitative immunoblot method [192], as well as with ELISA-like methods [193–195]. More research is needed to determine the biomarker potential of synaptic proteins in the CSF. Recent breakthroughs in ultra-sensitive immunochemical techniques may help in this regard [196, 197].

4.8 Other Protein Inclusions

Alpha-synuclein is the major component of intra-neuronal Lewy bodies, which are characteristic of Parkinson's disease (PD) and dementia with Lewy bodies [198]. Alpha-synuclein pathology is sometimes found together with Aβ plaques and neurofibrillary tangles in AD [199] and experimental studies show that Aβ42 enhances aggregation of α-synuclein [200]. In PD and other synucleinopathies CSF α-synuclein levels are typically reduced [201, 202], whilst in AD and CJD, the levels are elevated and correlate to T-tau, suggesting that α-synuclein may also be a non-specific marker of neurodegeneration [202–205]. Importantly, α-synuclein is highly expressed in red blood cells, a reason why blood contamination during sample collection may further limit any diagnostic value [206, 207].

4.9 AD Biomarkers in Blood

Whilst the most successful body fluid for finding biomarkers for AD has undoubtedly been CSF, probably because of its proximity to the brain and the pathologic processes of interest, the identification of one or more blood-based biomarkers would be highly advantageous for routine clinical use. However, despite much research in this field there is still no established blood-based biomarker for AD. Brain-derived proteins occur in lower concentrations in blood than in CSF, at least partly because of the blood-brain barrier which limits the transport of substances between blood vessels and the brain parenchyma, additional problems being binding of proteins of interest to plasma proteins in the blood and protein degradation. Analyses of Aβ peptides in blood have mainly shown similar levels in AD patients and controls [208]. Recent approaches using techniques where several biomarkers are analyzed simultaneously have identified some other promising biomarkers [209, 210], but the results have so far been hard to replicate [211, 212].

5   CSF Biomarkers in Relation to the Latest Clinical Trials

The CSF biomarkers reviewed above play several important roles in clinical trials of disease-modifying drug candidates against AD. They may be used as inclusion criteria to verify that the included patients have the pathological changes against which the drug is targeted [83]. They may also be used as pharmacodynamic markers or markers of target engagement to test if the drug had the desired biochemical effect in patients on active treatment [213]. From a regulatory perspective, the use of CSF Aβ42 and tau proteins for clinical trials in AD has been qualified by the European Medicines Agency (EMA) [214]. The EMA released qualification opinions in April 2011 and February 2012 stating that a pathological signature based on low CSF Aβ42 and high T-tau levels in subjects with MCI was useful for identifying those at increased risk of AD dementia. Given the high sensitivity and moderate specificity, EMA concluded that this CSF signature was useful for the purpose of enriching clinical trial populations [214]. The Food and Drug Administration (FDA) has recently released a draft guidance on clinical trials in subjects in the pre-dementia stages of AD (http://www.fda.gov/downloads/Drugs/Guidance ComplianceRegulatoryInformation/Guidances/UCM338287. pdf). According to this guidance document, there is not enough evidence that biomarkers can be used to predict clinical benefit although they could be used to support disease modification in combination with a clinical outcome measure.

In the context of targeted immunotherapy trials directed against Aβ pathology, two large phase III clinical trials in AD have recently been concluded, using the monoclonal antibodies bapineuzumab and solanezumab. Bapineuzumab is a humanized monoclonal IgG1 antibody against the Aβ N-terminus (Aβ1–5), based on the murine antibody 3D6, and was intended to promote brain Aβ clearance by binding to aggregated Aβ [215]. Solanezumab, on the other hand, is a humanized version of the mouse monoclonal antibody m266, raised against Aβ13–28 [216, 217], has little or no affinity for the fibrillar form, but binds soluble Aβ [218]. In phase II studies bapineuzumab had no clinical efficacy [215], and in the phase III study, despite reduced CSF tau levels, the drug failed to reach its primary, cognitive outcomes [219]. However, it is important to note that biomarker evidence of AD pathology was not a prerequisite for study entry; and that of those for whom biomarker evidence of AD pathology was available, 38 % did not have evidence of underlying AD. In the phase III study, solanezumab also did not reach its primary clinical endpoints [220], but in subgroup analyses, there was a small reduction in clinical progression in those with mild AD, although this was not associated with a reduction in CSF tau levels [220]. As discussed elsewhere in this book, there are multiple potential explanations for the many phase III failures of anti-AD drug candidates. However, most experts agree that it will be very important to ascertain that patients included in future clinical trials indeed have the pathology against which the drug is designed. Further, future phase I and II trials may benefit from using current and novel biomarkers in an attempt to demonstrate robust target engagement before later stage studies are embarked upon.

6   Standardisation Efforts

The clinical utility of CSF tests for T-tau, P-tau and Aβ42 is clear and their importance for selecting patients in pre-dementia stages of AD for clinical trials of disease-modifying drug candidates is undisputed [221]. However, most of the commercially available assays for these biomarkers are still of research grade, and there is a lack of common calibrators or certified reference measurement systems that can be used for standardisation [222]. This leads to a risk of bias in the biomarker measurements across different assay platforms. A recognisable consequence of this is that optimal CSF Aβ42 cut points for differentiating AD patients from control individuals vary from 192 ng/L [57] to around 550 ng/L [56, 223], depending on the assay format. Furthermore, even when the same assay is used, variation in biomarker measurements between laboratories is high, as can be seen in multicentre comparisons of measurements, including the Alzheimer's Association QC Programme for CSF Biomarkers [224, 225]. This programme includes around 90 participants around the globe and shows that the inter-laboratory coefficients of variation (CVs) for commercially available tau and Aβ assays are between 20 and 30 %, whereas intra-laboratory studies show that CVs of <10 % should be feasible.

Important pre-analytical sources of variation for the most variable AD biomarker, Aβ42, are storage tube type (polypropylene tubes are recommended but different brands seem to show different analyte adsorption [226]); sample aliquot volume [227]; the number of tube transfers of the collected CSF [228]; and blood contamination [229]. Analytical sources of variation include the composition of the diluent buffer—low concentrations of detergent increase the measured Aβ42 concentration, which has to be standardised [229]. Several additional factors may be important in an assay-specific manner and close adherence to kit inserts is recommended, as is participation in the Alzheimer's Association QC programme and other inter-laboratory comparison programmes to ensure that proper laboratory procedures are in place.

To help solve bias and variation problems, a number of standardisation efforts have been initiated, all aimed at facilitating the development of standard operating procedures for pre-analytical sample handling and assay procedures, as well as reference methods and materials for the key analytes. These initiatives include the Alzheimer's Association Global Consortium for Biomarker Standardization (GCBS) and the International Federation of Clinical Chemistry and Laboratory Medicine (IFCC) Working Group for CSF Proteins [230]. Standard operating procedures for CSF sampling and storage have been published [83] and selected reaction monitoring mass spectrometry-based candidate reference methods for Aβ1–42 have been described [231–233]. Strong collaborative efforts within GCBS are underway and updates are available on http://www.alz.org/research/funding/global_biomarker_consortium.asp.

7   Concluding Remarks

Three CSF biomarkers reflecting the core pathological features of AD are in common use: T-tau (broadly, but not entirely reflecting neurodegeneration), P-tau (reflecting tau hyperphosphorylation and tangle formation) and Aβ42 (which inversely correlates with plaque pathology). According to revised clinical criteria, these markers may help diagnose AD more accurately, and in a research setting open up the possibility of detecting pre-dementia stages of the disease. At present, their most obvious utility is in clinical trials of novel disease-modifying treatments against AD. In the future, they may help selecting the right treatment for individual patients by making it possible to assess which molecular pathology that is most likely to cause the patient's symptom at different stages of the disease. In addition, there is considerable promise that CSF biomarkers will be able to provide in vivo measurement of a range of additional pathophysiological processes in AD, including microglial activation and synapse loss.

Acknowledgements

We gratefully acknowledge the support of the Leonard Wolfson Experimental Neurology Centre. Work in the authors' laboratories is supported by the Swedish Research Council, the Knut and Alice

Wallenberg Foundation, Alzheimer's Association, Swedish State Support for Clinical Research, Alzheimer's Research UK and the NIHR Queen Square BRU in dementia. We wish to thank colleagues, patients and their families for generating the extensive literature that was reviewed here.

References

1. Alzheimer A, Stelzmann RA, Schnitzlein HN, Murtagh FR (1995) An English translation of Alzheimer's 1907 paper, "Uber eine eigenartige Erkankung der Hirnrinde". Clin Anat 8(6):429–431

2. Blennow K, De Leon MJ, Zetterberg H (2006) Alzheimer's disease. Lancet 368(9533): 387–403

3. Tomlinson BE, Blessed G, Roth M (1970) Observations on the brains of demented old people. J Neurol Sci 11(3):205–242

4. Katzman R (1986) Alzheimer's disease. N Engl J Med 314(15):964–973

5. Roth M, Tomlinson BE, Blessed G (1966) Correlation between scores for dementia and counts of 'senile plaques' in cerebral grey matter of elderly subjects. Nature 209(5018):109–110

6. Glenner GG, Wong CW (1984) Alzheimer's disease: initial report of the purification and characterization of a novel cerebrovascular amyloid protein. Biochem Biophys Res Commun 120(3):885–890

7. Masters CL, Simms G, Weinman NA, Multhaup G, Mcdonald BL, Beyreuther K (1985) Amyloid plaque core protein in Alzheimer disease and Down syndrome. Proc Natl Acad Sci U S A 82(12):4245–4249

8. Portelius E, Bogdanovic N, Gustavsson MK et al (2010) Mass spectrometric characterization of brain amyloid beta isoform signatures in familial and sporadic Alzheimer's disease. Acta Neuropathol 120(2):185–193

9. Grundke-Iqbal I, Iqbal K, Tung YC, Quinlan M, Wisniewski HM, Binder LI (1986) Abnormal phosphorylation of the microtubule-associated protein tau (tau) in Alzheimer cytoskeletal pathology. Proc Natl Acad Sci U S A 83(13):4913–4917

10. Nukina N, Ihara Y (1986) One of the antigenic determinants of paired helical filaments is related to tau protein. J Biochem 99(5): 1541–1544

11. Mandelkow EM, Mandelkow E (2012) Biochemistry and cell biology of tau protein in neurofibrillary degeneration. Cold Spring Harb Perspect Med 2(7):a006247

12. Kang J, Lemaire HG, Unterbeck A et al (1987) The precursor of Alzheimer's disease amyloid A4 protein resembles a cell-surface receptor. Nature 325(6106):733–736

13. Goldgaber D, Lerman MI, Mcbride OW, Saffiotti U, Gajdusek DC (1987) Characterization and chromosomal localization of a cDNA encoding brain amyloid of Alzheimer's disease. Science 235(4791): 877–880

14. Popovitch ER, Wisniewski HM, Barcikowska M et al (1990) Alzheimer neuropathology in non-Down's syndrome mentally retarded adults. Acta Neuropathol 80(4):362–367

15. Van Nostrand WE, Wagner SL, Suzuki M et al (1989) Protease nexin-II, a potent antichymotrypsin, shows identity to amyloid beta-protein precursor. Nature 341(6242):546–549

16. Nalivaeva NN, Turner AJ (2013) The amyloid precursor protein: a biochemical enigma in brain development, function and disease. FEBS Lett 587(13):2046–2054

17. Mullan M, Crawford F, Axelman K et al (1992) A pathogenic mutation for probable Alzheimer's disease in the APP gene at the N-terminus of beta-amyloid. Nat Genet 1(5):345–347

18. Van Duijn CM, Hendriks L, Cruts M, Hardy JA, Hofman A, Van Broeckhoven C (1991) Amyloid precursor protein gene mutation in early-onset alzheimer's disease. Lancet 337(8747):978

19. Chartier-Harlin MC, Crawford F, Houlden H et al (1991) Early-onset alzheimer's disease caused by mutations at codon 717 of the beta-amyloid precursor protein gene. Nature 353(6347):844–846

20. Selkoe DJ (2001) Alzheimer's disease: genes, proteins, and therapy. Physiol Rev 81(2): 741–766

21. Chavez-Gutierrez L, Bammens L, Benilova I et al (2012) The mechanism of gamma-Secretase dysfunction in familial Alzheimer disease. EMBO J 31(10):2261–2274

22. Walsh DM, Selkoe DJ (2007) A beta oligomers—a decade of discovery. J Neurochem 101(5):1172–1184

23. Hardy JA, Higgins GA (1992) Alzheimer's disease: the amyloid cascade hypothesis. Science 256(5054):184–185

24. Hardy J, Bogdanovic N, Winblad B et al (2014) Pathways to Alzheimer's disease. J Intern Med 275(3):296–303

25. Jonsson T, Atwal JK, Steinberg S et al (2012) A mutation in APP protects against Alzheimer's disease and age-related cognitive decline. Nature 488(7409):96–99

26. Blennow K, Wallin A (1992) Clinical heterogeneity of probable Alzheimer's disease. J Geriatr Psychiatry Neurol 5(2):106–113

27. Potter R, Patterson BW, Elbert DL et al. (2013) Increased in vivo amyloid-beta42 production, exchange, and loss in presenilin mutation carriers. Sci Transl Med 5(189):189ra177

28. Pedersen NL, Gatz M, Berg S, Johansson B (2004) How heritable is Alzheimer's disease late in life? Findings from Swedish twins. Ann Neurol 55(2):180–185

29. Gatz M, Reynolds CA, Fratiglioni L et al (2006) Role of genes and environments for explaining Alzheimer disease. Arch Gen Psychiatry 63(2):168–174

30. Holtzman DM, Herz J, Bu G (2012) Apolipoprotein E and apolipoprotein E receptors: normal biology and roles in Alzheimer disease. Cold Spring Harb Perspect Med 2(3):a006312

31. Lambert JC, Ibrahim-Verbaas CA, Harold D et al (2013) Meta-analysis of 74,046 individuals identifies 11 new susceptibility loci for Alzheimer's disease. Nat Genet 45(12): 1452–1458

32. Jones L, Holmans PA, Hamshere ML et al (2010) Genetic evidence implicates the immune system and cholesterol metabolism in the aetiology of Alzheimer's disease. PLoS ONE 5(11), e13950

33. Guerreiro R, Wojtas A, Bras J et al (2013) TREM2 variants in Alzheimer's disease. N Engl J Med 368(2):117–127

34. Jonsson T, Stefansson H, Steinberg S et al (2013) Variant of TREM2 associated with the risk of Alzheimer's disease. N Engl J Med 368(2):107–116

35. Fjell AM, Mcevoy L, Holland D, Dale AM, Walhovd KB (2013) Brain changes in older adults at very low risk for Alzheimer's disease. J Neurosci 33(19):8237–8242

36. Savva GM, Wharton SB, Ince PG, Forster G, Matthews FE, Brayne C (2009) Age, neuropathology, and dementia. N Engl J Med 360(22):2302–2309

37. Mattsson N, Rosen E, Hansson O et al (2012) Age and diagnostic performance of Alzheimer disease CSF biomarkers. Neurology 78(7): 468–476

38. Thal DR, Rub U, Orantes M, Braak H (2002) Phases of A beta-deposition in the human brain and its relevance for the development of AD. Neurology 58(12):1791–1800

39. Braak H, Zetterberg H, Del Tredici K, Blennow K (2013) Intraneuronal tau aggregation precedes diffuse plaque deposition, but amyloid-beta changes occur before increases of tau in cerebrospinal fluid. Acta Neuropathol 126(5):631–641

40. Nelson PT, Alafuzoff I, Bigio EH et al (2012) Correlation of Alzheimer disease neuropathologic changes with cognitive status: a review of the literature. J Neuropathol Exp Neurol 71(5):362–381

41. Wojtas A, Heggeli KA, Finch N et al (2012) C9ORF72 repeat expansions and other FTD gene mutations in a clinical AD patient series from Mayo Clinic. Am J Neurodegener Dis 1(1):107–118

42. Jin SC, Pastor P, Cooper B et al (2012) Pooled-DNA sequencing identifies novel causative variants in PSEN1, GRN and MAPT in a clinical early-onset and familial Alzheimer's disease Ibero-American cohort. Alzheimers Res Ther 4(4):34

43. Gottfries CG, Gottfries I, Roos BE (1969) Homovanillic acid and 5-hydroxyindoleacetic acid in the cerebrospinal fluid of patients with senile dementia, presenile dementia and parkinsonism. J Neurochem 16(9):1341–1345

44. Gottfries CG, Gottfries I, Roos BE (1970) Homovanillic acid and 5-hydroxyindoleacetic acid in cerebrospinal fluid related to rated mental and motor impairment in senile and presenile dementia. Acta Psychiatr Scand 46(2):99–105

45. Gottfries CG, Kjallquist A, Ponten U, Roos BE, Sundbarg G (1974) Cerebrospinal fluid pH and monoamine and glucolytic metabolites in Alzheimer's disease. Br J Psychiatry 124:280–287

46. Glenner GG, Wong CW (1984) Alzheimer's disease and Down's syndrome: sharing of a unique cerebrovascular amyloid fibril protein. Biochem Biophys Res Commun 122(3): 1131–1135

47. Haass C, Schlossmacher MG, Hung AY et al (1992) Amyloid beta-peptide is produced by cultured cells during normal metabolism. Nature 359(6393):322–325

48. Portelius E, Price E, Brinkmalm G et al (2011) A novel pathway for amyloid precursor protein processing. Neurobiol Aging 32(6):1090–1098

49. Motter R, Vigo-Pelfrey C, Kholodenko D et al (1995) Reduction of beta-amyloid peptide42 in the cerebrospinal fluid of patients with Alzheimer's disease. Ann Neurol 38(4):643–648

50. Rosen C, Hansson O, Blennow K, Zetterberg H (2013) Fluid biomarkers in Alzheimer's disease—current concepts. Mol Neurodegener 8:20

51. Strozyk D, Blennow K, White LR, Launer LJ (2003) CSF Abeta 42 levels correlate with amyloid-neuropathology in a population-based autopsy study. Neurology 60(4):652–656

52. Fagan AM, Mintun MA, Mach RH et al (2006) Inverse relation between in vivo amyloid imaging load and cerebrospinal fluid Abeta42 in humans. Ann Neurol 59(3):512–519

53. Forsberg A, Engler H, Almkvist O et al (2008) PET imaging of amyloid deposition in patients with mild cognitive impairment. Neurobiol Aging 29(10):1456–1465

54. Seppala TT, Nerg O, Koivisto AM et al (2012) CSF biomarkers for Alzheimer disease correlate with cortical brain biopsy findings. Neurology 78(20):1568–1575

55. Andreasen N, Minthon L, Vanmechelen E et al (1999) Cerebrospinal fluid tau and Abeta42 as predictors of development of Alzheimer's disease in patients with mild cognitive impairment. Neurosci Lett 273(1):5–8

56. Hansson O, Zetterberg H, Buchhave P, Londos E, Blennow K, Minthon L (2006) Association between CSF biomarkers and incipient Alzheimer's disease in patients with mild cognitive impairment: a follow-up study. Lancet Neurol 5(3):228–234

57. Shaw LM, Vanderstichele H, Knapik-Czajka M et al (2009) Cerebrospinal fluid biomarker signature in Alzheimer's disease neuroimaging initiative subjects. Ann Neurol 65(4):403–413

58. Visser PJ, Verhey F, Knol DL et al (2009) Prevalence and prognostic value of CSF markers of Alzheimer's disease pathology in patients with subjective cognitive impairment or mild cognitive impairment in the DESCRIPA study: a prospective cohort study. Lancet Neurol 8(7):619–627

59. Buchhave P, Minthon L, Zetterberg H, Wallin AK, Blennow K, Hansson O (2012) Cerebrospinal fluid levels of beta-amyloid 1-42, but not of tau, are fully changed already 5 to 10 years before the onset of Alzheimer dementia. Arch Gen Psychiatry 69(1):98–106

60. Skoog I, Davidsson P, Aevarsson O, Vanderstichele H, Vanmechelen E, Blennow K (2003) Cerebrospinal fluid beta-amyloid 42 is reduced before the onset of sporadic dementia: a population-based study in 85-year-olds. Dement Geriatr Cogn Disord 15(3):169–176

61. Fagan AM, Head D, Shah AR et al (2009) Decreased cerebrospinal fluid Abeta(42) correlates with brain atrophy in cognitively normal elderly. Ann Neurol 65(2):176–183

62. Gustafson DR, Skoog I, Rosengren L, Zetterberg H, Blennow K (2007) Cerebrospinal fluid beta-amyloid 1-42 concentration may predict cognitive decline in older women. J Neurol Neurosurg Psychiatry 78(5):461–464

63. Dubois B, Feldman HH, Jacova C et al (2014) Advancing research diagnostic criteria for Alzheimer's disease: the IWG-2 criteria. Lancet Neurol 13(6):614–629

64. Sjogren M, Gisslen M, Vanmechelen E, Blennow K (2001) Low cerebrospinal fluid beta-amyloid 42 in patients with acute bacterial meningitis and normalization after treatment. Neurosci Lett 314(1–2):33–36

65. Mattsson N, Axelsson M, Haghighi S et al (2009) Reduced cerebrospinal fluid BACE1 activity in multiple sclerosis. Mult Scler 15(4):448–454

66. Gisslen M, Krut J, Andreasson U et al (2009) Amyloid and tau cerebrospinal fluid biomarkers in HIV infection. BMC Neurol 9:63

67. Mattsson N, Bremell D, Anckarsater R et al (2010) Neuroinflammation in Lyme neuroborreliosis affects amyloid metabolism. BMC Neurol 10:51

68. Schoonenboom NS, Mulder C, Van Kamp GJ et al (2005) Amyloid beta 38, 40, and 42 species in cerebrospinal fluid: more of the same? Ann Neurol 58(1):139–142

69. Portelius E, Zetterberg H, Andreasson U et al (2006) An Alzheimer's disease-specific beta-amyloid fragment signature in cerebrospinal fluid. Neurosci Lett 409(3):215–219

70. Mattsson N, Portelius E, Rolstad S et al (2012) Longitudinal cerebrospinal fluid biomarkers over four years in mild cognitive impairment. J Alzheimers Dis 30(4):767–778

71. Vandermeeren M, Mercken M, Vanmechelen E et al (1993) Detection of tau proteins in normal and Alzheimer's disease cerebrospinal fluid with a sensitive sandwich enzyme-linked immunosorbent assay. J Neurochem 61(5):1828–1834

72. Blennow K, Wallin A, Agren H, Spenger C, Siegfried J, Vanmechelen E (1995) Tau protein in cerebrospinal fluid: a biochemical marker for axonal degeneration in Alzheimer disease? Mol Chem Neuropathol 26(3):231–245

73. Wang L, Fagan AM, Shah AR et al (2012) Cerebrospinal fluid proteins predict longitudinal hippocampal degeneration in early-stage dementia of the Alzheimer type. Alzheimer Dis Assoc Disord 26(4):314–321

74. Glodzik L, Mosconi L, Tsui W et al (2012) Alzheimer's disease markers, hypertension, and gray matter damage in normal elderly. Neurobiol Aging 33(7):1215–1227

75. Trojanowski JQ, Schuck T, Schmidt ML, Lee VM (1989) Distribution of tau proteins in the

normal human central and peripheral nervous system. J Histochem Cytochem 37(2): 209–215

76. Hesse C, Rosengren L, Andreasen N et al (2001) Transient increase in total tau but not phospho-tau in human cerebrospinal fluid after acute stroke. Neurosci Lett 297(3):187–190

77. Zetterberg H, Hietala MA, Jonsson M et al (2006) Neurochemical aftermath of amateur boxing. Arch Neurol 63(9):1277–1280

78. Wallin AK, Blennow K, Zetterberg H, Londos E, Minthon L, Hansson O (2010) CSF biomarkers predict a more malignant outcome in Alzheimer disease. Neurology 74(19):1531–1537

79. Sanchez-Juan P, Sanchez-Valle R, Green A et al (2007) Influence of timing on CSF tests value for Creutzfeldt-Jakob disease diagnosis. J Neurol 254(7):901–906

80. Saman S, Kim W, Raya M et al (2012) Exosome-associated tau is secreted in tauopathy models and is selectively phosphorylated in cerebrospinal fluid in early Alzheimer disease. J Biol Chem 287(6):3842–3849

81. Maia LF, Kaeser SA, Reichwald J et al. (2013) Changes in amyloid-beta and tau in the cerebrospinal fluid of transgenic mice overexpressing amyloid precursor protein. Sci Transl Med 5(194):194re192

82. Meredith JE Jr, Sankaranarayanan S, Guss V et al (2013) Characterization of Novel CSF Tau and ptau Biomarkers for Alzheimer's Disease. PLoS ONE 8(10), e76523

83. Blennow K, Hampel H, Weiner M, Zetterberg H (2010) Cerebrospinal fluid and plasma biomarkers in Alzheimer disease. Nat Rev Neurol 6(3):131–144

84. Uryu K, Chen XH, Martinez D et al (2007) Multiple proteins implicated in neurodegenerative diseases accumulate in axons after brain trauma in humans. Exp Neurol 208(2):185–192

85. Wischik CM, Novak M, Thogersen HC et al (1988) Isolation of a fragment of tau derived from the core of the paired helical filament of Alzheimer disease. Proc Natl Acad Sci U S A 85(12):4506–4510

86. Hampel H, Buerger K, Zinkowski R et al (2004) Measurement of phosphorylated tau epitopes in the differential diagnosis of Alzheimer disease: a comparative cerebrospinal fluid study. Arch Gen Psychiatry 61(1):95–102

87. Buerger K, Ewers M, Pirttila T et al (2006) CSF phosphorylated tau protein correlates with neocortical neurofibrillary pathology in Alzheimer's disease. Brain 129(Pt 11):3035–3041

88. Riemenschneider M, Wagenpfeil S, Vanderstichele H et al (2003) Phospho-tau/total tau ratio in cerebrospinal fluid discriminates Creutzfeldt-Jakob disease from other dementias. Mol Psychiatry 8(3):343–347

89. Skillback T, Rosen C, Asztely F, Mattsson N, Blennow K, Zetterberg H (2014) Diagnostic performance of cerebrospinal fluid total tau and phosphorylated tau in Creutzfeldt-Jakob disease: results from the Swedish Mortality Registry. JAMA Neurol 71(4):476–483

90. Mattsson N, Savman K, Osterlundh G, Blennow K, Zetterberg H (2009) Converging molecular pathways in human neural development and degeneration. Neurosci Res 66(3):330–332

91. Grahn A, Hagberg L, Nilsson S, Blennow K, Zetterberg H, Studahl M (2013) Cerebrospinal fluid biomarkers in patients with varicella-zoster virus CNS infections. J Neurol 260(7):1813–1821

92. Kondziella D, Zetterberg H (2008) Hyperphosphorylation of tau protein in superficial CNS siderosis. J Neurol Sci 273(1–2):130–132

93. Ikeda T, Noto D, Noguchi-Shinohara M et al (2010) CSF tau protein is a useful marker for effective treatment of superficial siderosis of the central nervous system: two case reports. Clin Neurol Neurosurg 112(1):62–64

94. Williams CT, Barnes BM, Richter M, Buck CL (2012) Hibernation and circadian rhythms of body temperature in free-living Arctic ground squirrels. Physiol Biochem Zool 85(4):397–404

95. Hartig W, Stieler J, Boerema AS et al (2007) Hibernation model of tau phosphorylation in hamsters: selective vulnerability of cholinergic basal forebrain neurons—implications for Alzheimer's disease. Eur J Neurosci 25(1):69–80

96. Whittington RA, Bretteville A, Dickler MF, Planel E (2013) Anesthesia and tau pathology. Prog Neuropsychopharmacol Biol Psychiatry 47:147–155

97. Johansson P, Mattsson N, Hansson O et al (2011) Cerebrospinal fluid biomarkers for Alzheimer's disease: diagnostic performance in a homogeneous mono-center population. J Alzheimers Dis 24(3):537–546

98. Mattsson N, Zetterberg H, Hansson O et al (2009) CSF biomarkers and incipient Alzheimer disease in patients with mild cognitive impairment. JAMA 302(4):385–393

99. Baumann TP, Duyar H, Sollberger M et al (2010) CSF-tau and CSF-Abeta(1-42) in

posterior cortical atrophy. Dement Geriatr Cogn Disord 29(6):530–533

100. Seguin J, Formaglio M, Perret-Liaudet A et al (2011) CSF biomarkers in posterior cortical atrophy. Neurology 76(21):1782–1788

101. Bibl M, Mollenhauer B, Lewczuk P et al (2011) Cerebrospinal fluid tau, p-tau 181 and amyloid-beta38/40/42 in frontotemporal dementias and primary progressive aphasias. Dement Geriatr Cogn Disord 31(1):37–44

102. Borroni B, Premi E, Agosti C et al (2011) CSF Alzheimer's disease-like pattern in corticobasal syndrome: evidence for a distinct disorder. J Neurol Neurosurg Psychiatry 82(8):834–838

103. Toledo JB, Xie SX, Trojanowski JQ, Shaw LM (2013) Longitudinal change in CSF tau and Abeta biomarkers for up to 48 months in ADNI. Acta Neuropathol 126(5):659–670

104. Mattsson N, Insel P, Nosheny R et al (2013) CSF protein biomarkers predicting longitudinal reduction of CSF beta-amyloid42 in cognitively healthy elders. Transl Psychiatry 3, e293

105. Moghekar A, Li S, Lu Y et al (2013) CSF biomarker changes precede symptom onset of mild cognitive impairment. Neurology 81(20):1753–1758

106. Zetterberg H, Pedersen M, Lind K et al (2007) Intra-individual stability of CSF biomarkers for Alzheimer's disease over two years. J Alzheimers Dis 12(3):255–260

107. Blennow K, Zetterberg H, Minthon L et al (2007) Longitudinal stability of CSF biomarkers in Alzheimer's disease. Neurosci Lett 419(1):18–22

108. Mattsson N, Rajendran L, Zetterberg H et al (2012) BACE1 inhibition induces a specific cerebrospinal fluid beta-amyloid pattern that identifies drug effects in the central nervous system. PLoS ONE 7(2), e31084

109. Lannfelt L, Blennow K, Zetterberg H et al (2008) Safety, efficacy, and biomarker findings of PBT2 in targeting Abeta as a modifying therapy for Alzheimer's disease: a phase IIa, double-blind, randomised, placebo-controlled trial. Lancet Neurol 7(9):779–786

110. May PC, Dean RA, Lowe SL et al (2011) Robust central reduction of amyloid-beta in humans with an orally available, non-peptidic beta-secretase inhibitor. J Neurosci 31(46): 16507–16516

111. Portelius E, Dean RA, Gustavsson MK et al (2010) A novel Abeta isoform pattern in CSF reflects gamma-secretase inhibition in Alzheimer disease. Alzheimers Res Ther 2(2):7

112. Gilman S, Koller M, Black RS et al (2005) Clinical effects of Abeta immunization (AN1792) in patients with AD in an interrupted trial. Neurology 64(9):1553–1562

113. Blennow K, Zetterberg H, Rinne JO et al (2012) Effect of immunotherapy with bapineuzumab on cerebrospinal fluid biomarker levels in patients with mild to moderate Alzheimer disease. Arch Neurol 69(8):1002–1010

114. Schott JM, Warren JD (2012) Alzheimer's disease: mimics and chameleons. Pract Neurol 12(6):358–366

115. Shim YS, Roe CM, Buckles VD, Morris JC (2013) Clinicopathologic study of Alzheimer's disease: Alzheimer mimics. J Alzheimers Dis 35(4):799–811

116. Andreasson U, Portelius E, Andersson ME, Blennow K, Zetterberg H (2007) Aspects of beta-amyloid as a biomarker for Alzheimer's disease. Biomark Med 1(1):59–78

117. Fukumoto H, Cheung BS, Hyman BT, Irizarry MC (2002) Beta-secretase protein and activity are increased in the neocortex in Alzheimer disease. Arch Neurol 59(9):1381–1389

118. Holsinger RM, Lee JS, Boyd A, Masters CL, Collins SJ (2006) CSF BACE1 activity is increased in CJD and Alzheimer disease versus other dementias. Neurology 67(4):710–712

119. Holsinger RM, Mclean CA, Collins SJ, Masters CL, Evin G (2004) Increased beta-Secretase activity in cerebrospinal fluid of Alzheimer's disease subjects. Ann Neurol 55(6):898–899

120. Zetterberg H, Andreasson U, Hansson O et al (2008) Elevated cerebrospinal fluid BACE1 activity in incipient Alzheimer disease. Arch Neurol 65(8):1102–1107

121. Mulder SD, Van Der Flier WM, Verheijen JH et al (2010) BACE1 activity in cerebrospinal fluid and its relation to markers of AD pathology. J Alzheimers Dis 20(1):253–260

122. Zhong Z, Ewers M, Teipel S et al (2007) Levels of beta-secretase (BACE1) in cerebrospinal fluid as a predictor of risk in mild cognitive impairment. Arch Gen Psychiatry 64(6):718–726

123. Rosen C, Andreasson U, Mattsson N et al (2012) Cerebrospinal fluid profiles of amyloid beta-related biomarkers in Alzheimer's disease. Neuromolecular Med 14(1):65–73

124. Olsson A, Hoglund K, Sjogren M et al (2003) Measurement of alpha- and beta-secretase cleaved amyloid precursor protein in cerebrospinal fluid from Alzheimer patients. Exp Neurol 183(1):74–80

125. Perneczky R, Tsolakidou A, Arnold A et al (2011) CSF soluble amyloid precursor proteins in the diagnosis of incipient Alzheimer disease. Neurology 77(1):35–38

126. Lewczuk P, Kamrowski-Kruck H, Peters O et al (2010) Soluble amyloid precursor proteins in the cerebrospinal fluid as novel potential biomarkers of Alzheimer's disease: a multicenter study. Mol Psychiatry 15(2):138–145

127. Lewczuk P, Popp J, Lelental N et al (2012) Cerebrospinal fluid soluble amyloid-beta protein precursor as a potential novel biomarkers of Alzheimer's disease. J Alzheimers Dis 28(1):119–125

128. Gabelle A, Roche S, Geny C et al (2010) Correlations between soluble alpha/beta forms of amyloid precursor protein and Abeta38, 40, and 42 in human cerebrospinal fluid. Brain Res 1357:175–183

129. Castellani RJ, Smith MA (2011) Compounding artefacts with uncertainty, and an amyloid cascade hypothesis that is 'too big to fail'. J Pathol 224(2):147–152

130. Walsh DM, Klyubin I, Fadeeva JV et al (2002) Naturally secreted oligomers of amyloid beta protein potently inhibit hippocampal long-term potentiation in vivo. Nature 416(6880):535–539

131. Zempel H, Thies E, Mandelkow E, Mandelkow EM (2010) Abeta oligomers cause localized Ca(2+) elevation, missorting of endogenous Tau into dendrites, Tau phosphorylation, and destruction of microtubules and spines. J Neurosci 30(36):11938–11950

132. Jin M, Shepardson N, Yang T, Chen G, Walsh D, Selkoe DJ (2011) Soluble amyloid beta-protein dimers isolated from Alzheimer cortex directly induce Tau hyperphosphorylation and neuritic degeneration. Proc Natl Acad Sci U S A 108(14):5819–5824

133. De Felice FG, Wu D, Lambert MP et al (2008) Alzheimer's disease-type neuronal tau hyperphosphorylation induced by A beta oligomers. Neurobiol Aging 29(9):1334–1347

134. Bruggink KA, Jongbloed W, Biemans EA et al (2013) Amyloid-beta oligomer detection by ELISA in cerebrospinal fluid and brain tissue. Anal Biochem 433(2):112–120

135. Shankar GM, Li S, Mehta TH et al (2008) Amyloid-beta protein dimers isolated directly from Alzheimer's brains impair synaptic plasticity and memory. Nat Med 14(8):837–842

136. Gao CM, Yam AY, Wang X et al (2010) Abeta40 oligomers identified as a potential biomarker for the diagnosis of Alzheimer's disease. PLoS ONE 5(12), e15725

137. Fukumoto H, Tokuda T, Kasai T et al (2010) High-molecular-weight {beta}-amyloid oligomers are elevated in cerebrospinal fluid of Alzheimer patients. FASEB J 24(8):2716–2726

138. Georganopoulou DG, Chang L, Nam JM et al (2005) Nanoparticle-based detection in cerebral spinal fluid of a soluble pathogenic biomarker for Alzheimer's disease. Proc Natl Acad Sci U S A 102(7):2273–2276

139. Pitschke M, Prior R, Haupt M, Riesner D (1998) Detection of single amyloid beta-protein aggregates in the cerebrospinal fluid of Alzheimer's patients by fluorescence correlation spectroscopy. Nat Med 4(7):832–834

140. Holtta M, Hansson O, Andreasson U et al (2013) Evaluating amyloid-beta oligomers in cerebrospinal fluid as a biomarker for Alzheimer's disease. PLoS ONE 8(6), e66381

141. Handoko M, Grant M, Kuskowski M et al (2013) Correlation of specific amyloid-beta oligomers with tau in cerebrospinal fluid from cognitively normal older adults. JAMA Neurol 70(5):594–599

142. Santos AN, Torkler S, Nowak D et al (2007) Detection of amyloid-beta oligomers in human cerebrospinal fluid by flow cytometry and fluorescence resonance energy transfer. J Alzheimers Dis 11(1):117–125

143. Blennow K, Wallin A, Fredman P, Karlsson I, Gottfries CG, Svennerholm L (1990) Blood-brain barrier disturbance in patients with Alzheimer's disease is related to vascular factors. Acta Neurol Scand 81(4):323–326

144. Wallin A, Blennow K, Rosengren L (1999) Cerebrospinal fluid markers of pathogenetic processes in vascular dementia, with special reference to the subcortical subtype. Alzheimer Dis Assoc Disord 13(Suppl 3): S102–S105

145. Tumani H, Nolker G, Reiber H (1995) Relevance of cerebrospinal fluid variables for early diagnosis of neuroborreliosis. Neurology 45(9):1663–1670

146. Chalbot S, Zetterberg H, Blennow K, Fladby T, Grundke-Iqbal I, Iqbal K (2010) Cerebrospinal fluid secretory Ca2+-dependent phospholipase A2 activity: a biomarker of blood-cerebrospinal fluid barrier permeability. Neurosci Lett 478(3):179–183

147. Zetterberg H, Andreasson U, Blennow K (2009) CSF antithrombin III and disruption of the blood-brain barrier. J Clin Oncol 27(13):2302–2303

148. Lee JM, Blennow K, Andreasen N et al (2008) The brain injury biomarker VLP-1 is increased in the cerebrospinal fluid of Alzheimer disease patients. Clin Chem 54(10):1617–1623

149. Paterson RW, Bartlett JW, Blennow K et al (2014) Cerebrospinal fluid markers including

trefoil factor 3 are associated with neurode-generation in amyloid-positive individuals. Transl Psychiatry 4, e419

150. Rosengren LE, Karlsson JE, Sjogren M, Blennow K, Wallin A (1999) Neurofilament protein levels in CSF are increased in dementia. Neurology 52(5):1090–1093

151. Agren-Wilsson A, Lekman A, Sjoberg W et al (2007) CSF biomarkers in the evaluation of idiopathic normal pressure hydrocephalus. Acta Neurol Scand 116(5):333–339

152. Wallin A, Sjogren M (2001) Cerebrospinal fluid cytoskeleton proteins in patients with subcortical white-matter dementia. Mech Ageing Dev 122(16):1937–1949

153. De Jong D, Jansen RW, Pijnenburg YA et al (2007) CSF neurofilament proteins in the differential diagnosis of dementia. J Neurol Neurosurg Psychiatry 78(9):936–938

154. Landqvist Waldo M, Frizell Santillo A, Passant U et al (2013) Cerebrospinal fluid neurofilament light chain protein levels in subtypes of frontotemporal dementia. BMC Neurol 13:54

155. Gisslen M, Hagberg L, Brew BJ, Cinque P, Price RW, Rosengren L (2007) Elevated cerebrospinal fluid neurofilament light protein concentrations predict the development of AIDS dementia complex. J Infect Dis 195(12):1774–1778

156. Skillbäck T, Zetterberg H, Blennow K, Mattsson N (2013) CSF biomarkers for Alzheimer's disease and subcortical axonal damage in 5542 clinical samples. Alzheimers Res Ther 5(5):47

157. Tortelli R, Ruggieri M, Cortese R et al (2012) Elevated cerebrospinal fluid neurofilament light levels in patients with amyotrophic lateral sclerosis: a possible marker of disease severity and progression. Eur J Neurol 19(12):1561–1567

158. Rosengren LE, Karlsson JE, Karlsson JO, Persson LI, Wikkelso C (1996) Patients with amyotrophic lateral sclerosis and other neurodegenerative diseases have increased levels of neurofilament protein in CSF. J Neurochem 67(5):2013–2018

159. Swardfager W, Lanctot K, Rothenburg L, Wong A, Cappell J, Herrmann N (2010) A meta-analysis of cytokines in Alzheimer's disease. Biol Psychiatry 68(10):930–941

160. Comi C, Carecchio M, Chiocchetti A et al (2010) Osteopontin is increased in the cerebrospinal fluid of patients with Alzheimer's disease and its levels correlate with cognitive decline. J Alzheimers Dis 19(4):1143–1148

161. Naude PJ, Nyakas C, Eiden LE et al (2012) Lipocalin 2: novel component of proinflammatory signaling in Alzheimer's disease. FASEB J 26(7):2811–2823

162. Rosen C, Mattsson N, Johansson PM et al (2011) Discriminatory analysis of biochip-derived protein patterns in CSF and plasma in neurodegenerative diseases. Front Aging Neurosci 3:1

163. Blennow K, Wallin A, Fredman P, Gottfries CG, Karlsson I, Svennerholm L (1990) Intrathecal synthesis of immunoglobulins in patients with Alzheimer's disease. Eur Neuropsychopharmacol 1(1):79–81

164. Rossor MN, Fox NC, Mummery CJ, Schott JM, Warren JD (2010) The diagnosis of young-onset dementia. Lancet Neurol 9(8): 793–806

165. Morrow JD, Roberts LJ (1997) The isoprostanes: unique bioactive products of lipid peroxidation. Prog Lipid Res 36(1):1–21

166. Brys M, Pirraglia E, Rich K et al (2009) Prediction and longitudinal study of CSF biomarkers in mild cognitive impairment. Neurobiol Aging 30(5):682–690

167. De Leon MJ, Desanti S, Zinkowski R et al (2006) Longitudinal CSF and MRI biomarkers improve the diagnosis of mild cognitive impairment. Neurobiol Aging 27(3):394–401

168. Grossman M, Farmer J, Leight S et al (2005) Cerebrospinal fluid profile in frontotemporal dementia and Alzheimer's disease. Ann Neurol 57(5):721–729

169. Montine TJ, Beal MF, Cudkowicz ME et al (1999) Increased CSF F2-isoprostane concentration in probable AD. Neurology 52(3):562–565

170. Montine TJ, Markesbery WR, Morrow JD, Roberts LJ 2nd (1998) Cerebrospinal fluid F2-isoprostane levels are increased in Alzheimer's disease. Ann Neurol 44(3):410–413

171. Ringman JM, Younkin SG, Pratico D et al (2008) Biochemical markers in persons with preclinical familial Alzheimer disease. Neurology 71(2):85–92

172. Duits FH, Kester MI, Scheffer PG et al (2013) Increase in cerebrospinal fluid F2-isoprostanes is related to cognitive decline in APOE epsilon4 carriers. J Alzheimers Dis 36(3):563–570

173. Gackowski D, Rozalski R, Siomek A et al (2008) Oxidative stress and oxidative DNA damage is characteristic for mixed Alzheimer disease/vascular dementia. J Neurol Sci 266(1–2):57–62

174. Podlesniy P, Figueiro-Silva J, Llado A et al (2013) Low cerebrospinal fluid concentration of mitochondrial DNA in preclinical Alzheimer disease. Ann Neurol 74(5):655–668

175. Renkema GH, Boot RG, Au FL et al (1998) Chitotriosidase, a chitinase, and the 39-kDa human cartilage glycoprotein, a chitin-binding lectin, are homologues of family 18 glycosyl hydrolases secreted by human macrophages. Eur J Biochem 251(1–2):504–509

176. Hollak CE, Van Weely S, Van Oers MH, Aerts JM (1994) Marked elevation of plasma chitotriosidase activity. A novel hallmark of Gaucher disease. J Clin Invest 93(3):1288–1292

177. Watabe-Rudolph M, Song Z, Lausser L et al (2012) Chitinase enzyme activity in CSF is a powerful biomarker of Alzheimer disease. Neurology 78(8):569–577

178. Hakala BE, White C, Recklies AD (1993) Human cartilage gp-39, a major secretory product of articular chondrocytes and synovial cells, is a mammalian member of a chitinase protein family. J Biol Chem 268(34):25803–25810

179. Craig-Schapiro R, Perrin RJ, Roe CM et al (2010) YKL-40: a novel prognostic fluid biomarker for preclinical Alzheimer's disease. Biol Psychiatry 68(10):903–912

180. Olsson B, Hertze J, Lautner R et al (2013) Microglial markers are elevated in the prodromal phase of Alzheimer's disease and vascular dementia. J Alzheimers Dis 33(1):45–53

181. Sokolova A, Hill MD, Rahimi F, Warden LA, Halliday GM, Shepherd CE (2009) Monocyte chemoattractant protein-1 plays a dominant role in the chronic inflammation observed in Alzheimer's disease. Brain Pathol 19(3):392–398

182. Westin K, Buchhave P, Nielsen H, Minthon L, Janciauskiene S, Hansson O (2012) CCL2 is associated with a faster rate of cognitive decline during early stages of Alzheimer's disease. PLoS ONE 7(1), e30525

183. Correa JD, Starling D, Teixeira AL, Caramelli P, Silva TA (2011) Chemokines in CSF of Alzheimer's disease patients. Arq Neuropsiquiatr 69(3):455–459

184. Galimberti D, Schoonenboom N, Scheltens P et al (2006) Intrathecal chemokine levels in Alzheimer disease and frontotemporal lobar degeneration. Neurology 66(1):146–147

185. Galimberti D, Schoonenboom N, Scheltens P et al (2006) Intrathecal chemokine synthesis in mild cognitive impairment and Alzheimer disease. Arch Neurol 63(4):538–543

186. Mattsson N, Tabatabaei S, Johansson P et al (2011) Cerebrospinal fluid microglial markers in Alzheimer's disease: elevated chitotriosidase activity but lack of diagnostic utility. Neuromolecular Med 13(2):151–159

187. Blasko I, Lederer W, Oberbauer H et al (2006) Measurement of thirteen biological markers in CSF of patients with Alzheimer's disease and other dementias. Dement Geriatr Cogn Disord 21(1):9–15

188. Yin GN, Jeon H, Lee S, Lee HW, Cho JY, Suk K (2009) Role of soluble CD14 in cerebrospinal fluid as a regulator of glial functions. J Neurosci Res 87(11):2578–2590

189. Engelborghs S, De Brabander M, De Cree J et al (1999) Unchanged levels of interleukins, neopterin, interferon-gamma and tumor necrosis factor-alpha in cerebrospinal fluid of patients with dementia of the Alzheimer type. Neurochem Int 34(6):523–530

190. Terry RD, Masliah E, Salmon DP et al (1991) Physical basis of cognitive alterations in Alzheimer's disease: synapse loss is the major correlate of cognitive impairment. Ann Neurol 30(4):572–580

191. Davidsson P, Puchades M, Blennow K (1999) Identification of synaptic vesicle, pre- and postsynaptic proteins in human cerebrospinal fluid using liquid-phase isoelectric focusing. Electrophoresis 20(3):431–437

192. Thorsell A, Bjerke M, Gobom J et al (2010) Neurogranin in cerebrospinal fluid as a marker of synaptic degeneration in Alzheimer's disease. Brain Res 1362:13–22

193. Kvartsberg H, Portelius E, Andreasson U et al (2015) Characterization of the postsynaptic protein neurogranin in paired cerebrospinal fluid and plasma samples from Alzheimer's disease patients and healthy controls. Alzheimers Res Ther 7(1):40

194. Kvartsberg H, Duits FH, Ingelsson M et al (2015) Cerebrospinal fluid levels of the synaptic protein neurogranin correlates with cognitive decline in prodromal Alzheimer's disease. Alzheimers Dement 11(10):1180–1190

195. De Vos A, Jacobs D, Struyfs H et al (2015) C-terminal neurogranin is increased in cerebrospinal fluid but unchanged in plasma in Alzheimer's disease. Alzheimers Dement 11(12):1461–1469

196. Chang L, Rissin DM, Fournier DR et al (2012) Single molecule enzyme-linked immunosorbent assays: theoretical considerations. J Immunol Methods 378(1–2):102–115

197. Hartung HP, Steinman L, Goodin DS et al (2013) Interleukin 17F level and interferon beta response in patients with multiple sclerosis. JAMA Neurol 70(8):1017–1021

198. Mollenhauer B, El-Agnaf OM, Marcus K, Trenkwalder C, Schlossmacher MG (2010) Quantification of alpha-synuclein in cerebrospinal fluid as a biomarker candidate: review of the literature and considerations for future studies. Biomark Med 4(5):683–699

199. Guo JL, Covell DJ, Daniels JP et al (2013) Distinct alpha-synuclein strains differentially promote tau inclusions in neurons. Cell 154(1):103–117

200. Pletnikova O, West N, Lee MK et al (2005) Abeta deposition is associated with enhanced cortical alpha-synuclein lesions in Lewy body diseases. Neurobiol Aging 26(8):1183–1192

201. Hall S, Ohrfelt A, Constantinescu R et al (2012) Accuracy of a panel of 5 cerebrospinal fluid biomarkers in the differential diagnosis of patients with dementia and/or parkinsonian disorders. Arch Neurol 69(11):1445–1452

202. Mollenhauer B, Locascio JJ, Schulz-Schaeffer W, Sixel-Doring F, Trenkwalder C, Schlossmacher MG (2011) alpha-Synuclein and tau concentrations in cerebrospinal fluid of patients presenting with parkinsonism: a cohort study. Lancet Neurol 10(3):230–240

203. Tateno F, Sakakibara R, Kawai T, Kishi M, Murano T (2012) Alpha-synuclein in the cerebrospinal fluid differentiates synucleinopathies (Parkinson Disease, dementia with Lewy bodies, multiple system atrophy) from Alzheimer disease. Alzheimer Dis Assoc Disord 26(3):213–216

204. Wennstrom M, Surova Y, Hall S et al (2013) Low CSF levels of both alpha-synuclein and the alpha-synuclein cleaving enzyme neurosin in patients with synucleinopathy. PLoS ONE 8(1), e53250

205. Ohrfelt A, Grognet P, Andreasen N et al (2009) Cerebrospinal fluid alpha-synuclein in neurodegenerative disorders-a marker of synapse loss? Neurosci Lett 450(3):332–335

206. Barbour R, Kling K, Anderson JP et al (2008) Red blood cells are the major source of alpha-synuclein in blood. Neurodegener Dis 5(2):55–59

207. Hong Z, Shi M, Chung KA et al (2010) DJ-1 and alpha-synuclein in human cerebrospinal fluid as biomarkers of Parkinson's disease. Brain 133(Pt 3):713–726

208. Irizarry MC (2004) Biomarkers of Alzheimer disease in plasma. NeuroRx 1(2):226–234

209. Doecke JD, Laws SM, Faux NG et al (2012) Blood-based protein biomarkers for diagnosis of Alzheimer disease. Arch Neurol 69(10):1318–1325

210. Ray S, Britschgi M, Herbert C et al (2007) Classification and prediction of clinical Alzheimer's diagnosis based on plasma signaling proteins. Nat Med 13(11):1359–1362

211. Bjorkqvist M, Ohlsson M, Minthon L, Hansson O (2012) Evaluation of a previously suggested plasma biomarker panel to identify Alzheimer's disease. PLoS ONE 7(1), e29868

212. Soares HD, Chen Y, Sabbagh M, Roher A, Schrijvers E, Breteler M (2009) Identifying early markers of Alzheimer's disease using quantitative multiplex proteomic immunoassay panels. Ann N Y Acad Sci 1180:56–67

213. Hampel H, Lista S, Teipel SJ et al (2014) Perspective on future role of biological markers in clinical therapy trials of Alzheimer's disease: a long-range point of view beyond 2020. Biochem Pharmacol 88(4):426–449

214. Isaac M, Vamvakas S, Abadie E, Jonsson B, Gispen C, Pani L (2011) Qualification opinion of novel methodologies in the predementia stage of Alzheimer's disease: cerebro-spinal-fluid related biomarkers for drugs affecting amyloid burden—regulatory considerations by European Medicines Agency focusing in improving benefit/risk in regulatory trials. Eur Neuropsychopharmacol 21(11):781–788

215. Salloway S, Sperling R, Gilman S et al (2009) A phase 2 multiple ascending dose trial of bapineuzumab in mild to moderate Alzheimer disease. Neurology 73(24):2061–2070

216. Seubert P, Vigo-Pelfrey C, Esch F et al (1992) Isolation and quantification of soluble Alzheimer's beta-peptide from biological fluids. Nature 359(6393):325–327

217. Siemers ER, Friedrich S, Dean RA et al (2010) Safety and changes in plasma and cerebrospinal fluid amyloid beta after a single administration of an amyloid beta monoclonal antibody in subjects with Alzheimer disease. Clin Neuropharmacol 33(2):67–73

218. Seubert P, Barbour R, Khan K et al (2008) Antibody capture of soluble Abeta does not reduce cortical Abeta amyloidosis in the PDAPP mouse. Neurodegener Dis 5(2):65–71

219. Salloway S, Sperling R, Fox NC et al (2014) Two phase 3 trials of bapineuzumab in mild-to-moderate Alzheimer's disease. N Engl J Med 370(4):322–333

220. Doody RS, Thomas RG, Farlow M et al (2014) Phase 3 trials of solanezumab for mild-to-moderate Alzheimer's disease. N Engl J Med 370(4):311–321

221. Hampel H, Frank R, Broich K et al (2010) Biomarkers for Alzheimer's disease: academic, industry and regulatory perspectives. Nat Rev Drug Discov 9(7):560–574

222. Mattsson N, Zegers I, Andreasson U et al (2012) Reference measurement procedures for Alzheimer's disease cerebrospinal fluid biomarkers: definitions and approaches with focus on amyloid beta42. Biomark Med 6(4):409–417

223. Duits FH, Teunissen CE, Bouwman FH et al (2014) The cerebrospinal fluid "Alzheimer

profile": Easily said, but what does it mean? Alzheimers Dement 10(6):713–723.e2

224. Mattsson N, Andreasson U, Persson S et al (2011) The Alzheimer's Association external quality control program for cerebrospinal fluid biomarkers. Alzheimers Dement 7(4):386–395, e386

225. Mattsson N, Andreasson U, Persson S et al (2013) CSF biomarker variability in the Alzheimer's Association quality control program. Alzheimers Dement 9(3):251–261

226. Perret-Liaudet A, Pelpel M, Tholance Y et al (2012) Risk of Alzheimer's disease biological misdiagnosis linked to cerebrospinal collection tubes. J Alzheimers Dis 31(1):13–20

227. Toombs J, Paterson RW, Lunn MP et al (2013) Identification of an important potential confound in CSF AD studies: aliquot volume. Clin Chem Lab Med 51(12): 2311–2317

228. Toombs J, Paterson RW, Schott JM, Zetterberg H (2014) Amyloid-beta 42 adsorption following serial tube transfer. Alzheimers Res Ther 6(1):5

229. Bjerke M, Portelius E, Minthon L et al (2010) Confounding factors influencing amyloid Beta concentration in cerebrospinal fluid. Int J Alzheimers Dis 2010

230. Carrillo MC, Blennow K, Soares H et al (2013) Global standardization measurement of cerebral spinal fluid for Alzheimer's disease: An update from the Alzheimer's Association Global Biomarkers Consortium. Alzheimers Dement 9(2):137–140

231. Pannee J, Portelius E, Oppermann M et al (2013) A selected reaction monitoring (SRM)-based method for absolute quantification of Abeta38, Abeta40, and Abeta42 in cerebrospinal fluid of Alzheimer's disease patients and healthy controls. J Alzheimers Dis 33(4):1021–1032

232. Leinenbach A, Pannee J, Dulffer T et al (2014) Mass spectrometry-based candidate reference measurement procedure for quantification of amyloid-beta in cerebrospinal fluid. Clin Chem 60(7):987–994

233. Korecka M, Waligorska T, Figurski M et al (2014) Qualification of a surrogate matrix-based absolute quantification method for amyloid-beta(4)(2) in human cerebrospinal fluid using 2D UPLC-tandem mass spectrometry. J Alzheimers Dis 41(2):441–451

Chapter 12

Volumetric MRI as a Diagnostic Tool in Alzheimer's Disease

Eric Westman, Lena Cavalin, and Lars-Olof Wahlund

Abstract

Brain atrophy is one of the key features of Alzheimer's disease (AD), and neuroimaging techniques, such as computer tomography (CT) and magnetic resonance imaging (MRI), have made it possible to study this pathological process in vivo. However, the use of clinical imaging in dementia evaluation is often suboptimal. Evidence supports the role of regional and global atrophy as well as white matter changes as markers of disease in dementia. There is an urgent need to apply this knowledge to optimize clinical imaging practice. In the following chapter we describe different methods to measure or estimate brain structures and white matter changes. Methods to judge the presence and distribution of cerebral microbleeds are also discussed. We describe both methods that are used in clinical practice today and methods that are still only applied in research or in clinical trials. The more advanced automated methods to estimate brain atrophy as well as other changes will hopefully be implemented in clinical practice in the future.

Key words Magnetic resonance imaging, Volumetry, Medial temporal lobe atrophy, Dementia, Alzheimer's disease, Multivariate analyses

1 Introduction

Since the first description of Alzheimer's disease (AD) by Alois Alzheimer, in the beginning of last century, it has been known that one of the key features in the disease is an atrophy of the brain. Since the advent of neuroimaging techniques, such as computer tomography (CT) and magnetic resonance imaging (MRI), possibilities to study the atrophy process in the disease has increased enormously. For many years MRI and CT were used to detect other courses for the cognitive impairment, such as tumors, bleedings and normal pressure hydrocephalus. However, the knowledge about the pathophysiology behind the disease has increased and the technique has improved. The atrophy process that is more specific for AD has been possible to study. The atrophy starts in the same place as where the first histopathological signs appear, namely in the entorhinal cortex and hippocampus area of the medial temporal lobe [1]. Subsequently, other areas such as the temporal and

Martin Ingelsson and Lars Lannfelt (eds.), *Immunotherapy and Biomarkers in Neurodegenerative Disorders*, Methods in Pharmacology and Toxicology, DOI 10.1007/978-1-4939-3560-4_12, © Springer Science+Business Media New York 2016

parietal lobes, and—in later disease stages—sometimes also the frontal lobe are affected.

The presence of medial temporal lobe atrophy in subjects with early memory problems has been shown to be an early sign of Alzheimer's disease [2, 3]. However atrophy in the medial temporal lobe is not unique for this disorder as it can also be found in frontotemporal dementia, vascular dementia and Lewy body dementia [4, 5]. There are several ways of estimating the atrophy. The earliest and most commonly used ones are visual rating scales and—for medial temporal atrophy—the Scheltens rating scale [6]. There are also rating scales for global atrophy and for atrophy in the posterior parts of the brain [7, 8].

Evidence supports the role of regional and global atrophy as well as white matter changes as markers of disease in dementia. There is an urgent need to apply this knowledge to optimize clinical imaging practice. The increasing knowledge regarding these issues has also been put into clinical practice with the Scheltens rating scale used for evaluation of medial temporal lobe atrophy. Modern MR-technique and image analysis have made it possible to make more sophisticated measurements as compared to visual rating alone [9]. By these developments it is now possible to measure the cortical thickness of regions in the brain as well as volumes of regions by using fully automated methods. Although these techniques have to be validated before they can be used in clinical practice they represent promising tools to detect very early atrophic changes, which might have a future impact on the diagnostic procedure. By using fully automated methods it is also possible to repeat measurements and detect subtle changes in volume, something that can be of great importance in clinical trials where the degree of atrophy is one outcome measurement.

In the first clinical trials using immunotherapy against AD it was evident that treatment led to an increase of Aβ42 in cerebral blood vessels, which paralleled the decreased concentration of Aβ42 in plaques. An increased concentration of Aβ40 was also noticed in the immunized compared to the non-immunized subjects. Also in the treated subjects a significantly increased number of cerebral microbleeds (CMB) or micro hemorrhages (MH) were found [10]. Cerebral microbleeds are small rounded areas in the brain that can be detected with MRI and specific iron sensitive sequences (susceptibility weighted images SWI). Those areas represent signs of old bleedings and are caused by the presence of hemosiderin in macrophages. It has been hypothesized that the transfer of Aβ from plaques to the blood may be the underlying event causing cerebral amyloid angiopathy (CAA) related hemorrhages. Vasogenic edema is another side effect caused by immunotherapy and the first clinical trial was stopped due to an unforeseen side effect of autoimmune inflammation in the brain, called vasogenic edema [11]. The term amyloid related imaging abnormalities ARIA was coined in 2011 by a workgroup convened by the Alzheimer Association Research Roundtable to describe vasogenic edema and microhemorrhages as seen on MRI in connection to amyloid modifying therapeutic approaches [12]. One other goal of the work group was to develop recommendations regarding how to conduct AD clinical trials in the setting of ARIA, inclusion/exclusion criteria, and safety monitoring.

In the following sections we describe different methods to measure or estimate brain structures. Also methods to judge the presence and distribution of cerebral microbleeds are presented. We describe both methods that are used in clinical practice and methods that are still only applied in research or in clinical trials.

2 Visual Assessment

Volumetric calculation and measurement of cortical thickness are, in daily clinical practice, too time consuming. The need for faster, but still reliable, tools for assessing atrophy in both MRI and CT started a cascade of different visual rating scales in the 1990s. The proved connection between hippocampal atrophy and Alzheimer's disease made it even more urgent to create visual rating scales suitable for clinical practice [13, 14]. Visual assessment of brain atrophy is a standardized method to evaluate a brain region just by looking at it without any measurement at all. Visual assessment of brain atrophy can be divided into different areas of interest:

– MTA, medial temporal lobe atrophy, with hippocampus in focus.

– GCA, global cortical atrophy with whole brain or regional brain atrophy.

– PA, posterior or parietal and occipital atrophy with precuneus and posterior gyrus cinguli atrophy in focus.

The method for visual assessment of medial temporal lobe atrophy, MTA, was described in 1992 by Philip Scheltens et al. [6, 15]. For this scale, a good compliance with volumetric calculations has been reported [16]. The assessment is performed on coronal or 3D T1 weighted images, on MRI or coronal CT, with an angulation along the dorsal border of the brainstem or perpendicular to the anterior commissure–posterior commissure (AC-PC). A visual estimation of the height of hippocampus, the width of the temporal horn of lateral ventricle and the width of choroid fissure, creates a 5-grade visual rating scale (Fig. 1).

In MTA 0, the hippocampus height is normal and neither the choroid fissure nor the temporal horn of lateral ventricle can be seen. In MTA1, hippocampus is still normal, but the choroid fissure and temporal horn is starting to get visible. In MTA 2 a slight

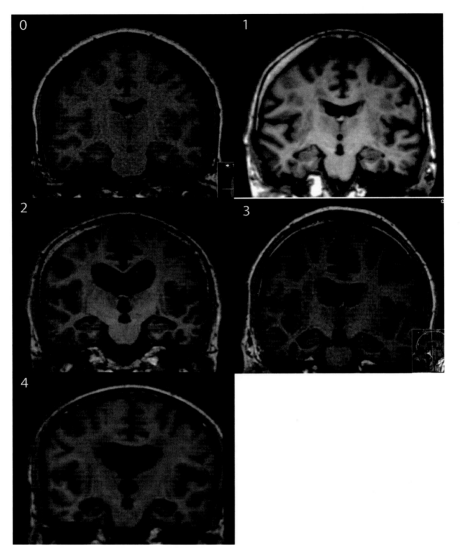

Fig. 1 Scheltens scale for medial temporal lobe atrophy (MTA), where 0 represents no atrophy and 4 end stage atrophy

atrophy of hippocampus is seen as the height of hippocampus is decreasing and the width of the choroid fissure and temporal horn is increasing. In MTA 3, these changes progress further. In MTA 4, end-stage-atrophy, a pronounced atrophy of hippocampus and a marked dilatation of surrounding liquor spaces of the choroid fissures and temporal horns can be seen. Whereas MTA grade 0 and 1 can be considered normal, MTA 2 is pathological when found in persons below 70 years of age. Similarly, MTA 3 is considered pathological when present in subjects below 80 years of age and MTA 4 is always considered pathological (although it can be found in cognitively healthy very old individuals) [16]. In addition to

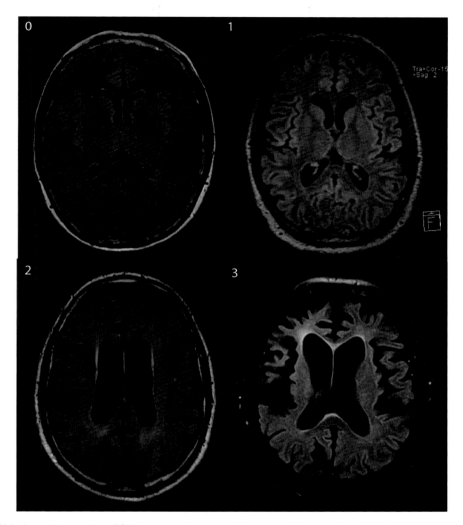

Fig. 2 Global cortical atrophy (GCA), where 0 represents no atrophy and 3 end stage atrophy

age, also other factors such as disease onset and ApoE genotype, need to be considered when defining the cutoffs for MTA [17].

Global cortical atrophy, GCA, a scale developed by Pasquier et al. in 1996 [8], is based on a visual assessment of widening of sulci and reduction of cortical thickness. It is a 4-graded scale where no widening of sulci and no cortical atrophy can be defined as GCA 0. In GCA 1 the sulci is beginning to widen and GCA 2 implies a reduction of cortical thickness and a progression of sulci width. Finally, GCA 3 is the end stage of cortical atrophy (Fig. 2). In a healthy population, GCA 0-1 is regarded as normal. For persons over 80 years of age, GCA 2 is normal, whereas GCA3 is always considered to be pathological. Whole brain atrophy of GCA 1 and GCA2 can be seen, but GCA 3 is usually just seen in a small region, or in a few gyri.

A rather new visual rating scale is based on visual assessment of atrophy in posterior regions, PA. This rating scale was published in 2011 by Koedam et al. [7]. Atrophy in parietal and occipital lobes have an association to AD in middle-aged and elderly subjects with a disease onset before the age of 65 [7, 18]. The visual rating is based on MRI or CT images in all three dimensions (axial, coronal, and sagittal). In MRI, the assessment uses a FLAIR sequence for axial images and a T1 weighted sequence for sagittal and coronal images. As for GCA, the estimation of width of the sulci and reduction of cortical thickness is the base for the 4-graded scale. Anatomic regions for investigation of PA are posterior cingulate sulcus, precuneus, parieto-occipital sulcus, and the cortex of parietal lobes. In PA 0 there is no visible atrophy. PA 1 indicates mild widening of sulci without volume loss of gyri and PA 2 represents substantial widening of sulci and volume loss of gyri. PA 3 means severe end-stage-atrophy. Both PA 0 and 1 are considered to be normal. As opposed to the MTA scale, no age-related cutoff values for pathological PA 2 and PA 3 have been published. There are also scales for rating of the presence and severity of white matter lesions in the brain.

Visual rating scales are of importance in the recruitment process for clinical trials in AD. For example, it is crucial to use these scales to decrease the risk of including subjects with vascular cognitive impairment.

Visual rating scales for white matter lesions are numerous. Some are easy to perform, but most of them are difficult and with low intra- and inter-rater agreement. There is one scale validated for rating WML both on CT and MRI scans [19], which gives a regional distribution of the lesions [12]. The scale can be used in clinical trials as an outcome measure parameter.

One of the most used white matter scales in clinical practice is the Fazekas simplified 4 grade rating scale, originating from 1987 [20, 21]. MRI with an axial or 3D FLAIR sequence is the preferred method. In Fazekas 0, no white matter spots can been found. Fazekas 1 means there is one, or several punctate white spots. Fazekas 2 implies that there are many punctate white matter lesions that are grouped and linked by no more than connecting bridges. In Fazekas 3, there are confluent hyper intense white matter areas (Fig. 3). Fazekas 2–3 are considered to be pathological for persons over 60 years of age, but can be considered normal in subjects over 80. When performing visual rating of age-related WML, the differentiations towards MS-plaque, edema/gliosis of tumors, intracerebral bleedings, brain infarcts, infections, and trauma must be clarified before rating.

There are two validated rating scales for detection and evaluation of the distribution of CMBs, Brain Observer MicroBleed scale BOMBS and the Microbleed Anatomical Rating scale [22, 23]. In both scales microbleeds are detected and counted, both to give an

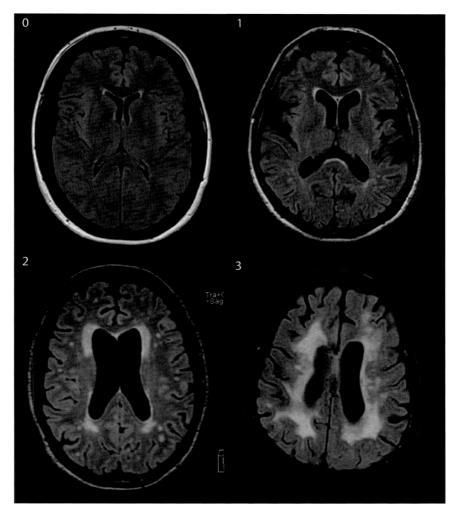

Fig. 3 Fazekas scale for white matter lesions. 0 represents a lack of lesions and 3 is the most severely affected form

overall and regional estimate (Fig. 4). There are also guidelines for how to avoid structures mimicking CMB. Both scales report fairly good intra and inter reliability. Detailed rating procedures and rating forms can be found in the previously published studies [22, 23].

3 Amyloid Related Imaging Abnormalities (ARIAs)

The ARIA work group has written recommendations for monitoring ARIAs in clinical trials [12]. In these recommendations both vasogenic edema and microhemorraghes are considered.

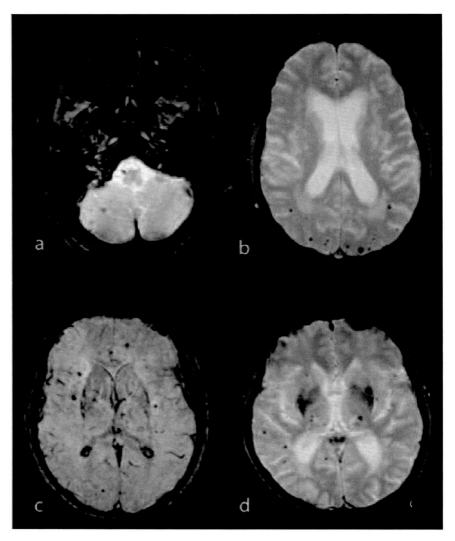

Fig. 4 Images of cerebral microbleeds. These are seen as *small black rounded spots* and represent accumulated hemosiderin. T2* (**a**, **b**, **d**) and SWI (**c**) weighted images

A minimum standard MR protocol is suggested and magnetic field strengths of 1.5T or more are recommended. Moreover, a susceptibility sensitive sequence is needed; either T2* or SWI to detect bleedings or T2 FLAIR to detect edema. The work group recognizes that there still are limited data available regarding the risks in patients with evidence of CMB at baseline—both with respect to amyloid modifying and amyloid lowering therapies. Nevertheless, they recommend that four or more CMBs at baseline should be an exclusion criterion for such trials.

4   Manual Outlining

Manual outlining has for a long time been considered as the most accurate way of measuring the volume of different structures in the brain and it is still regarded as the golden standard [24]. A manual evaluation can be performed in several ways and the most common form is to draw a line around the region of interest in all the contiguous slices where the region can be observed in the 3D MR image. Other methods, such as stereological point counting techniques, can also be used [25]. The main limitations with manual outlining are that it is very time-consuming and requires a skilled tracer. Due to the anatomical variations in individual brain structures the operator needs to be very experienced. There can also be significant differences between different raters. Therefore, intra- and inter-rater reliability has to be carefully calculated to ensure high quality volumetric measures.

Many validated protocols for manual segmentation exist for different regions involved in AD, such as entorhinal cortex [26], hippocampus [27], and intracranial volume [28]. Entorhinal cortex is thought be affected at an early stage, probably earlier than hippocampus, but volumetric measurements of this region are not likely to provide any additional information [29]. With the increasing availability of high fields MRI scanners (3T and 7T), even smaller structures can be measured such as the subfields in hippocampus (e.g., CA1, CA4, dentate gyrus, and subiculum). Evidence points at a selective vulnerability of hippocampal subfield in AD [30]. However, diagnostic use of measuring subfields is probably limited to small selective samples and the clinical relevance of these measures is still unclear [31].

Hippocampal volumetry is today the most established volumetric biomarker used for the AD diagnosis and it has also been shown to predict future conversion from MCI to AD with high accuracy [32]. By using manually delineated hippocampal volumes a clear separation between healthy individuals and AD subjects with a volume reduction of up 40 % have consistently been observed. Clear reductions have also been seen in MCI subjects compared to healthy individuals, albeit less pronounced [33, 34]. Due to the time-consuming nature of the method and other problems mentioned above, it is not likely to become a tool routinely used in clinical practice. However, the measurement of hippocampal volumes has the potential to be used in diagnostic studies, clinical trials, and to validate automated algorithms for hippocampal segmentation.

Different protocols for hippocampal segmentation exist in the literature. These protocols are developed in different research environments, following heterogeneous procedures. The consequence is that slightly different volumetric measurements are obtained due to the use of different anatomical boundaries. This makes it difficult to compare results across studies and validate automated segmentation algorithms. To solve this problem an effort has been launched to harmonize hippocampal segmentation by leading international specialists. The resulting protocol (EADC-ADNI (European Alzheimer's Disease Consortium-Alzheimer's Disease Neuroimaging Initiative) Harmonized Hippocampal Protocol) will be used as gold standard [35]. Further, the European Medicine Agency (EMA) has endorsed a qualification process for enrichment of study samples with the help of low hippocampal volume as a biomarker. Due to the consistent findings which have been observed in both AD dementia and prodromal AD [36], reduction of hippocampal volume, as measured by MRI, is now included in both the International Working Group (IWG) criteria and the National Institute of Ageing (NIA) and the Alzheimer's Association (AA) criteria as one of the most important biomarkers for AD. The assessment of hippocampal volume has now been used as a secondary endpoint [36] in several clinical trials on potential disease modifiers, including muscarinic receptor antagonists [37], glutamate modulators [38], and immunotherapy [39].

5 Automated Measures

In recent years, many automated and semi-automated techniques have been developed and enhanced for analyzing high-resolution structural MRI data to detect regional and global changes in brain structure. Software packages such as FreeSurfer (http://surfer.nmr.mgh.harvard.edu/), FSL (http://fsl.fmrib.ox.ac.uk/), and SPM (http://www.fil.ion.ucl.ac.uk/spm/) are advanced tools for analyzing structural changes. These software are today mainly used in research, but there are also automated programs which have already been approved to be marketed as medical devices by the US Food and Drug Administration (FDA).

The main purpose of these advanced methods is to quantify different measures of the brain, such as size, shape, volume, and thickness. The output can vary from single voxels, to regions of interest (ROIs) from cortical to subcortical structures, or whole brain. The measures should be accurate with as little manual intervention as possible and reflect the most relevant disease patterns. These methods consist of several steps for image-processing and statistical analysis and they provide a wide range of potential applications. The most common techniques produce volumetric and thickness measurement or morphometric assessments.

Many of these methods are hypothesis driven approaches [40–42] which focus on selective regions, such as the hippocampus (Fig. 5), entorhinal cortex, and other medial temporal lobe structures as well as other regions across the brain. Both automated

a   b

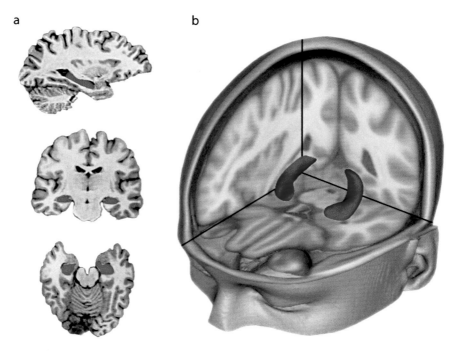

Fig. 5 Automatically generated volume of hippocampus (**a**) sagittal, coronal, and axial views (**b**) 3D view. Image kindly provided by Daniel Ferreira

segmentation of multiple brain regions as well as single region assessments can be performed. For example, automated analyses of hippocampus have been shown to produce similar diagnostic sensitivity/specificity and anatomic accuracy compared to what can be seen with manual measures [31]. There are also automated segmentation algorithms for segmenting the subfield of hippocampus [43] but, as mentioned previously, the clinical relevance of these are still unclear. Further, since the hippocampus has been shown to be affected in many neurodegenerative disorders purely volumetric measurements may not help to differentiate between the different diseases. For this purpose purely data-driven methods have been developed to investigate the shape of regions rather than the total volume. It has been demonstrated that with the help of shape analysis it is possible to differentiate between different disorders where no absolute differences in volume could be observed [44]. However, choosing software focusing on single regions may not be optimal. It may potentially be better to choose software which allow the automated parcellation of multiple anatomic regions across the brain. Such an approach is better modeling the typical pattern of AD atrophy, which spread from the medial temporal structures to the temporoparietal neocortex. In addition, it is more likely to also detect changes in AD patients with a more atypical pattern of atrophy, with minimal involvement of the hippocampus [45]. In recent years, software for automated segmentation of

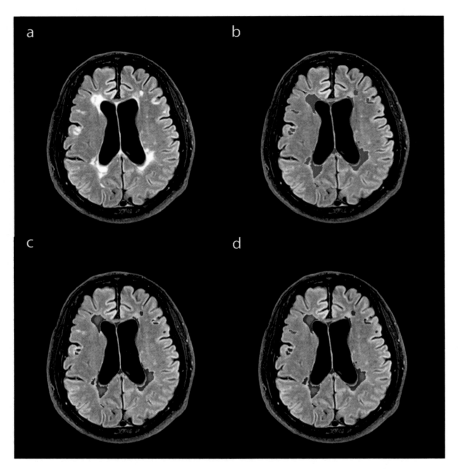

Fig. 6 White matter lesions. (**a**) original FLAIR image (**b**) manual traced white matter lesions, (**c**) automated segmentation of white matter lesions using CASADE, (**d**) comparison between manual and automated segmentation. As can be observed, there is a good agreement between manual and automated measures. Image kindly provided by Soheil Damangir

white matter lesions (Fig. 6) have also been developed [46]. Further, more advanced and novel imaging methods, may potentially allow us to measure the volume of the cholinergic nuclei of the basal forebrain or the *locus coeruleus* are under development. A selective involvement of these subcortical regions has been suggested in AD [31, 36].

Several additional techniques describe and distinguish the macroscopic shape and neuroanatomical differences between different brains and have been used to study structural differences between groups (voxel-based morphometry (VBM), deformation-based morphometry (DBM), or tensor-based morphometry (TBM)). For example, VBM in its simplest form is a voxel-wise statistical method that computes differences in the local brain structure between two groups of subjects [40]. Most commonly, differences in gray matter are investigated, but differences in white matter and CSF can be calculated as well. VBM has still not been validated in respect of the underlying neurobiological changes, but the method has been widely used and similar results have been observed in different studies. The typical AD pattern of cortical atrophy in the medial and lateral cortices has been consistently reported. Further, this analysis technique seems to be robust even if different scanners and processing approaches are used [31].

Not only measurements of hippocampal volumes have been used in clinical trials. Whole brain volume has also been used as a secondary endpoint [39, 47], although this measure has become less common nowadays with the development of regional and specific measurements. Longitudinal measures of atrophy patterns have also begun to be used in clinical trials [48].

6   Patterns of Atrophy and Disease

Modern neuroimaging, with the development of automated tools for the generation of multiple volumetric and cortical thickness measures or other types of high dimensional data, has great potential. However, these methods produce large amounts of data which have to be analyzed in an efficient way. Therefore, different multivariate and machine learning techniques have been developed. The methods provide the opportunity to analyze many variables simultaneously and observe inherent patterns in the data, which are difficult to observe with traditional statistical methods. Further, it is important to take advantage of all the information that is generated. Research has for many years focused on studying or searching for a single region/measure, such as the volume of hippocampus. Due to the complexity and heterogeneity of AD and other neurodegenerative disorders this is probably not enough. For this reason, many recent neuroimaging studies have focused on finding patterns of atrophy, based on the assumption that neurodegeneration is associated with systematic changes in brain structure. Analyzing patterns of disease, utilizing information from the entire brain and combining the different brain regions, have shown promising results both for AD classification and for predicting conversion from mild cognitive impairment (MCI) to AD [49–52]. These methods allow us to separate groups, determine the factors that cause the separation, and make predictive models of disease. Such models can potentially be used for early diagnosis, to monitor disease progression, or as an outcome measure in clinical trials to ensure an optimal recruitment of subjects for clinical trials.

Many different methods have been used and developed for multivariate data analysis and machine learning. The most commonly used technique in the AD literature is support vector machines (SVM) [53, 54], but there are many other methods which has been utilized such as orthogonal partial least squares to latent structures (OPLS) [55] and linear discriminant analysis (LDA) [56]. However, it seems that most techniques are sufficient for the different problems and produce similar results [57] The limitations are probably a cause of the input data for analysis such as image quality, image segmentation, the cohort studied, and the clinical diagnosis [57].

Several studies have shown that multivariate data analysis and machine learning can predict future conversion from MCI to AD. Such data indicate that AD can be detected already at the prodromal stages of the disease, before clinical manifestation. These techniques can also be used to combine different imaging techniques and to combine imaging data with different biomarkers measured in blood and cerebrospinal fluid (CSF). Further, clinical data and information from neuropsychological test can also be incorporated, which means the analysis can be extended from investigating pattern of atrophy to patterns of disease. Several studies have combined different biomarkers, e.g., MRI measures, CSF markers, and positron emission tomography (PET) measures [54, 55, 58]. To combine different biomarkers investigating patterns of disease may prove to be useful since the different biomarkers reflect different but connected aspects of AD. It is however important to investigate the optimal combination of biomarkers, particularly for predicting future MCI conversion to AD. Further, incorporation of clinical and neuropsychological test measures has to be done in a proper way to avoid circularity and over-fitting. It is also very important that the different multivariate/machine learning techniques are carefully validated and tested against conventional diagnostics in a clinical setting where the population is more heterogeneous than in a research cohort with strict inclusion and exclusion criteria. Several studies have utilized multivariate techniques to create indices or scores to describe pattern of disease, which can potentially be very useful and serves as a diagnostic aid in clinical practice or to target homogeneous population for clinical trials [51, 59]. Heterogeneous populations may be one potential factor for the failure of many clinical trials. Several treatment strategies are currently being explored with the goal to significantly slow down and prevent the disease. Due to the complexity and heterogeneity of AD and other neurodegenerative disorders it is probably not enough to use a battery of cognitive tests for early episodic memory impairment as inclusion criteria for clinical trials. A combination of different biomarkers, possibly condensed to an index, which reflects different aspects of the disease may be needed to include a more homogenous group. For this reason, multivariate techniques applied to structural MRI in combination with other biomarkers are interesting and potentially exciting avenues to consider in the future.

7 Conclusions

Structural neuroimaging is today an integrated part in routine clinical work and is included in the new diagnostic criteria for AD [60, 61]. Neuroimaging is also a key component in clinical trials and it can be used to target the right population, for safety monitoring as well as an outcome measure. The role of visual assessment will probably only be used for safety monitoring (microbleeds) or as an inclusion/exclusion criterion (white matter lesions), since the scales for brain atrophy are probably to crude to use in clinical trials. Volumetry has already been used as a secondary endpoint in several clinical trials. Automated measures of hippocampus and brain atrophy patterns are likely to become more common in the near future as primary or secondary endpoints in disease modifying clinical trials. The changes which can be observed using MRI are today much more sensitive and small changes can be observed in volumes and cortical thickness The structural imaging markers are closely associated with the underlying changes of neuronal integrity [62]. For this reason they will play an important role in the search for biological markers for disease modification.

References

1. Braak H, Braak E (1991) Neuropathological stageing of Alzheimer-related changes. Acta Neuropathol 82(4):239–259

2. Jack CR Jr, Petersen RC, Xu Y et al (1998) Rate of medial temporal lobe atrophy in typical aging and Alzheimer's disease. Neurology 51(4):993–999

3. Jack CR Jr, Petersen RC, Xu YC et al (1997) Medial temporal atrophy on MRI in normal aging and very mild Alzheimer's disease. Neurology 49(3):786–794

4. de Souza LC, Chupin M, Bertoux M et al (2013) Is hippocampal volume a good marker to differentiate Alzheimer's disease from frontotemporal dementia? J Alzheimers Dis 36(1):57–66. doi:10.3233/JAD-122293

5. Laakso MP, Partanen K, Riekkinen P et al (1996) Hippocampal volumes in Alzheimer's disease, Parkinson's disease with and without dementia, and in vascular dementia: An MRI study. Neurology 46(3):678–681

6. Scheltens P, Leys D, Barkhof F et al (1992) Atrophy of medial temporal lobes on MRI in "probable" Alzheimer's disease and normal ageing: diagnostic value and neuropsychological correlates. J Neurol Neurosurg Psychiatry 55(10):967–972

7. Koedam EL, Lehmann M, van der Flier WM et al (2011) Visual assessment of posterior atrophy development of a MRI rating scale. Eur Radiol 21(12):2618–2625. doi:10.1007/s00330-011-2205-4

8. Pasquier F, Leys D, Weerts JG et al (1996) Inter- and intraobserver reproducibility of cerebral atrophy assessment on MRI scans with hemispheric infarcts. Eur Neurol 36(5):268–272

9. Westman E, Cavallin L, Muehlboeck JS et al (2011) Sensitivity and specificity of medial temporal lobe visual ratings and multivariate regional MRI classification in Alzheimer's disease. PLoS ONE 6(7), e22506. doi:10.1371/journal.pone.0022506, PONE-D-11-06805 [pii]

10. Boche D, Zotova E, Weller RO et al (2008) Consequence of Abeta immunization on the vasculature of human Alzheimer's disease brain. Brain 131(Pt 12):3299–3310. doi:10.1093/brain/awn261

11. Orgogozo JM, Gilman S, Dartigues JF et al (2003) Subacute meningoencephalitis in a subset of patients with AD after Abeta42 immunization. Neurology 61(1):46–54

12. Sperling RA, Jack CR Jr, Black SE et al (2011) Amyloid-related imaging abnormalities in amyloid-modifying therapeutic trials: recommendations from the Alzheimer's Association Research Roundtable Workgroup. Alzheimers

Dement 7(4):367–385. doi:10.1016/j.jalz.2011.05.2351

13. Wahlund LO, Julin P, Johansson SE et al (2000) Visual rating and volumetry of the medial temporal lobe on magnetic resonance imaging in dementia: a comparative study. J Neurol Neurosurg Psychiatry 69(5):630–635

14. Wahlund LO, Julin P, Lindqvist J et al (1999) Visual assessment of medical temporal lobe atrophy in demented and healthy control subjects: correlation with volumetry. Psychiatry Res 90(3):193–199

15. Scheltens P, Launer LJ, Barkhof F et al (1995) Visual assessment of medial temporal lobe atrophy on magnetic resonance imaging: interobserver reliability. J Neurol 242(9):557–560

16. Cavallin L, Bronge L, Zhang Y et al (2012) Comparison between visual assessment of MTA and hippocampal volumes in an elderly, non-demented population. Acta Radiol 53(5):573–579. doi:10.1258/ar.2012.110664

17. Pereira JB, Cavallin L, Spulber G et al (2013) Influence of age, disease onset and ApoE4 on visual medial temporal lobe atrophy cut-offs. J Intern Med. doi:10.1111/joim.12148

18. Karas G, Scheltens P, Rombouts S et al (2007) Precuneus atrophy in early-onset alzheimer's disease: a morphometric structural MRI study. Neuroradiology 49(12):967–976. doi:10.1007/s00234-007-0269-2

19. Wahlund LO, Barkhof F, Fazekas F et al (2001) A new rating scale for age-related white matter changes applicable to MRI and CT. Stroke 32(6):1318–1322. doi:10.1161/01.str.32.6.1318

20. Fazekas F, Chawluk JB, Alavi A et al (1987) MR signal abnormalities at 1.5 T in Alzheimer's dementia and normal aging. Am J Roentgenol 149(2):351–356. doi:10.2214/ajr.149.2.351

21. Inzitari D, Pracucci G, Poggesi A et al. (2009) Changes in white matter as determinant of global functional decline in older independent outpatients: three year follow-up of LADIS (leukoaraiosis and disability) study cohort. BMJ 339:b2477. doi:10.1136/bmj.b2477

22. Cordonnier C, Potter GM, Jackson CA et al (2009) Improving interrater agreement about brain microbleeds: development of the Brain Observer MicroBleed Scale (BOMBS). Stroke 40(1):94–99. doi:10.1161/STROKEAHA.108.526996

23. Gregoire SM, Chaudhary UJ, Brown MM et al (2009) The microbleed anatomical rating scale (MARS): reliability of a tool to map brain microbleeds. Neurology 73(21):1759–1766. doi:10.1212/WNL.0b013e3181c34a7d

24. Hampel H, Bürger K, Teipel SJ et al (2008) Core candidate neurochemical and imaging biomarkers of Alzheimer's disease. Alzheimers Dement 4(1):38–48

25. Howard MA, Roberts N, Garcia-Finana M et al (2003) Volume estimation of prefrontal cortical subfields using MRI and stereology. Brain Res Brain Res Protoc 10(3):125–138

26. Goncharova II, Dickerson BC, Stoub TR et al (2001) MRI of human entorhinal cortex: a reliable protocol for volumetric measurement. Neurobiol Aging 22(5):737–745

27. Jack CR Jr, Theodore WH, Cook M et al (1995) MRI-based hippocampal volumetrics: data acquisition, normal ranges, and optimal protocol. Magn Reson Imaging 13(8):1057–1064

28. Eritaia J, Wood SJ, Stuart GW et al (2000) An optimized method for estimating intracranial volume from magnetic resonance images. Magn Reson Med 44(6):973–977

29. Teipel SJ, Pruessner JC, Faltraco F et al (2006) Comprehensive dissection of the medial temporal lobe in AD: measurement of hippocampus, amygdala, entorhinal, perirhinal and parahippocampal cortices using MRI. J Neurol 253(6):794–800. doi:10.1007/s00415-006-0120-4

30. Giannakopoulos P, Kovari E, Gold G et al (2009) Pathological substrates of cognitive decline in Alzheimer's disease. Front Neurol Neurosci 24:20–29. doi:10.1159/000197881

31. Teipel SJ, Grothe M, Lista S et al (2013) Relevance of magnetic resonance imaging for early detection and diagnosis of Alzheimer disease. Med Clin N Am 97(3):399–424. doi:10.1016/j.mcna.2012.12.013, http://dx.doi.org

32. Jack CR Jr, Petersen RC, Xu YC et al (1999) Prediction of AD with MRI-based hippocampal volume in mild cognitive impairment. Neurology 52(7):1397–1403

33. Convit A, De Leon MJ, Tarshish C et al (1997) Specific hippocampal volume reductions in individuals at risk for Alzheimer's disease. Neurobiol Aging 18(2):131–138

34. Killiany RJ, Moss MB, Albert MS et al (1993) Temporal lobe regions on magnetic resonance imaging identify patients with early Alzheimer's disease. Arch Neurol 50(9):949–954

35. Frisoni GB, Jack CR (2011) Harmonization of magnetic resonance-based manual hippocampal segmentation: a mandatory step for wide clinical use. Alzheimers Dement 7(2):171–174. doi:10.1016/j.jalz.2010.06.007

36. Hampel H, Lista S, Teipel SJ et al (2014) Perspective on future role of biological markers in clinical therapy trials of Alzheimer's disease: a long-range point of view beyond 2020. Biochem Pharmacol 88(4):426–449. doi:10.1016/j.bcp.2013.11.009

37. Jack CR, Slomkowski M, Gracon S et al (2003) MRI as a biomarker of disease progression in a therapeutic trial of milameline for AD. Neurology 60(2):253–260. doi:10.1212/01.wnl.0000042480.86872.03

38. Wilkinson D, Fox NC, Barkhof F et al (2012) Memantine and brain atrophy in Alzheimer's disease: a 1-year randomized controlled trial. J Alzheimers Dis 29(2):459–469. doi:10.3233/JAD-2011-111616

39. Fox NC, Black RS, Gilman S et al (2005) Effects of Aβ immunization (AN1792) on MRI measures of cerebral volume in Alzheimer disease. Neurology 64(9):1563–1572. doi:10.1212/01.wnl.0000159743.08996.99

40. Ashburner J, Friston KJ (2000) Voxel-based morphometry—the methods. Neuroimage 11(6 Pt 1):805–821. doi:10.1006/nimg.2000.0582

41. Desikan RS, Ségonne F, Fischl B et al (2006) An automated labeling system for subdividing the human cerebral cortex on MRI scans into gyral based regions of interest. Neuroimage 31(3):968–980

42. Fischl B, van der Kouwe A, Destrieux C et al (2004) Automatically parcellating the human cerebral cortex. Cereb Cortex 14(1):11–22

43. Hanseeuw BJ, Van Leemput K, Kavec M et al (2011) Mild cognitive impairment: differential atrophy in the hippocampal subfields. Am J Neuroradiol 32(9):1658–1661. doi:10.3174/ajnr.A2589

44. Lindberg O, Walterfang M, Looi JC et al (2012) Hippocampal shape analysis in Alzheimer's disease and frontotemporal lobar degeneration subtypes. J Alzheimers Dis 30(2):355–365. doi:10.3233/JAD-2012-112210

45. Whitwell JL, Dickson DW, Murray ME et al (2012) Neuroimaging correlates of pathologically defined subtypes of Alzheimer's disease: a case-control study. Lancet Neurol 11(10):868–877. doi:10.1016/S1474-4422(12)70200-4

46. Damangir S, Manzouri A, Oppedal K et al (2012) Multispectral MRI segmentation of age related white matter changes using a cascade of support vector machines. J Neurol Sci 322(1-2):211–216. doi:10.1016/j.jns.2012.07.064

47. Smith AD, Smith SM, de Jager CA et al (2010) Homocysteine-lowering by B vitamins slows the rate of accelerated brain atrophy in mild cognitive impairment: a randomized controlled trial. PLoS One 5(9), e12244. doi:10.1371/journal.pone.0012244

48. Douaud G, Refsum H, de Jager CA et al (2013) Preventing Alzheimer's disease-related gray matter atrophy by B-vitamin treatment. Proc Natl Acad Sci U S A 110(23):9523–9528. doi:10.1073/pnas.1301816110

49. Cuingnet R, Gerardin E, Tessieras J et al (2011) Automatic classification of patients with Alzheimer's disease from structural Magnetic Resonance Imaging (MRI): a comparison of ten methods using the ADNI database. Neuroimage 56(2):766–781. doi:10.1016/j.neuroimage.2010.06.013, doi:S1053-8119(10)00857-8 [pii]

50. Davatzikos C, Bhatt P, Shaw LM et al. (2011) Prediction of MCI to AD conversion, via MRI, CSF biomarkers, and pattern classification. Neurobiol Aging. doi:S0197-4580(10)00237-X [pii], 10.1016/j.neurobiolaging.2010.05.023

51. Spulber G, Simmons A, Muehlboeck JS et al (2013) An MRI-based index to measure the severity of Alzheimer's disease-like structural pattern in subjects with mild cognitive impairment. J Intern Med 273(4):396–409. doi:10.1111/joim.12028

52. Westman E, Simmons A, Muehlboeck JS et al (2011) AddNeuroMed and ADNI: similar patterns of Alzheimer's atrophy and automated MRI classification accuracy in Europe and North America. Neuroimage 58(3):818–828. doi:10.1016/j.neuroimage.2011.06.065, doi:S1053-8119(11)00711-7 [pii]

53. Davatzikos C, Fan Y, Wu X et al (2008) Detection of prodromal Alzheimer's disease via pattern classification of magnetic resonance imaging. Neurobiol Aging 29(4):514–523. doi:10.1016/j.neurobiolaging.2006.11.010, doi:S0197-4580(06)00429-5 [pii]

54. Zhang D, Wang Y, Zhou L et al (2011) Multimodal classification of Alzheimer's disease and mild cognitive impairment. Neuroimage 55(3):856–867

55. Westman E, Muehlboeck JS, Simmons A (2012) Combining MRI and CSF measures for classification of Alzheimer's disease and prediction of mild cognitive impairment conversion. Neuroimage 62(1):229–238. doi:10.1016/j.neuroimage.2012.04.056, doi:S1053-8119(12)00452-1 [pii]

56. McEvoy LK, Fennema-Notestine C, Roddey JC et al. (2009) Alzheimer disease: quantitative structural neuroimaging for detection and prediction of clinical and structural changes in mild cognitive impairment. Radiology:2511080924. doi:10.1148/radiol.2511080924

57. Falahati F, Westman E, Simmons A (2014) Multivariate data analysis and machine learning in Alzheimer's disease with a focus on structural magnetic resonance imaging. J Alzheimers Dis 41(3):685–708. doi:10.3233/JAD-131928

58. Walhovd KB, Fjell AM, Brewer J et al (2010) Combining MR imaging, positron-emission tomography, and CSF biomarkers in the diagnosis and prognosis of Alzheimer disease. Am J Neuroradiol 31(2):347–354. doi:10.3174/ajnr.A1809, doi:ajnr.A1809 [pii]

59. Mattila J, Koikkalainen J, Virkki A et al (2011) A disease state fingerprint for evaluation of Alzheimer's disease. J Alzheimers Dis 27(1):163–176. doi:10.3233/JAD-2011-110365

60. Dubois B, Feldman HH, Jacova C et al (2007) Research criteria for the diagnosis of Alzheimer's disease: revising the NINCDS-ADRDA criteria. Lancet Neurol 6(8):734–746

61. McKhann GM, Knopman DS, Chertkow H et al (2011) The diagnosis of dementia due to Alzheimer's disease: recommendations from the National Institute on Aging-Alzheimer's Association workgroups on diagnostic guidelines for Alzheimer's disease. Alzheimers Dement 7(3):263–269. doi:10.1016/j.jalz.2011.03.005, doi:S1552-5260(11)00101-4 [pii]

62. Zarow C, Vinters HV, Ellis WG et al (2005) Correlates of hippocampal neuron number in Alzheimer's disease and ischemic vascular dementia. Ann Neurol 57(6):896–903. doi:10.1002/ana.20503

Chapter 13

PET Imaging as a Diagnostic Tool in Alzheimer's Disease

Juha O. Rinne

Abstract

There is a long presymptomatic period during which a person may have biomarker evidence of Alzheimer's disease (AD) pathophysiology but still be cognitively intact. It is yet unclear which additional factors that ultimately will determine progression to mild cognitive impairment and eventually to AD dementia. Amyloid-β (Aβ) and tau imaging reveal in vivo the key protein aggregates seen in the AD brain and will help in early diagnosis. However, a considerable proportion of elderly individuals are Aβ PET positive while being cognitively intact. With FDG PET, a typical pattern of hypometabolism can be found in both AD and FTD, which reflects the disease progression and can be used to aid in the differential diagnostics. Moreover, tau, neurotransmitter, and neuroinflammation ligands help to understand the pathophysiology of AD, but further studies are needed to understand how they can be applied in the diagnostic process. Which combination of these biomarkers that eventually will turn out to be the most sensitive and best predictor of AD remains to be determined.

Key words Alzheimer's disease, Amyloid, Dementia, Diagnosis, Diagnostic, FDG, Neuroinflammation, Neurotransmitter, PET, Positron emission tomography, Tau

1 Introduction

Positron emission tomography (PET) is a functional imaging technique for the versatile investigation of various brain functions such as blood flow, glucose metabolism, neurotransmitter function, and neuroinflammation. In addition, PET allows visualization of protein aggregates (such as amyloid-β (Aβ) and tau).

In Alzheimer's disease (AD) PET can be used to help in the diagnostics and differential diagnostics of different dementing diseases, to investigate the pathophysiology, to follow disease progression, to identify individuals at an asymptomatic stage, and to monitor treatment effects.

Clinically, AD is characterized by progressive impairment of episodic memory. Gradually there is also impairment of other cognitive domains leading to impairment in the activities of daily living. The typical pathological hallmarks of the disease are extracellular Aβ plaques and intraneuronal paired helical filaments

Martin Ingelsson and Lars Lannfelt (eds.), *Immunotherapy and Biomarkers in Neurodegenerative Disorders*, Methods in Pharmacology and Toxicology, DOI 10.1007/978-1-4939-3560-4_13, © Springer Science+Business Media New York 2016

Table 1
The potential use of PET in Alzheimer's disease

Pathophysiology
Diagnostics/differential diagnostics
Follow-up
Detection of asymptomatic cases
Development of treatment
– Proof-of-concept
– Dose selection
– Selection of study participants
Evaluation of treatment effects

(neurofibrillary tangles) that contain hyperphosphorylated tau. These changes have a typical order of temporal and anatomical progression [1–3]. Other pathophysiological processes in the AD brain include inflammation, astrocytosis, microgliosis, apoptosis, and necrosis. These processes finally lead to synaptic and neuronal dysfunction followed by neuronal death. The exact relationship and interplay between these processes is unclear at present. According to some theories, brain amyloid accumulation is considered to be an early pathological event of the AD process and the earliest changes are found even years before the onset of symptoms [4, 5].

The diagnostic workup of an individual with memory complaint includes clinical investigation, cognitive testing, laboratory examinations, and structural brain imaging (computerized tomography (CT) or magnetic resonance imaging (MRI)). In special situations cerebrospinal fluid (CSF) investigation or functional brain imaging (single photon emission tomography (SPET) or PET) may be used.

The characteristic clinical course and the typical pathological changes have been guiding the search for PET imaging markers to enable early detection of the pathophysiological process in AD The potential use of PET in AD is listed in Table 1.

2 Glucose Metabolism

Fluorodeoxyglucose (2-[^{18}F] fluoro-2-deoxy-d-glucose, FDG) is an [^{18}F] labeled analog of glucose which enters neurons by glucose transporter molecules. In neurons, FDG is converted by hexokinase enzyme to FDG-6-phosphate which has a structure that prevents it from entering the next steps of glycolysis.

Thus FDG "gets trapped" into metabolically active cells as FDG-6-phosphate which can be detected by PET. Since neurons use glucose as their main source of energy, FDG uptake is an indirect reflection of neuronal and synaptic functioning. In AD reduced FDG uptake is thought to reflect loss of synaptic activity and density [6, 7]. In a baboon study [8] in vivo glucose metabolism evaluated by PET was associated with post mortem levels of synaptophysin, which is a marker of synaptic density. In FDG PET patients with AD typically show symmetrical temporo-parietal hypometabolism [9–12]. In earlier studies the presence of early hippocampal hypometabolism was controversial, partly due to the small size of the structure and other technical issues. The use of different co-registration and/or anatomical masking techniques to explore hippocampus has revealed early hypometabolism in AD [10, 13–15]. Figure 1 shows a typical pattern of hypometabolism in a patient with AD. Similar changes have been detected also in patients with mild cognitive impairment (MCI) and in healthy individuals carrying the apolipoprotein E epsilon 4 (ApoEε4) allele, especially in ApoEε4 homozygotes [16, 17] and in healthy

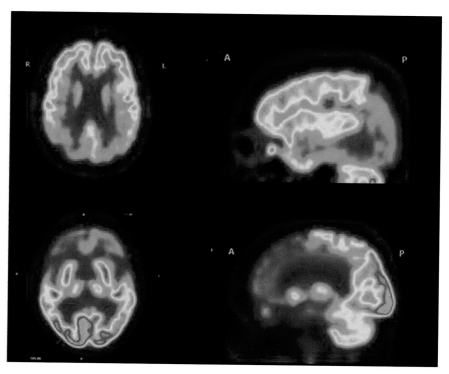

Fig. 1 Examples of axial (*left*) and sagittal (*right*) [^{18}F]FDG images in a patient with Alzheimer's disease (AD, *upper panel*) and in a patient with frontotemporal dementia (FTD, *lower panel*). Note the temporal-parietal hypometabolism in the AD patient and the frontal (and to some extent anterior temporal) hypometabolism in the patient with FTD. *A* anterior, *P* posterior, *R* right, *L* left

elderly individuals with familial (especially maternal) history for AD [18]. This kind of hypometabolism in brain areas typically affected in AD in healthy elderly has been shown to predict future cognitive decline [13, 19].

The largest study with *postmortem* neuropathological verification of diagnosis [20]. included 138 patients (97 had AD, 23 had other degenerative dementia and 18 had no degenerative dementia). The presence of cortical hypometabolism had an 88 % accuracy to identify AD (sensitivity 94 %, specificity 73 %). In addition, similar figures were obtained in a subpopulation of patients who had questionable or mild dementia [20].

In other dementing disease the regional pattern of hypometabolism is different. In frontotemporal dementia (FTD) hypometabolism is more severe in the frontal and anterior and/or mesiotemporal structures as compared to the parietotemporal cortex. Moreover, the primary visual and sensorimotor cortices are usually preserved. This prominent "frontal" pattern of hypometabolism in FTD as compared to the primarily "posterior" (parieto-temporal) hypometabolism in AD (12, 21, 22, Fig. 1) has led to the approval by the Food and Drug Administration (FDA) of FDG PET for the differential diagnostics between FTD and AD.

In dementia with Lewy bodies (DLB) FDG PET deficits in general resemble those seen in AD, but with additional involvement of the occipital primary cortex and cerebellum [23–26] (Fig. 2). A study showed that neuropathologically confirmed DLB cases had clear hypometabolism in the occipital cortex, especially in the primary visual cortex, a region which is relatively spared in AD [24]. The regional differences in PET FDG retention could discriminate AD from DLB with 90 % sensitivity and 80 % specificity [23].

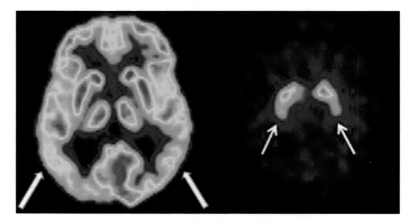

Fig. 2 An example of axial [¹⁸F]FDG PET (*left*) and DATSCAN (dopamine transporter) SPET (*right*) in a patient with dementia with Lewy bodies (DLB). Note the bilateral occipital hypometabolism (*thick arrows*) and reduced striatal dopamine transporter function, especially in the putamina (*thin arrows*)

In vascular dementia there is no specific pattern of hypometabolism, since the location of hypometabolic areas depends on the location of ischemic changes. Therefore, the hypometabolism in vascular dementia is usually "patchy" or diffuse and also often involves subcortical and cerebellar areas, which are usually spared in AD [27, 28]. A metabolic ratio between the regions typically affected in AD to those typically non-affected in AD was found to separate AD and vascular dementia with 75 % sensitivity and 53 % specificity [28].

Parkinson's disease (PD) is often accompanied by cognitive problems and a vast majority of patients show at least some degree of impairment with a prevalence of dementia four to six times higher than in healthy controls [29, 30]. At 15 years follow-up cognitive decline was present in 84 % and 48 % fulfilled the criteria for dementia. At 20 years follow-up dementia was present in 83 % of remaining participants [30, 31]. In general, PD patients with MCI (PD-MCI) show hypometabolism as compared to healthy controls and the reduction in FDG uptake is more severe and widespread in demented PD patients [32–36]. As compared to healthy controls a decreased FDG uptake in the frontal lobe and, to a lesser extent, also in parietal areas has been reported among PD-MCI subjects [36]. Furthermore, patients with PD-dementia show hypometabolism in the parietal, occipital, and temporal areas and a less severe reduction in the frontal lobes compared with both healthy controls and PD-MCI patients. This hypometabolism was found to be associated with impairments in visuospatial, memory, and executive functions [36].

3   Neurotransmitter Function

Impairment of brain cholinergic function is the most common and consistent neurochemical abnormality seen in the brains of patients with AD and can, to a smaller degree, be seen already at the MCI stage [37–39]. However, although AD patients show impaired activity of the acetylcholinesterase enzyme (AChE) with PET, PD dementia patients can show an even greater reduction in AChE activity [40].

There are also deficiencies of other neurotransmitters, such as serotonin, noradrenalin, and glutamate, in the AD brain (for a review see Refs. [41–43]. On the other hand various kinds of neurotransmitter deficiencies are also seen in patients with other dementing diseases. Thus, the neurotransmitter system deficits seen with PET in AD are not specific for AD. For this reason, neurotransmitter PET studies are mainly used in research settings and their diagnostic or differential diagnostic value is limited, with the exception of dopamine transporter imaging.

The dopamine transporter (DAT) is a membrane protein that takes part in the presynaptic reuptake of dopamine. Dopamine transporter imaging, either with PET or single photon emission tomography (SPET), is a sensitive method to visualize dopaminergic hypofunction [44, 45]. Apart from PD, there is a clear reduction in nigrostriatal dopaminergic function also in DLB (46, 47, Fig. 2) whereas in AD, typically no changes are found. Therefore, DAT imaging seems to be useful in the differential diagnostics between AD and DLB, which may sometimes be clinically challenging. In a large multicenter study [48], including 326 patients with clinical diagnoses of probable ($n=94$) or possible ($n=57$) DLB or non-DLB dementia ($n=147$), DAT-scan was found to have a mean sensitivity of 77.7 % for detecting clinically probable DLB, with a specificity of 90.4 % for excluding non-DLB dementia (predominantly due to AD). One study showed that the sensitivity and specificity of DAT imaging to differentiate DLB from AD was 88 % and 100 %, as compared to the neuropathological diagnoses [49].

4   Amyloid and Tau Imaging

4.1   Amyloid

The realization that different protein aggregates (Aβ and tau) play a central role in AD pathogenesis prompted investigators to develop in vivo imaging markers to visualize these pathological changes. The first successful human amyloid imaging with PET was published in 2004 and clearly demonstrated that AD patients had a stronger retention of the amyloid-specific ligand [11C]PIB (11C-6-OH-BTA or 11C-Pittsburgh Imaging Compound B) [50]. Subsequent studies have corroborated that patients with AD show a clear increase in [11C]PIB uptake in frontal, parietal, temporal cortices and in the posterior cingulate gyrus in AD [51–57]. At the AD stage there is a relatively small increase (0–3.4 % annually in different studies) in brain Aβ PET ligand uptake [53–57]. The progression of Aβ accumulation in AD patients was influenced by ApoEε4 allele, the progression being highest in ApoEε4 homozygotes [56].

Patients with amnestic MCI have shown signs of either increased or normal levels of Aβ PET tracer uptake [54, 58–60]. Follow-up studies have shown that increased brain Aβ burden at baseline predicts conversion to AD [61], which occurs earlier in individuals with higher Aβ level at baseline [62].

Studies have revealed that, with advancing age, also elderly cognitively normal individuals show an increased Aβ PET tracer uptake in cortex [51, 63–66]. Thus, positive amyloid imaging in an elderly individual indicates the presence of brain amyloidosis, but does not necessarily predict cognitive decline. Thus, it is good to keep in mind that positive amyloid imaging in an elderly individual does not necessarily imply AD. Recently, a published meta-analysis of 2914 individuals with normal cognition showed that Aβ positivity increases from 10 % at the age of 55 years to 44 % at the age of 90 years [67]. Moreover, carriers of the ApoEε4 allele had two to three times higher prevalence estimates than noncarriers.

Since the development of [11C]PIB several new ligands have been developed, also with an ^{18}F label. Labeling the PET tracer with ^{18}F has some practical advantages. The half-life of ^{18}F (around 109 min) is much longer than that for 11C (around 20 min). Therefore, it is possible to manufacture the ligand at one site and ship it to remotely located imaging sites. In addition, it enables cost-saving investigation of several subjects using one synthesis batch. During the last few years three [^{18}F] labeled Aβ imaging tracers, [^{18}F]florbetapir [68], [^{18}F]florbetaben [69], [^{18}F]flutemetamol [70] have been approved by FDA and the European Medicines Agency (EMA) for the diagnostics of AD (an example of [^{18}F]flutemetamol PET scan in a patient with AD and in a healthy control is shown in Fig. 3). One study, using [^{18}F]NAV4694 (former [^{18}F]AZD4694), showed low white matter retention and the cortical binding had a good correlation with that of [11C]PIB

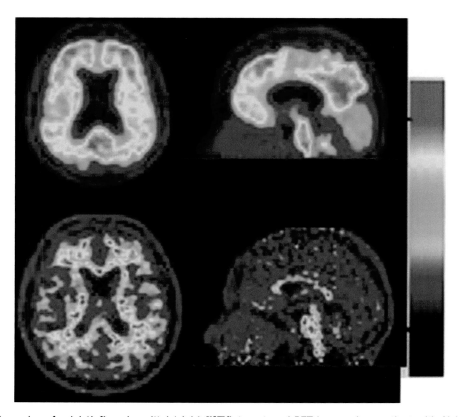

Fig. 3 Examples of axial (*left*) and sagittal (*right*) [^{18}F]flutemetamol PET images in a patient with Alzheimer's disease (AD, *upper panel*) and in a healthy control (*lower panel*). Note the widespread cortical [^{18}F]flutemetamol accumulation in the AD patient (*red color*) and virtual absence of cortical uptake in a healthy age matched volunteer

[71]. Importantly, [^{18}F]NAV4694 was also found to separate AD patients from healthy controls [71, 72].

Another ligand, [^{18}F]FDDNP is a napthol derivative which binds both to Aβ plaques and intracellular tau and has demonstrated increased binding in patients with MCI and AD in relation to healthy controls [73, 74]. In addition, an increased uptake of this ligand has been demonstrated in several neurodegenerative disorders, including primary tauopathies like chronic traumatic encephalopathy, frontotemporal degeneration, or progressive supranuclear palsy (for a review see Refs. 75, 76). However, further studies are needed to determine the ability of FDDNP to discriminate between different neurodegenerative disorders.

It is important to keep in mind that the current Aβ imaging PET tracers bind preferentially or solely to fibrillar Aβ. However, oligomeric or profibrillar forms of Aβ are probably more important species in the pathophysiology of AD and to date there are no PET imaging ligands available to directly visualize these soluble forms of Aβ.

Appropriate criteria for the clinical use of amyloid PET has been published [77] listing indications where amyloid imaging is justified. These include: (1) persistent or unexplained MCI, (2) signs of possible AD with unclear clinical presentation, an atypical clinical course or etiologically mixed presentation, (3) a progressive dementia atypical early age of onset (usually defined as 65 years of age or younger).

4.2 Tau

There are several tau imaging ligands available, for which the clinical utility is under investigation (reviewed in Refs. 76, 78). Of the "THK tau tracer family," [^{18}F]THK5105 and [^{18}F]THK5117 have shown cortical uptake in AD, which is in agreement with the suggested anatomical pattern of tau pathology [79, 80]. The uptake was increased in AD brain as compared to healthy controls and the retention signals were associated with the degree of dementia and the severity of cortical atrophy [79]. Moreover, a higher retention than [11C]PIB could be seen in the medial temporal cortex [80]. Preliminary findings suggest that [^{18}F]THK5351 seems to have faster kinetics and better signal to noise ratio than its predecessors [81]. Another ligand, [^{18}F]T807 was found to show relatively low white matter binding and about 25-fold selectivity for tau over Aβ [82, 83]. Yet another ligand, [^{18}F]T808 has been reported to show more faster kinetics and reaches a steady state concentration during the imaging period [78]. Moreover, the [11C]PBB3 ligand has also shown uptake in the AD hippocampus, which is consistent with the known location of tau deposits [84]. In addition, a patient with corticobasal degeneration showed increased uptake suggesting that this ligand also could visualize tau pathology in non-AD tauopathies.

Development of PET imaging tracers for tau represents a great new achievement in the research of degenerative brain disorders. The present ligands look promising but more studies will be required to evaluate their usefulness in the diagnosis of AD and other non-AD tauopathies.

5 Other Targets

Neuroinflammation may have a central pathogenic role in many neurodegenerative diseases (reviewed in Ref. 85). Microglia may have a dual role in neurodegeneration since they seem to mediate both beneficial and detrimental effects. The most commonly used PET tracers of microglial pathology bind to the translocator protein (TSPO), which is expressed in the outer mitochondrial membrane of activated microglia. Results based on the use of TSPO PET-ligands have so far been conflicting. Some studies have demonstrated an increased signal in frontal, temporal, parietal, occipital, and posterior cingulate cortical areas [86–88], whereas no differences have been detected in other studies [89].

Another ligand, [11C]deuterium-deprenyl [11C]DED, is a marker of monoaminooxidase (MAO) activity, a common enzymatic reaction in astrocytes [90, 91]. In one study [11C]DED binding increased bilaterally in the frontal and parietal cortices of MCI patients, but not in AD patients, as compared to controls. These findings suggest that increased MAO activity may be an early phenomenon in the AD process [92]. Studies regarding neuroinflammation and astrocytosis are important to help us understand the complex pathophysiology of AD, but these processes are nonspecific which may limit their relevance for diagnostic imaging of AD and other neurodegenerative disorders.

6 New Research Criteria for AD

Increasing knowledge of cognitive and biomarker changes in the continuum from normal aging to MCI and AD has lead to suggestions of new clinical criteria for AD, which include the use of biomarkers in the diagnostic algorithm. According to the hypothetical model of biomarker dynamics, the earliest abnormalities in AD process are changes in Aβ and tau [4]. These changes start to develop several years, if not decades, before the first clinical symptoms as suggested by findings in the AIBL study cohort [93].

The two main suggested new clinical research criteria for AD are the International Working Group (IWG-2) criteria [94] and the National Institute on Aging—Alzheimer's Association (NIA-AA) workgroup diagnostic guidelines [95]. These two criteria aim at separating the AD pathophysiological process (that can be detected earlier) from clinical AD dementia. Both criteria are currently meant for research purposes only. There are some differences between the IWG-2 and NIA-AA criteria regarding terminology, required biomarker abnormalities and their application. According to the IWG-2 criteria AD could be diagnosed when a clinical AD phenotype (typical or atypical) is present, together with biomarkers consistent with AD pathology (positive amyloid PET or decreased Aβ and increased tau or phospho tau in cerebrospinal fluid (CSF)). According to these criteria, volumetric changes in brain MRI or changes in FDG PET are regarded as "progression markers" and are considered to better reflect clinical severity and disease progression. Contrary to the IWG-2 criteria, the NIA-AA criteria refer to "AD" as a pathological process regardless of whether the disease is in a symptomatic or asymptomatic stage, In addition, the NIA-AA criteria retain the term "MCI" (whereas the IWG-2 criteria instead use the term "prodromal AD"). According to the NIA-AA criteria, biomarker abnormalities can be used to support the clinical diagnosis, but they are not mandatory. Moreover, these criteria make a distinction between those biomarkers which reflect Aβ pathology (PET or CSF Aβ) and those that reflect neuronal injury (CSF tau, FDG PET, structural MRI). By applying the NIA-AA criteria, individuals can be characterized into three stages. At stage 1 an individual has only abnormal Aβ markers. At stage 2 both Aβ and neuronal injury markers are positive and at stage 3 an individual show positive Aβ and neuronal injury marker accompanied with cognitive impairment. There have also been attempts to harmonize between the different suggested new criteria [96].

Recently the prognostic value of these criteria to predict conversion from MCI to AD has been investigated. In a study including 73 individuals with MCI evaluated amyloidosis (CSF Aβ) or neurodegeneration (hippocampal atrophy in MRI, FDG PET, CSF tau), the best predictor of conversion to AD turned out to be a combined measure of Aβ and any marker of neurodegeneration biomarkers (either positive CSF tau or positive FDG PET or hippocampal atrophy in MRI) [97]. Of the individual biomarkers FDG PET showed the best prediction. In another multicenter study a large number ($n = 1607$) of individuals with MCI were identified and followed up to 3 years [98]. It was then found that using both Aβ and neuronal injury markers, as proposed by the NIA-AA criteria, resulted in the most accurate prognosis. However, more studies with longer follow-up periods are needed to determine the relative predictive value of the different suggested diagnostic criteria. For instance it may take longer for an individual with MCI with only abnormal Aβ biomarker at baseline to convert to AD than for an individual with both abnormal Aβ and abnormal neuronal injury biomarkers.

Amyloid, tau, neurotransmitter, and neuroinflammation PET ligands help to understand the pathophysiology of AD and multi-tracer studies will give further information about the temporal relationships between these processes. Amyloid imaging is very promising, but must be interpreted in relation to the patient's cognitive status and its changes over time. Positive amyloid imaging in an elderly individual does not necessarily imply AD, but its prognostic value of is high in individuals with a progressive episodic memory decline. The role of tau, neurotransmitter, and neuroinflammation imaging in the diagnostics of AD deserves further study.

References

1. Braak H, Braak E (1991) Neuropathological staging of Alzheimer-related changes. Acta Neuropathol (Berl) 82:239–259

2. Braak H, Braak E (1997) (1997). Frequency of stages of Alzheimer-related lesions in different age categories. Neurobiol Aging 18(4):351–357

3. Thal DR, Rub U, Orantes M, Braak H (2002) Phases of A beta-deposition in the human brain and its relevance for the development of AD. Neurology 58:1791–1800

4. Jack CR Jr, Knopman DS, Jagust WJ et al (2013) Tracking pathophysiological processes in Alzheimer's disease: an updated hypothetical model of dynamic biomarkers. Lancet Neurol 12(2):207–216

5. Choi SH, Kim YH, Hebisch M et al (2014) A three-dimensional human neural cell culture model of Alzheimer's disease. Nature 515(7526):274–278

6. Herholz K (2003) PET studies in dementia. Ann Nucl Med 17:79–89

7. Mielke R, Kessler J, Szelies B et al (1998) Normal and pathological aging—findings of positron-emission-tomography. J Neural Transm 105:821–837

8. Rocher AB, Chapon F, Blaizot X et al (2004) Resting-state brain glucose utilization as measured by PET is directly related to regional synaptophysin levels: a study in baboons. Neuroimage 20:1894–1898

9. Minoshima S, Giordani B, Berent S et al (1997) Metabolic reduction in the posterior cingulate cortex in very early Alzheimer's disease. Ann Neurol 42:85–94

10. De Santi S, de Leon MJ, Rusinek H et al (2001) Hippocampal formation glucose metabolism and volume losses in MCI and AD. Neurobiol Aging 22:529–539

11. Nestor PJ, Fryer TD, Smielewski P, Hodges JR (2003) Limbic hypometabolism in Alzheimer's disease and mild cognitive impairment. Ann Neurol 54:343–351

12. Mosconi L, Tsui WH, Herholz K et al (2008) Multicenter standardized ^{18}F-FDG PET diagnosis of mild cognitive impairment, Alzheimer's disease, and other dementias. J Nucl Med 49(3):390–398

13. de Leon MJ, Convit A, Wolf OT et al (2001) Prediction of cognitive decline in normal elderly subjects with 2-[(18)F]fluoro-2-deoxy-D-glucose/positron-emission tomography (FDG/PET). Proc Natl Acad Sci U S A 98(19):10966–10971

14. Mosconi L (2005) Brain glucose metabolism in the early and specific diagnosis of Alzheimer's disease. FDG-PET studies in MCI and AD. Eur J Nucl Med Mol Imaging 32:486–510

15. Li Y, Rinne JO, Mosconi L et al (2008) Regional analysis of FDG and PIB-PET images in normal aging, mild cognitive impairment, and Alzheimer's disease. Eur J Nucl Med Mol Imaging 35(12):2169–2181

16. Reiman EM, Caselli RJ, Yun LS et al (1996) Preclinical evidence of Alzheimer's disease in persons homozygous for the epsilon 4 allele for apolipoprotein E. N Engl J Med 334(12):752–758

17. Small GW, Ercoli LM, Silverman DH et al (2000) Cerebral metabolic and cognitive decline in persons at genetic risk for Alzheimer's disease. Proc Natl Acad Sci U S A 97(11):6037–6042

18. Mosconi L, Rinne JO, Tsui WH et al (2013) Amyloid and metabolic positron emission

tomography imaging of cognitively normal adults with Alzheimer's parents. Neurobiol Aging 34(1):22–34

19. Jagust W, Gitcho A, Sun F et al (2006) Brain imaging evidence of Alzheimer's disease in normal aging. Ann Neurol 59:673–681

20. Silverman DHS, Small GW, Chang CY et al (2001) Positron emission tomography in evaluation of dementia: regional brain metabolism and long-term outcome. JAMA 286:2120–2127

21. Santens P, De Bleecker J, Goethals P et al (2001) Differential regional cerebral uptake of ¹⁸F-fluoro-2-deoxy-D-glucose in Alzheimer's disease and frontotemporal dementia at initial diagnosis. Eur Neurol 45:19–27

22. Foster NL, Heidebrink JL, Clark CM et al (2007) FDG-PET improves accuracy in distinguishing frontotemporal dementia and Alzheimer's disease. Brain 130(Pt 10):2616–2635

23. Minoshima S, Foster NL, Sima AA et al (2001) Alzheimer's disease versus dementia with Lewy bodies: cerebral metabolic distinction with autopsy confirmation. Ann Neurol 50:358–365

24. Albin RL, Minoshima S, DAmato CJ et al (1996) Fluoro-deoxyglucose positron emission tomography in diffuse Lewy body disease. Neurology 47:462–466

25. Higuchi M, Tashiro M, Arai H et al (2000) Glucose hypometabolism and neuropathological correlates in brains of dementia with Lewy bodies. Exp Neurol 162:247–256

26. Ishii K, Imamura T, Sasaki M et al (1998) Regional cerebral glucose metabolism in dementia with Lewy bodies and Alzheimer's disease. Neurology 51:125–130

27. Barber R, Ballard C, McKeith IG, Gholkar A, O'Brien JT (2000) MRI volumetric study of dementia with Lewy bodies: a comparison with AD and vascular dementia. Neurology 54:1304–1309

28. Szelies B, Mielke R, Herholz K, Heiss W-D (1994) Quantitative topographical EEG compared to FDG PET for classification of vascular and degenerative dementia. Electroencephalogr Clin Neurophysiol 91:131–139

29. Aarsland D, Kurz MW (2010) The epidemiology of dementia associated with Parkinson disease. J Neurol Sci 289(1-2):18–22. doi:10.1016/j.jns.2009.08.034

30. Hely MA, Morris JG, Reid WG, Trafficante R (2005) Sydney Multicenter Study of Parkinson's disease: non-L-dopa-responsive problems dominate at 15 years. Mov Disord 20(2):190–199

31. Hely MA, Reid WG, Adena MA, Halliday GM, Morris JG (2008) The Sydney multicenter study of Parkinson's disease: the inevitability of dementia at 20 years. Mov Disord 23(6):837–844. doi:10.1002/mds.21956

32. Jokinen P, Scheinin N, Aalto S et al (2010) [(11)C]PIB-, [(18)F]FDG-PET and MRI imaging in patients with Parkinson's disease with and without dementia. Parkinsonism Relat Disord 16(10):666–670

33. Lyoo CH, Jeong Y, Ryu YH, Rinne JO, Lee MS (2010) Cerebral glucose metabolism of Parkinson's disease patients with mild cognitive impairment. Eur Neurol 64(2):65–73. doi:10.1159/000315036

34. Bohnen NI, Koeppe RA, Minoshima S, Giordani B, Albin RL, Frey KA, Kuhl DE (2011) Cerebral glucose metabolic features of Parkinson disease and incident dementia: longitudinal study. J Nucl Med 52(6):848–855. doi:10.2967/jnumed.111.089946

35. Edison P, Ahmed I, Fan Z et al (2013) Microglia, amyloid, and glucose metabolism in Parkinson's disease with and without dementia. Neuropsychopharmacology 38(6):938–949. doi:10.1038/npp.2012.255

36. Garcia-Garcia D, Clavero P, Gasca Salas C et al (2012) Posterior parietooccipital hypometabolism may differentiate mild cognitive impairment from dementia in Parkinson's disease. Eur J Nucl Med Mol Imaging 39(11):1767–1777

37. Iyo M, Namba H, Fukushi K et al (1997) Measurement of acetylcholinesterase by positron emission tomography in the brain of healthy controls and patients with Alzheimer's disease. Lancet 349:1805–1809

38. Kuhl DE, Koeppe RA, Minoshima S et al (1999) In vivo mapping of cerebral acetylcholinesterase activity in aging and Alzheimer's disease. Neurology 52:691–699

39. Rinne JO, Kaasinen V, Järvenpää T et al (2003) Brain acetycholinesterase activity in mild cognitive impairment and early Alzheimer's disease. J Neurol Neurosurg Psychiatry 74:113–115

40. Bohnen NI, Kaufer DI, Ivanco L et al (2003) Cortical cholinergic function is more severely affected in Parkinsonian dementia than in Alzheimer's Disease: an in vivo PET Study. Arch Neurol 60:1745–1748

41. Francis PT, Webster MT, Chessell IP et al (1993) Neurotransmitters and second messengers in aging and Alzheimer's disease. Ann N Y Acad Sci 695:19–26

42. Xu Y, Yan J, Zhou P et al (2012) Neurotransmitter receptors and cognitive

dysfunction in Alzheimer's disease and Parkinson's disease. Prog Neurobiol 97(1):1–13. doi:10.1016/j.pneurobio.2012.02.002

43. Lanari A, Amenta F, Silvestrelli G, Tomassoni D, Parnetti L (2006) Neurotransmitter deficits in behavioural and psychological symptoms of Alzheimer's disease. Mech Ageing Dev 127(2):158–165

44. Booij J, Habraken JB, Bergmans P et al (1998) Imaging of dopamine transporters with iodine-123-FP-CIT SPECT in healthy controls and patients with Parkinson's disease. J Nucl Med 39(11):1879–1884

45. Rinne JO, Nurmi E, Ruottinen HM et al (2001) [(18)F]FDOPA and [(18)F]CFT are both sensitive PET markers to detect presynaptic dopaminergic hypofunction in early Parkinson's disease. Synapse 40(3):193–200

46. Walker Z, Jaros E, Walker RW et al (2007) Dementia with Lewy bodies: a comparison of clinical diagnosis, FP-CIT single photon emission computed tomography imaging and autopsy. J Neurol Neurosurg Psychiatry 78(11):1176–1181

47. Koeppe RA, Gilman S, Junck L, Wernette K, Frey KA (2008) Differentiating Alzheimer's disease from dementia with Lewy bodies and Parkinson's disease with (+)-[11C]dihydrotetrabenazine positron emission tomography. Alzheimers Dement 4(1 Suppl 1):S67–S76. doi:10.1016/j.jalz.2007.11.016

48. McKeith I, O'Brien J, Walker Z et al (2007) Sensitivity and specificity of dopamine transporter imaging with ^{123}I-FP-CIT SPECT in dementia with Lewy bodies: a phase III, multicentre study. Lancet Neurol 6:305–313

49. Walker Z, Costa DC, Walker RWH et al (2002) Differentiation of dementia with Lewy bodies from Alzheimer's disease using a dopaminergic presynaptic ligand. J Neurol Neurosurg Psychiatry 73:134–140

50. Klunk WE, Engler H, Nordberg A et al (2004) Imaging brain amyloid in Alzheimer's disease with Pittsburgh compound-B. Ann Neurol 55:306–319

51. Mintun MA, Larossa GN, Sheline YI et al (2006) [11C]PIB in a nondemented population: potential antecedent marker of Alzheimer disease. Neurology 67:446–452

52. Rowe CC, Ng S, Ackermann U et al (2007) Imaging beta-amyloid burden in aging and dementia. Neurology 68:1718–1725

53. Engler H, Forsberg A, Almkvist O et al (2006) Two-year follow-up of amyloid deposition in patients with Alzheimer's disease. Brain 129(Pt 11):2856–2866

54. Jack CR Jr, Lowe VJ, Weigand SD et al (2009) Serial PIB and MRI in normal, mild cognitive impairment and Alzheimer's disease: implications for sequence of pathological events in Alzheimer's disease. Brain 132(Pt 5): 1355–1365

55. Scheinin NM, Aalto S, Koikkalainen J et al (2009) Follow-up of [11C]PIB uptake and brain volume in patients with Alzheimer disease and controls. Neurology 73(15):1186–1192

56. Grimmer T, Tholen S, Yousefi BH et al (2010) Progression of cerebral amyloid load is associated with the apolipoprotein E ε4 genotype in Alzheimer's disease. Biol Psychiatry 68(10):879–884

57. Villemagne VL, Pike KE, Chételat G et al (2011) Longitudinal assessment of Aβ and cognition in aging and Alzheimer disease. Ann Neurol 69(1):181–192

58. Kemppainen NM, Aalto S, Wilson IA et al (2007) PET amyloid ligand [11C]PIB uptake is increased in mild cognitive impairment. Neurology 68(19):1603–1606

59. Forsberg A, Engler H, Almkvist O et al (2008) PET imaging of amyloid deposits in patients with mild cognitive impairment. Neurobiol Aging 29:1456–1465

60. Wolk DA, Price JC, Saxton JA et al (2009) Amyloid imaging in mild cognitive impairment subtypes. Ann Neurol 65(5):557–568. doi:10.1002/ana.21598

61. Nordberg A, Carter SF, Rinne J et al (2013) A European multicentre PET study of fibrillar amyloid in Alzheimer's disease. Eur J Nucl Med Mol Imaging 40:104–114

62. Okello A, Koivunen J, Edison P et al (2009) Conversion of amyloid positive and negative MCI to AD over 3 years. An 11C-PIB PET study. Neurology 73(10):754–760

63. Pike KE, Savage G, Villemagne VL et al (2007) Beta-amyloid imaging and memory in non-demented individuals: evidence for preclinical Alzheimer's disease. Brain 130:2837–2844

64. Villain N, Chetelat G, Grassiot B et al (2012) Regional dynamics of amyloid-beta deposition in healthy elderly, mild cognitive impairment and Alzheimer's disease: a voxelwise PiB-PET longitudinal study. Brain 135(Pt 7):2126–2139

65. Rowe CC, Ellis KA, Rimajova M et al (2010) Amyloid imaging results from the Australian Imaging, Biomarkers and Lifestyle (AIBL) study of aging. Neurobiol Aging 31:1275–1283

66. Scheinin NM, Wikman K, Jula A et al (2014) Cortical ^{11}C-PIB uptake is associated with age,

APOE genotype, and gender in "healthy aging". J Alzheimers Dis 41(1):193–202

67. Jansen WJ, Ossenkoppele R, Knol DL et al (2015) Prevalence of cerebral amyloid pathology in persons without dementia: a meta-analysis. JAMA 313(19):1924–1938. doi:10.1001/jama.2015.4668

68. Joshi AD, Pontecorvo MJ, Clark CM et al (2012) Performance characteristics of amyloid PET with florbetapir F 18 in patients with Alzheimer's disease and cognitively normal subjects. J Nucl Med 53:378–384

69. Rowe CC, Ackerman U, Browne W et al (2008) Imaging of amyloid beta in Alzheimer's disease with ^{18}F-BAY94-9172, a novel PET tracer: proof of mechanism. Lancet Neurol 7: 129–135

70. Vandenberghe R, Van Laere K, Ivanoiu A et al (2010) ^{18}F-Flutemetamol Amyloid Imaging in Alzheimer Disease and Mild Cognitive Impairment A Phase 2 Trial. Ann Neurol 68:319–329

71. Rowe CC, Pejoska S, Mulligan RS et al (2013) (2013) Head-to-head comparison of 11C-PiB and ^{18}F-AZD4694 (NAV4694) for β-amyloid imaging in aging and dementia. J Nucl Med 54(6):880–886. doi:10.2967/jnumed.112.114785

72. Cselényi Z, Jönhagen ME, Forsberg A et al (2012) Clinical validation of ^{18}F-AZD4694, an amyloid-β-specific PET radioligand. J Nucl Med 53(3):415–424. doi:10.2967/jnumed.111.094029

73. Shoghi-Jadid K, Small GW, Agdeppa ED et al (2002) (2002) Localization of neurofibrillary tangles and beta-amyloid plaques in the brains of living patients with Alzheimer disease. Am J Geriatr Psychiatr 10:24–35

74. Small GW, Kepe V, Ercoli LM et al (2006) PET of brain amyloid and tau in mild cognitive impairment. N Engl J Med 355:2652–2663

75. Shin J, Kepe V, Barrio JR, Small GW (2011) The merits of FDDNP-PET imaging in Alzheimer's disease. J Alzheimers Dis 26(Suppl 3):135–145

76. Zwan MD, Okamura N, Fodero-Tavoletti MT et al (2014) Voyage au bout de la nuit: Aβ and tau imaging in dementias. Q J Nucl Med Mol Imaging 58(4):398–412

77. Johnson KA, Minoshima S, Bohnen NI et al (2013) Appropriate use criteria for amyloid PET: A report of the amyloid imaging task force, the society of nuclear medicine and molecular imaging, and the Alzheimer's association. J Nucl Med 54(3):476–490

78. Okamura N, Harada R, Furumoto S et al (2014) Tau PET imaging in Alzheimer's dis-

ease. Curr Neurol Neurosci Rep 14(11):500. doi:10.1007/s11910-014-0500-6

79. Okamura N, Furumoto S, Fodero-Tavoletti MT et al (2014) Non-invasive assessment of Alzheimer's disease neurofibrillary pathology using ^{18}F-THK5105 PET. Brain 137(Pt 6):1762–1771. doi:10.1093/brain/awu064

80. Harada R, Okamura N, Furumoto S et al (2015) [(18)F]THK-5117 PET for assessing neurofibrillary pathology in Alzheimer's disease. Eur J Nucl Med Mol Imaging 42(7):1052–1061. doi:10.1007/s00259-015-3035-4

81. Okamura N, Furumoto S, Harada R et al (2014) Characterization of [^{18}F]THK-5351, a novel PET tracer for imaging tau pathology in Alzheimer's disease. Eur J Nucl Med Mol Imaging 41:S260

82. Chien DT, Bahri S, Szardenings AK, Walsh JC, Mu F, Su MY (2013) Early clinical PET imaging results with the novel PHF-tau radioligand [F-18]-T807. J Alzheimers Dis 34:457–468

83. Chien DT, Szardenings AK, Bahri S et al (2014) Early clinical PET imaging results with the Novel PHF-Tau radioligand [F18]-T808. J Alzheimers Dis 38:171–184

84. Maruyama M, Shimada H, Suhara T et al (2013) Imaging of tau pathology in a tauopathy mouse model and in Alzheimer patients compared to normal controls. Neuron 79: 1094–1108

85. Jacobs AH, Tavitian B; INMiND consortium (2012) Noninvasive molecular imaging of neuroinflammation. J Cereb Blood Flow Metab 32(7):1393–1415. doi:10.1038/jcbfm.2012.53

86. Cagnin A, Brooks DJ, Kennedy AM et al (2001) In-vivo measurement of activated microglia in dementia. Lancet 358(9280): 461–467

87. Edison P, Archer HA, Gerhard A et al (2008) Microglia, amyloid, and cognition in Alzheimer's disease: An [11C](R)PK11195-PET and [11C]PIB-PET study. Neurobiol Dis 32(3):412–419. doi:10.1016/j.nbd.2008.08.001

88. Kreisl WC, Lyoo CH, McGwier M et al (2013) Biomarkers Consortium PET Radioligand Project Team. In vivo radioligand binding to translocator protein correlates with severity of Alzheimer's disease. Brain 136(Pt 7):2228–2238. doi:10.1093/brain/awt145

89. Wiley CA, Lopresti BJ, Venneti S et al (2009) Carbon 11-labeled Pittsburgh Compound B and carbon 11-labeled (R)-PK11195 positron emission tomographic imaging in Alzheimer disease. Arch Neurol 66(1):60–67

90. Fowler JS, Logan J, Volkow ND, Wang GJ (2005) Translational neuroimaging: positron emission tomography studies of monoamine oxidase. Mol Imaging Biol 7:377–387

91. Saura J, Bleuel Z, Ulrich J et al (1996) Molecular neuroanatomy of human monoamine oxidases A and B revealed by quantitative enzyme radio-autography and in situ hybridization histochemistry. Neuroscience 70:755–774

92. Carter SF, Schöll M, Almkvist O et al (2012) Evidence for astrocytosis in prodromal Alzheimer disease provided by 11C-deuterium-L-deprenyl: a multitracer PET paradigm combining 11C-Pittsburgh compound B and ^{18}F-FDG. J Nucl Med 53(1):37–46

93. Villemagne VL, Burnham S, Bourgeat P et al (2013) Amyloid β deposition, neurodegeneration, and cognitive decline in sporadic Alzheimer's disease: a prospective cohort study. Lancet Neurol 12(4):357–367

94. Dubois B, Feldman HH, Jacova C et al (2014) Advancing research diagnostic criteria for Alzheimer's disease: the IWG-2 criteria. Lancet Neurol 13(6):614–629

95. McKhann GM, Knopman DS, Chertkow H et al (2011) The diagnosis of dementia due to Alzheimer's disease: recommendations from the National Institute on Aging-Alzheimer's Association workgroups on diagnostic guidelines for Alzheimer's disease. Alzheimers Dement 7(3):263–269

96. Morris JC, Blennow K, Froelich L et al (2014) Harmonized diagnostic criteria for Alzheimer's disease: recommendations. J Intern Med 275(3):204–213. doi:10.1111/joim.12199

97. Prestia A, Caroli A, Wade SK et al (2015) Prediction of AD dementia by biomarkers following the NIA-AA and IWG diagnostic criteria in MCI patients from three European memory clinics. Alzheimers Dement 11(10):1191–1201, pii: S1552-5260 (14)02890-8

98. Vos SJ, Verhey F, Frölich L et al (2015) Prevalence and prognosis of Alzheimer's disease at the mild cognitive impairment stage. Brain 138(Pt 5):1327–1338. doi:10.1093/brain/awv029

Chapter 14

Alpha-Synuclein as a Diagnostic Biomarker for Parkinson's Disease

Joakim Bergström and Martin Ingelsson

Abstract

The development of new biomarkers for Parkinson's disease has been focused on the analyses of the α-synuclein protein in cerebrospinal fluid and plasma. Although significant differences in the levels of total α-synuclein have been found between patients and controls, none of these markers have been proven clinically useful as there has been a substantial overlap between the groups. Instead, assessment of toxic prefibrillar α-synuclein species has shown promising results, but further studies are needed to prove their diagnostic usefulness. In addition to analyses of body fluids, detection of α-synuclein in peripheral tissues—such as subcolonic mucosa and parotid gland—seem to offer novel interesting diagnostic possibilities.

Key words ELISA, α-Synuclein, Plasma, Cerebrospinal fluid, Colon mucosa, Parotid gland

1 Introduction

Parkinson's disease (PD), dementia with Lewy bodies (DLB) and multiple system atrophy (MSA) are the three most prevalent disorders with deposition of α-synuclein in the brain. In PD, pathological α-synuclein accumulates as Lewy bodies in the brain stem and, with increased disease duration, also in other brain regions [1]. In DLB, there is typically Lewy body pathology in widespread neocortical areas already early in the disease [2] and in MSA, pathological α-synuclein mainly accumulates in oligodendroglial cells of the brain stem, cerebellum, and the nigrostriatal area (reviewed in [3]).

Parkinson's disease is characterized by tremor, hypokinesia, or rigidity to various degrees, whereas in DLB, the patients suffer from early memory impairment or other cognitive dysfunctions (reviewed in [4]). However, also PD patients may have cognitive disabilities—ranging from mild impairment at early stages [5] to various degrees of dementia later during the disease course—and DLB patients also typically develop varying degrees of motor

Martin Ingelsson and Lars Lannfelt (eds.), *Immunotherapy and Biomarkers in Neurodegenerative Disorders*, Methods in Pharmacology and Toxicology, DOI 10.1007/978-1-4939-3560-4_14, © Springer Science+Business Media New York 2016

abnormalities (reviewed in [6]). Clinically, patients with MSA manifest with autonomic failure associated with various degrees of parkinsonism and cerebellar dysfunction. The diverse clinical picture has led to a subclassification of MSA into MSA-P and MSA-C, depending on whether the parkinsonian or the cerebellar symptoms are dominating (reviewed in [7]). Thus, apart from identifying early forms of PD and DLB it is important to differentiate the α-synucleinopathies from each other.

As of today, the diagnoses of disorders with α-synuclein pathology are mainly based on clinical examination, although imaging by Single-Photon Emission Computed Tomography (SPECT), Positron Emission Tomography (PET), and Magnetic Resonance Imaging (MRI) can aid the physician in the diagnostic process. In particular, the use of DAT-scan, a SPECT-marker for the dopamine transporter protein, has proven useful for the in vivo detection of nigrostriatal neuronal degeneration in the brain stem (reviewed in [8]).

As of non-imaging biomarkers, there has been a focus on trying to develop useful α-synuclein assays for assessment of plasma and cerebrospinal fluid (CSF). Although it was originally believed that α-synuclein was exclusively expressed in the central nervous system (CNS), it is now well known that the protein also is present in several cell types as well as in extracellular compartments. In fact, the concentration of α-synuclein has been shown to be higher in blood and plasma than in cerebrospinal fluid (CSF) [9].

It has already for some time been acknowledged that α-synuclein pathology appears in a hierarchical pattern in the PD brain. The initially affected areas, such as the dorsal motor nucleus of the glossopharyngeal/vagal nerves and the anterior olfactory nucleus, are followed by Lewy body pathology in substantia nigra pars compacta and other brain stem areas [10]. Subsequently, the pathology spreads to the anteromedial temporal mesocortex and, with increased disease duration, also to neocortical regions [10]. Moreover, recent findings indicate that α-synuclein pathology may even start outside the CNS with the finding of early pathological changes in the mesenteric plexus of the gut [11]. Moreover, a recently published experimental study on rats suggested that initial deposition of α-synuclein in such locations may act like a seed that can be transported retrogradely to interconnecting CNS regions and subsequently to areas corresponding to the main disease symptoms [12].

The identification of affected peripheral tissues offers novel possibilities to sample biopsies that can be analyzed for diagnostic purposes. In the following we describe the current status of the field, highlighting both studies on plasma/CSF and the efforts to explore biopsied patient tissues for the development of novel biomarkers for PD and related disorders.

2   Alpha-Synuclein in CSF

Alpha-synuclein has been studied extensively as a potential biomarker for both PD and DLB. However, the results have so far been somewhat inconsistent. A reduction of α-synuclein levels in cerebrospinal fluid (CSF) compared to control groups has been reported in numerous studies [13–31], whereas no significant differences between the groups could be observed in other studies [32–43] (Table 1). In contrast, only one study has reported increased CSF levels of α-synuclein in DLB [44]. Most of these investigations have measured total α-synuclein and thus not discriminated between different molecular forms of the protein. Recent studies, however, have specifically targeted post translationally modified α-synuclein, such as phosphorylated or oligomeric forms [16, 33, 45–47]. Initial findings indicate that these forms of α-synuclein indeed seem to be present in CSF and most studies have indicated higher levels in PD patients compared to controls [16, 33, 45].

Early studies, using western blot analysis with antibodies targeting the C-terminal part of the protein, failed to detect α-synuclein in human CSF [48]. However, Borghi and colleagues became the first group to identify a monomeric 19 kDa α-synuclein band in CSF by applying an immunoprecipation protocol followed by western blot [40]. However, when they analyzed twelve patients with idiopathic PD and ten age matched controls by this method, the amount of immunoreactive α-synuclein material did not differ significantly between the two groups.

The first study to show a significant decrease of α-synuclein levels in CSF was performed by Tokuda et al. [13], adopting a sandwich ELISA using the syn 211 monoclonal antibody (recognizing epitopes 121–125 [49]) as detection antibody and the polyclonal FL-140 antibody (Santa Cruz Biotechnology, Santa Cruz, CA) as detection antibody. In idiopathic PD patients ($n = 33$) they found mean α-synuclein CSF levels of 18.16 ng/ml, whereas the control subjects ($n = 38$) had a twofold higher mean concentration of α-synuclein. However, the authors raised some issues that could have affected the study outcome, including the fact that CSF had to be concentrated fivefold during sample preparation to enable detection. Furthermore, since α-synuclein can be found at high concentrations in red blood cells [50] ($26,200 \pm 1300$ ng/ml), a small potential contamination from such a source could not be ruled out.

In a follow up study, Mollenhauer and colleagues could unequivocally show the presence of α-synuclein in CSF using both mass spectrometry and a second generation ELISA using a custom developed rabbit polyclonal antibody (mSA-1 raised against mouse α-synuclein) as capture antibody and syn-1 (Clone 42, recognizing epitopes 91–99, BD Transduction Laboratories) as a

Table 1
Studies on α-synuclein in CSF

Study	Diagnoses	Target	Results	References
Borghi et al. (2000)	PD vs. controls	Total α-syn	Unchanged levels in PD	[40]
Tokuda et al. (2006)	PD vs. controls	Total α-syn	Lower levels in PD	[13]
Mollenhauer et al. (2008)	PD/DLB vs. controls	Total α-syn	Lower levels in PD/DLB	[14]
Van Geel et al. (2008)	PD vs. controls	Total α-syn	Lower levels in PD	[23]
Öhrfelt et al. (2009)	PD/DLB vs. controls	Total α-syn	Unchanged levels in PD	[34]
Noguchi-Shinohara (2009)	DLB vs. AD	Total α-syn	Unchanged levels in DLB	[35]
Spies et al. (2009)	DLB vs. controls	Total α-syn	Unchanged levels in DLB	[36]
Hong et al. (2010)	PD vs. controls	Total α-syn	Lower levels in PD	[20]
Tokuda et al. (2010)	PD vs. controls	Total α-syn, oligomeric α-syn	Unchanged levels of total α-syn in PD, oligomeric α-syn increased in PD	[45]
Kasuga et al. (2010)	PD vs. AD	Total α-syn	Lower levels in PD	[37]
Reesink et al. (2012)	PD/DLB vs. AD	Total α-syn, oligomeric α-syn	Unchanged levels in PD/ DLB	[38]
Parnetti et al. (2011)	PD/DLB vs. controls	Total α-syn	Lower levels in PD/DLB	[18]
Mollenhauer et al. (2011)	PD/DLB vs. controls	Total α-syn	Lower levels in PD/DLB	[15]
Shi et al. (2011)	PD vs. controls	Total α-syn	Lower levels in PD	[22]
Park et al. (2011)	PD vs. controls	Total α-syn, oligomeric α-syn	Unchanged levels of total α-syn in PD, oligomeric α-syn increased in PD	[33]
Aerts et al. (2012)	PD/DLB vs. controls	Total α-syn	Unchanged levels in PD	[32]
Bidinosti et al. (2012)	PD vs. controls	Total α-syn	Unchanged levels in PD	[24]
Hall et al. (2012)	PD/DLB vs. controls	Total α-syn	Lower levels in PD/DLB	[26]
Tateno et al. (2012)	PD/DLB vs. controls	Total α-syn	Lower levels in PD/DLB	[17]
Wennström et al. (2012)	DLB vs. controls	Total α-syn	Unchanged levels in PD	[39]

(continued)

Table 1
(continued)

Study	Diagnoses	Target	Results	References
Wang et al. (2012)	PD vs. controls	Total α-syn, phosphorylated α-syn	Lower levels of total α-syn in PD, Higher levels of phosphorylated α-syn in PD	[16]
Kapaki et al. (2013)	DLB vs. controls	Total α-syn	Higher levels of total α-syn in DLB	[44]
Kang et al. (2013)	PD vs. controls	Total α-syn	Lower levels in PD	[27]
Mollenhauer et al. (2013)	PD vs. controls	Total α-syn	Lower levels in PD	[19]
Wennström et al. (2013)	PD/DLB vs. controls	Total α-syn	Lower levels in PD/DLB	[64]
Aasly et al. (2014)	PD vs. controls	Total α-syn	Unchanged levels in PD	[46]
Hansson et al. (2014)	PD vs. controls	Oligomeric α-syn	Higher levels of oligomeric α-syn in PD	[47]
Mondello et al. (2014)	PD/DLB vs. controls	Total α-syn	Lower levels in PD/DLB	[28]
Parnetti et al. (2014)	PD vs. controls	Total α-syn, oligomeric α-syn	Lower levels of total α-syn in PD, Higher levels of oligomeric α-syn in PD	[29]
Slaets et al. (2014)	PD/DLB vs. controls	Total α-syn	Unchanged levels in PD/DLB	[41]
Unterberger et al. (2014)	DLB vs. controls	Total α-syn	Lower levels in PD	[30]
Van Dijk et al. (2014)	PD vs. controls	Total α-syn	Lower levels in PD	[21]
Buddhala et al. (2015)	PD vs. controls	Total α-syn	Lower levels in PD	[31]
Compta et al. (2015)	PD/PDD vs. controls	Total α-syn, oligomeric α-syn	Higher levels in PDD but not in PD	[42]
Magdalinou et al. (2015)	PD vs. controls	Total α-syn	Unchanged levels in PD	[43]

biotinylated detection antibody [14]. This was the first cross sectional study performed and it showed slightly lower mean levels CSF α-synuclein in PD patients ($n = 8$, 3 ng/ml $\pm$ 1.3) compared to controls ($n = 13$, 6.0 ± 5.73 ng/ml).

Since these pioneering studies, numerous investigations measuring total levels of α-synuclein have been performed, adopting ELISA and bead-based flow cytometric assays using various monoclonal bodies (usually targeting the C-terminal part of the protein). Most of these studies have reported a decrease of CSF α-synuclein in PD patients compared to controls [13–22].

For example, Parnetti and colleagues used an ELISA based on the combination of syn 211 antibody and the polyclonal FL-140 antibody [18]. They could show that mean α-synuclein levels in CSF were significantly lower among PD patients ($n = 38$) compared to age-matched controls ($n = 32$). However, CSF α-synuclein alone did not provide a relevant basis for a PD diagnosis as the specificity in the study was low (25 %) [18].

Mollenhauer et al. used a previously published sandwich ELISA together with a newly developed ELISA based on the pairing of a mice monoclonal capture antibody (epitope, amino acids 103–107) and a rabbit monoclonal detection antibody (epitope, amino acids 118–123) [19]. The mean levels of CSF α-synuclein in the two assays were decreased in PD patients ($n = 78$, 1.40 ± 0.24 ng/ml) compared to healthy controls ($n = 48$, 1.51 ± 0.34 ng/ml). The new ELISA showed a sensitivity value of 0.91 at a specificity of 0.25 for the diagnosis of PD.

Hong and colleagues applied a bead-based Luminex assay using the syn 211 antibody and could show that PD patients ($n = 117$) had significantly reduced CSF α-synuclein levels compared to controls ($n = 132$) [20]. However, in this study samples with high hemoglobin (>200 ng/ml) were omitted, thus highlighting α-synuclein from red blood cells as a potential source for false positive results.

By applying a time-resolved Förster's resonance energy transfer assay using the phage display developed α-synuclein antibodies SynBa2-Tb and SynBa3-d2, Van Dijk et al. measured the concentration of CSF α-synuclein in PD patients ($n = 53$) and controls ($n = 50$) [21]. Mean α-synuclein levels were significantly lower in the patient group (1.48 ± 0.41 ng/ml) compared to controls (1.70 ± 0.47 ng/ml), although there was a large overlap between groups. In their study, the sensitivity and specificity values for distinguishing PD patients from controls were 56 % and 74 %, respectively.

Yet other studies have shown no differences between PD patients and controls. For example, Aaerts and colleagues could not find any significant changes between PD patients ($n = 58$, 26.0 ng/ml) and controls ($n = 57$, 25.0 ng/ml) using the syn 211/ FL-140 sandwich ELISA [32]. Moreover, in another study the same ELISA setup was used and also here no significant differences could be found between a cohort of drug naïve PD patients ($n = 23$) and a control group ($n = 29$) [33].

Many factors might have contributed to the discordance observed between the different studies. For example, differences in the patient cohorts regarding age, disease duration and disease severity may have influenced the results. Other potential confounding factors include differences in sample handling and storage, specificities and affinities of the antibodies used, as well as differences in the applied immunological assays. Recently, a study was performed on validating a quantitative CSF α-synuclein ELISA in 18 participating laboratories [51]. Although preanalytical sample handling and lot-to-lot variability were minimized by the study design, a high variation in absolute α-synuclein CSF levels could be identified even when the same samples and the same assay setup (a sandwich ELISA α-synuclein kit (Cat.-# SIG-38974, Covance, Dedham, MA) was applied. Despite the variation, the quantitative results from the different laboratories were comparable suggesting that such an assay, with further standardization, could be used to reliably compare α-synuclein CSF levels between different laboratories [51].

Several studies have shown that α-synuclein CSF levels are significantly lower in PD compared to AD [15, 17, 22]. However, among the α-synucleinopathies, most studies have not found any significant change in α-synuclein levels between PD, DLB and MSA patients [17, 18, 32, 52]. Attempts to link decreased levels of total α-synuclein to disease severity and disease duration in PD patients have in general been unsuccessful [16, 20, 22, 45, 52]. However, Kang and colleagues found that lower levels of α-synuclein correlated with worse performance on the Unified Parkinson's Disease Rating Scale (UPDRS) part III motor scores among PD patients ($n = 63$) [27]. Accordingly, Tokuda et al. found an inverse correlation between total α-synuclein levels in CSF and Hoehn and Yahr scale performance in PD patients ($n = 33$) [13].

Recently, three meta-analysis studies have been performed to investigate α-synuclein as a biomarker for PD and other α-synucleinopathies. Gao and colleagues evaluated 17 studies, including 3311 patients, and found a significantly lower mean CSF α-synuclein level in PD patients compared to controls with a weight mean difference (WMD) of −0.31 ($p < 0.0001$) [53]. Whereas there was no difference in mean α-synuclein levels between PD and DLB patients (WMD −0.03, $p = 0.58$), or between PD and MSA patients (WMD 0.05, $p = 0.25$), there was a significant difference between PD and AD patients (WMD −0.15, p weight mean difference <0.0001). In this meta-analysis, the sensitivity and specificity of CSF α-synuclein levels to accurately diagnose PD was 0.88 (95 % CI, 0.84–0.91) and 0.40 (95 % CI, 0.35–0.45), respectively [53].

Sako and colleagues performed another meta-analysis investigating nine studies involving 843 PD, 130 MSA and 537 control patients [54]. They found reduced α-synuclein levels in CSF in PD compared to normal controls or disease controls (standardized mean difference (SMD) −0.67, $p < 0.00001$). Similarly, they found no difference in CSF α-synuclein between PD and MSA patients (SMD 0.17, $p = 0.11$) [54].

In addition, Zetterberg and colleagues performed a meta-analysis of 18 independent studies and, although several studies did not show any significant differences, the overall result showed a certain reduction of α-synuclein levels in CSF between PD patients and controls [55].

As α-synuclein oligomers have been proposed to be the most harmful α-synuclein species in vivo [56, 57], they could potentially be developed as a powerful biomarker, offering a better estimate of disease progression. To date there have been seven studies showing the presence of α-synuclein oligomers in CSF and several of those have showed that the concentration is higher in PD patients compared to controls [30, 33, 45–47, 58, 59]. In four of these studies, the monoclonal syn 211 antibody was used as both capture and (biotinylated) reporter antibody [13, 14, 16, 17]. Such an ELISA design avoids detection of monomeric protein but measures everything from dimers to larger oligomers/protofibrils. However, none of the conducted studies could determine a true concentration of such species, as no oligomeric standard curve was included in the respective assays. However, as the pool of α-synuclein oligomers in CSF most likely are heterogeneous in size, generating similar oligomeric species in vitro would be very challenging, thus making direct quantifications difficult.

The first study on oligomeric α-synuclein in CSF was conducted by Tokuda and colleagues, who could show that among PD patients ($n = 32$) both levels of α-synuclein oligomers and the ratio of α-synuclein oligomers vs. total α-synuclein were significantly increased compared to neurologically normal control subjects ($n = 28$) [45]. The increased levels of α-synuclein oligomers had a sensitivity of 75.0 % and a specificity of 87.5 % for a correct diagnosis of PD, whereas the ratio of oligomeric vs. total α-synuclein levels of the protein both had greater sensitivity (89.3 %) and specificity (90.6 %) [45].

Park et al. compared drug naïve PD patients ($n = 23$) with age- and sex-matched neurological controls and showed that increased CSF levels of α-synuclein oligomers were observed in PD patients [33]. However, a limitation of the study was the sizable overlap among the patient group with respect to the amount of CSF α-synuclein oligomers.

As mutations in the leucine-rich repeat kinase 2 (LRRK2) gene is the most common form of familial PD [60], Aasly and colleagues hypothesized that the levels of α-synuclein oligomers in CSF may differ between LRRK2 carriers and sporadic PD patients [46]. They could show that both sporadic PD patients ($n = 35$) and asymptomatic LRRK carriers ($n = 20$) had elevated oligomeric levels with a sensitivity of 65.0 % and 63.0 % and a specificity of 83.0 and 74.0 %, respectively. However, they found no significant difference in the levels of oligomeric α-synuclein between symptomatic LRRK2 carriers and healthy controls. These results could possibly be due to a lack of power, since there was a lower number of individuals in the patient group ($n = 13$) compared to the control group ($n = 42$) or, alternatively, that oligomeric levels only are elevated in the early disease phases in LRRK2-related PD. Furthermore, the study showed an inverse correlation between disease duration/severity of the disease and α-synuclein oligomers in CSF, but only in the sporadic PD group.

Hansson and colleagues were able to show that the concentration of α-synuclein oligomers in CSF was higher in PD patients with dementia (PDD) ($n = 30$), but not in DLB patients ($n = 71$), as compared to healthy controls ($n = 98$) [47]. However, both CSF α-synuclein oligomers and α-synuclein oligomers vs. total-α-synuclein levels could distinguish PDD and DLB patients from AD patients ($n = 48$) with a sensitivity of 75 % and 64 %, respectively. Another study measuring oligomeric α-synuclein in CSF could show increased levels in PDD patients ($n = 20$), but not in non-demented PD patients ($n = 21$) compared to controls [42]. Measurements of total α-synuclein did not differ between patients groups and neither did the oligomeric-total ration of α-synuclein. Also in this study, a large overlap between groups was observed for oligomeric α-synuclein.

To enhance the possibility of detecting α-synuclein oligomers, an increased attention has been given to the development of new binders (e.g., monoclonal antibodies, nanobodies) with higher affinity for oligomeric assemblies of the protein, as well as to the development of novel and more sensitive techniques. However, these proof of concept studies have not investigated larger sample sets. For example, Sierks and colleagues linked a nanobody with high specificity for α-synuclein oligomers to an electronic biosensor and were able to detect oligomers in human CSF [58]. In addition, Brännström and colleagues could detect α-synuclein oligomers in CSF from PD patients using a newly developed oligomer-selective antibody (ASyO2) both for capture and detection in a sandwich ELISA [59]. Also, it could be shown that the monoclonal 5G4 antibody, which displayed high affinity for aggregated forms of α-synuclein in immunohistochemical studies, could detect higher levels of disease associated α-synuclein in CSF from PD ($n = 2$) and DLB ($n = 5$) compared to controls ($n = 9$) when used as the capture antibody in a sandwich ELISA [30].

Several different post translational modifications have been found for α-synuclein when present in LBs, including N-terminal acetylation, N-terminal ubiquination, C-terminal truncations, and C-terminal phosphorylation [61]. The most common form of α-synuclein phosphorylation occurs at the Ser129 residue

(PS-129), as 90 % of α-synuclein in Lewy bodies has this modification [62]. By using a Luminex assay specifically targeting PS-129 α-synuclein, Wang et al. showed that PD patients ($n=93$) had higher levels of PS-129 α-synuclein (79.22 ± 23.22 pg/ml) in comparison to both controls ($n=78$, 69.61 ± 17.25 pg/ml) and MSA patients ($n=16$, 58.12 ± 20.24 pg/ml) [16]. In this study, the authors could also observe a weak correlation between PS-129 α-synuclein levels and disease severity, as judged by the UPDRS motor score, in the PD group. In a follow up study, also utilizing the Luminex technique, Stewart et al. could show a significant increase in UPDRS motor scores with higher PS-129 α-synuclein CSF values in late stage PD patients ($n=164$), but not in those with early stage PD ($n=69$) [63].

In contrast to the study by Wang et al. an earlier study by Foulds and colleagues failed to detect any differences in the concentration of PS-129 α-synuclein between PD patients ($n=39$) and controls ($n=18$) [52]. That study also investigated oligomeric forms of PS-129 α-synuclein, but also here no significant differences between PD patients and controls could be detected. Interestingly, a small cohort of MSA patients ($n=6$) had significantly higher levels of oligomeric PS-129 α-synuclein compared to both PD patients and controls.

Further studies are thus warranted to evaluate whether PS-129 α-synuclein in either its monomeric or oligomeric form could serve as a diagnostic marker for PD, or other synucleinopathies, and whether any of these measures potentially could correlate to disease severity and disease duration.

Taken together, the majority of studies, including recent meta-analyses, indicate that α-synuclein CSF levels are indeed reduced in PD. However, the diagnostic usefulness is not obvious since most studies have indicated a substantial overlap between patients and controls. Initial studies suggesting increased CSF levels of oligomeric forms of α-synuclein need to be replicated before we can better evaluate their diagnostic value. Moreover, the use of novel binders and more sensitive techniques could allow future development of better α-synuclein based markers that not only could distinguish patients from healthy subjects, but also mirror the disease course and thereby offer a possibility to follow both disease progression and the effects of therapeutic interventions.

3 Alpha-Synuclein in Blood

3.1 Plasma and Serum

To date, about a dozen studies on the quantification of α-synuclein in either plasma or serum have been reported—with conflicting results. Whereas four studies have reported increased levels of α-synuclein among PD patients as compared to healthy controls,

Table 2
Studies on α-synuclein in plasma

Study	Diagnoses	Target	Results	Reference
El-Agnaf et al. (2006)	PD/DLB vs. controls	Oligomeric α-syn	Increased levels in PD	[66]
Lee et al. (2006)	PD/MSA vs. controls	Total α-syn	Increased levels in PD	[67]
Duran et al. (2010)	PD vs. controls	Total α-syn, phospho α-syn	Increased levels in PD	[68]
Foulds et al. (2011)	PD vs. controls	Total α-syn, oligomeric α-syn, phospho α-syn	Increased phospho α-syn levels in PD. Total α-syn and oligomeric α-syn were unchanged	[52]
Li et al. (2007)	PD vs. controls	Total α-syn	Decreased levels in PD	[70]
Laske et al. (2011)	DLB vs. controls	Total α-syn	Decreased levels in DLB	[71]
Gorostidi et al. (2012)	PD vs. controls	Total α-syn, oligomeric α-syn	Decreased levels of total α-syn in PD, oligomeric α-syn was unchanged	[72]
Shi et al. (2010)	PD vs. controls	Total α-syn	Unchanged levels in PD	[73]
Park et al. (2011)	PD vs. controls	Total α-syn, oligomeric α-syn	Unchanged levels in PD	[33]
Mata et al. (2010)	PD vs. controls	Total α-syn	Unchanged levels in PD	[74]
Besong-Agbo et al. (2013)	PD vs. controls	Total α-syn	Unchanged levels in PD	[75]

three investigations did not find any differences among the groups. In yet four other studies there were decreased levels in patient samples than in non-affected individuals (Table 2).

In a pioneering study, El-Agnaf et al. applied immunoprecipitation to detect α-synuclein in plasma from patients with PD and DLB [65]. Subsequently, the same research group published the first study comparing the levels of plasma α-synuclein between PD cases and healthy controls [66]. As described above for the CSF studies, using an ELISA that adopts the same monoclonal antibody (mAb211, Santa Cruz Biotechnology, Santa Cruz, CA, USA) for both capture and detection only α-synuclein in dimers or higher molecular weight oligomers were targeted. With this assay the authors could report increased levels of such oligomeric α-synuclein species in plasma from PD patients compared to healthy controls, although with a large interindividual variation and a considerable overlap between the two groups [66]. Although the number of subjects investigated were rather small (PD 34, C 27), the results encouraged other groups to conduct similar studies.

In the first ensuing study, Lee and colleagues included samples from both PD, DLB and MSA patients and found a small, but significantly different, increase in α-synuclein plasma levels in both PD (79.9 ± 4.0 pg/ml) and MSA (78.1 ± 3.5 pg/ml) compared to controls (76.1 ± 3.9 pg/ml) [67]. In addition, the difference in α-synuclein levels between PD and MSA cases was statistically significant whereas the levels among DLB patients did not differ compared to controls.

In a study by Duran et al. it was investigated whether PD patients have different levels of plasma α-synuclein at various stages of the disease [68]. The authors compared two groups of patients—those that had been newly diagnosed and were drug-naïve ($n = 53$) and those that had been under treatment for at least one year ($n = 42$). Like in the previous studies, PD patients displayed higher α-synuclein levels than healthy controls, but there were no differences in levels between the two different PD groups [68]. Thus, neither disease duration nor anti-parkinsonian treatment (with L-dopa, dopamine-receptor agonists, and COMT-inhibitors) seemed to affect the plasma concentration of α-synuclein.

In yet another study, investigators were analyzing several different species of α-synuclein in plasma from 32 PD cases and 30 age-matched healthy control subjects. Apart from measuring total α-synuclein with the same antibody setup as used in previous studies (monoclonal 211 as capture and monoclonal FL-140 as detection antibodies), also oligomeric α-synuclein (211 as capture and biotinylated 211 as detection antibodies) and phosphorylated α-synuclein (polyclonal N-19 as capture and monoclonal p-129 as detection antibodies) species were measured with the help of separate assays [52]. Whereas this study demonstrated similar levels of both total and oligomeric (measuring dimers and larger oligomers) α-synuclein between the groups, the levels of phosphorylated α-synuclein turned out to be slightly higher among the PD patients.

Thus, contrary to the three previous investigations, the study by Foulds et al. did not find any increase neither in total nor in oligomeric α-synuclein among PD patients, but instead a small increase in the levels of α-synuclein phosphorylated at serine 129 [52]. This post-translational modification seems to be of pathogenic significance, since an increase in staining of P129-α-synuclein normally can be found in the brains of PD patients, but—because of the small sample sizes and the significant group overlap—it is still unclear whether measurement of this α-synuclein species in plasma could be diagnostically relevant.

In the study by Foulds et al. each PD patient had been sampled at three different time points over 2–3 years, allowing for longitudinal analyses of the plasma levels. It could then be found that whereas levels differed greatly among individuals, all three α-synuclein read-outs were relatively stable over time [69]. In a follow-up study, a larger number of PD patients (189 cases) had been followed with plasma sampling every six months for up to 20 years. A statistically significant increase in total α-synuclein levels over time could then be observed, but the levels of P-129 α-synuclein remained constant during the observation period. The authors thus conclude that whereas plasma levels of phosphorylated α-synuclein can be diagnostically useful, total plasma α-synuclein might serve as a marker for disease progression [69].

In contrast to the above mentioned studies, Li et al. was the first study to report decreased α-synuclein levels in plasma from PD patients—with a more marked decrease among those with a lower age at disease onset [70]. Instead of using ELISA, the investigators adopted a strategy in which they immunoprecipitated α-synuclein with the 97/8 antibody—recognizing an epitope in the protein's C-terminus—and visualized the bands by western blot. The results from this study should be interpreted with caution as the number of subjects was small (27 PD cases and 11 healthy controls). However, in yet another study—that was based on a larger number of subjects—Laske et al. reported a decrease in α-synuclein among patients with DLB ($n = 40$), as compared to AD patients ($n = 80$) and healthy controls ($n = 40$). Instead of plasma, this study was carried out on serum and a commercially available kit for total α-synuclein measurement was used (Invitrogen, Immunoassay kit KHB0061) [71]. Yet another study tested the interesting hypothesis that *LRRK2* mutation carriers would display altered levels of α-synuclein in plasma. Among mutation carriers, lower levels of total plasma α-synuclein could be seen, whereas oligomeric α-synuclein was found to be unchanged between the groups [72].

Thus, although most initial studies found a small, but statistically significant increase in plasma levels of α-synuclein between patients with Lewy body disorders and controls several subsequent studies have reported lower levels among patients. Moreover, yet other studies have not been able to find any differences between the diagnostic groups. For example, Shi et al. reported that there were no significant differences in plasma α-synuclein levels between PD patients ($n = 117$), AD patients ($n = 33$) and control subjects ($n = 95$) [73]. Their measurements were based on a bead-based flow cytometry assay (Luminex), using the two monoclonal anti α-synuclein antibodies LB509 and 211 for capture and detection, respectively.

In an ELISA-based study by Park et al. there was also no difference in plasma α-synuclein between PD patients ($n = 23$) and controls ($n = 29$) [33]. In addition, three other studies have also failed to show any significant differences between diseased and healthy control subjects [74–76].

3.2 Blood Cells   As most of the above studies have assessed the free fraction of α-synuclein in either plasma or serum, a number of studies have investigated whether analysis of certain blood cells could be more informative. However, when leucocytes, lymphomonocytes, mononuclear cells, or platelets have been analyzed separately almost all studies have failed to show any alteration in α-synuclein levels between patients and controls (reviewed in [77]).

3.3 Plasma Exosomes   The discouraging outcome of most CSF and plasma based studies has prompted researchers to seek new methods to detect α-synuclein in biological samples. In 2014, Shi and colleagues aimed at isolating CNS-derived exosomes from human plasma and compared the levels of total α-synuclein in such preparations between 267 PD and 215 healthy control samples [78]. The authors utilized a magnetic bead-based capture assay, in which the beads were conjugated with a monoclonal antibody against the neural cell adhesion molecule L1CAM. Thus, they aimed to specifically enrich vesicles with a CNS origin under the assumption that the content of such vesicles would more closely mirror the situation in the brain.

The three day protocol is based on an overnight incubation of L1CAM antibody (10 μg, clone UJ127, Abcam, Cambridge, MA) together with 300 μl of plasma, which has previously been centrifuged sequentially at 2000 and $15,000 \times g$ to get rid of cell debris and larger protein aggregates. Upon incubation, beads are thoroughly washed and the remaining bead-antibody-vesicle complex is lysed with 1 % Triton-X [78]. Upon measuring the resulting lysate by a Luminex ELISA, the PD samples displayed statistically significantly higher levels of total α-synuclein ($p < 0.001$). In parallel, the free fraction of α-synuclein was measured in the plasma of the same subjects and did not show any group differences. Moreover, CSF was available from a subset (PD = 100, C = 100) of the subjects and displayed the expected decrease in α-synuclein concentration among PD patients [78]. Interestingly, no correlation was found between the increase of α-synuclein in L1CAM positive plasma exosomes and the decrease of α-synuclein in CSF, indicating that these compartments do not influence each other with respect to α-synuclein biology. Taken together, these data seem to suggest that α-synuclein detected in CSF and in CNS-derived plasma exosomes may reflect different pools of the protein.

4 Alpha-Synuclein in Other Body Fluids

4.1 Saliva   In the search for easily accessible biomarkers, researchers have also tried to assess the presence of α-synuclein in saliva. In the only published study, 24 PD patients were included and compared to a similarly sized group of healthy controls, but no differences in α-synuclein levels could be found [79].

5   Alpha-Synuclein in Peripheral Tissues

A thorough *post mortem* investigation, aimed at characterizing the presence of α-synuclein in different tissues and organs, demonstrated that the protein is widely expressed also throughout the peripheral nervous system and that it seemed to be more frequently displayed in PD [80].

5.1   Colonic Mucosa

In 2006, it was described that α-synuclein could be detected in the Meissner and Auerbach plexa of the enteric nervous system in PD patients [11] and additional studies highlighted the possibility to examine α-synuclein in patient biopsies [81]. The finding of pathological protein deposits in the wall of the gut thus offered an attractive patho-anatomical correlate to the well-described early constipation symptoms that PD patients often suffer from. In a study from 2010 colon mucosa samples were biopsied from subjects with and without PD [82]. In that study it could be demonstrated that 72 % of PD patients (21/29) were positive for α-synuclein pathology, whereas none of the included healthy controls (0/10) displayed any presence of aggregated α-synuclein. Moreover, it was found that patients who were positive for α-synuclein had a decreased L-dopa repsonsiveness as well as an increased constipation risk [82]. In a study on archived tissues, Shannon et al. described that nine out of ten PD patients displayed α-synuclein reactivity in the colonic submucosa, whereas all ten controls were negative for this marker [83]. Interestingly, one study indicated that different parts of the colon seem to be differently affected by α-synuclein pathology [84]. Although the sensitivity was lower than in previous studies, ranging from 23 % in rectum to 65 % in the ascending colon, the specificity remained high as none of the control subjects displayed any α-synuclein in neither of these regions [84]. In a separate study by the same investigator it could be shown that both the mucosa and the submucosa could be affected by α-synuclein pathology [85].

5.2   Ventricular Mucosa

The presence of α-synuclein does not seem to be restricted to one part of the gastrointestinal tract. For example, it could previously be shown that the protein also can be detected in the ventricular mucosa [86] and a recent study investigated the correlation between disease status and the presence of α-synuclein [87]. The biopsies on PD patients were taken during gastroscopy performed as a part of the procedure of initiating levodopa (l-dopa) therapy, whereas control biopsies were taken during the diagnostic procedure on patients with symptoms such as gastroesophageal reflux and unclear abdominal pain. Intriguingly, positive staining for α-synuclein could be found in 60.7 % (17/28) of the PD patients, but only in 4.3 % (1/23) of the control subjects [87].

5.3 Submandibular Gland

Upon systematically assessing the levels of α-synuclein in different parts of the peripheral nervous system it was found that the submandibular gland displayed the highest concentration [88]. Moreover, this *post mortem* study revealed that 100 % (28/28) of the investigated PD cases were positive for α-synuclein in the submandibular gland whereas only 6 % (3/50) of individuals with other neurodegenerative disorders had detectable α-synuclein in this tissue. Among non-neurological control subjects, none (0/50) displayed any α-synuclein in their *post mortem* biopsies [88]. In another study on archived tissues, another investigator demonstrated similar findings. In this study, 9/9 PD cases, 2/3 DLB cases, but 0/19 control subjects displayed α-synuclein reactivity [89].

As this organ is easily accessible for biopsies it could provide a new potential source for diagnostic material. One study, in which living individuals were biopsied, found that 75 % (9/12) of PD patients were positive for α-synuclein. Although no healthy controls were included in this study, the findings do suggest that α-synuclein detection in submandibular gland tissue could be a useful diagnostic marker for PD.

5.4 Skin

A good biomarker should be easily accessible and preferentially not require too invasive procedures. For this reason, a skin biopsy would be an attractive way source for diagnostic information. In a recent study, it was demonstrated that α-synuclein could be detected in all (21/21) analyzed skin biopsies from PD patients whereas none (0/30) of the control subjects displayed any such reactivity [90]. In this study, the authors compared different biopsy locations and found that those containing skin nerve fibers corresponding to the cervical dermatomes were most useful in discriminating diseased from healthy subjects. Moreover, the presence of α-synuclein was found to correlate with decreased skin innervation, indicating that protein deposition also interfered with normal nervous function [90].

5.5 Other Parts of the Peripheral Nervous System

In a *post mortem* study by Mu et al. α-synuclein was assessed in the pharyngeal plexus, a cervical part of the vagus nerve, and it was found that all ten PD patients but none of the four controls displayed α-synuclein reactivity [91]. However, due to its invasive nature, such a biomarker does not seem feasible for future routine diagnostic use.

5.6 Heart

Several studies have been published, in which a higher frequency of α-synuclein has been found in cardiac tissue from deceased PD patients as compared to controls (reviewed in [77]). Also in this case, it does not seem feasible to believe that α-synuclein in heart biopsied material could serve as a future diagnostic marker for PD or other Lewy body disorders.

6 Summary and Conclusions

A large number of studies have now been conducted, in which α-synuclein has been assessed as a novel biomarker. Whereas most CSF-based studies have shown a slight decrease in total α-synuclein among PD and DLB patients, the differences do not seem to be robust enough to be diagnostically useful. Moreover, it can be concluded that there do not seem to be any consistent change in α-synuclein in plasma- or serum-based investigations. However, a more recent study—based on measurement of plasma exosomes—has indicated a robust increase of α-synuclein in PD cases, but needs to be replicated before we know the usefulness of this approach.

Promising findings have been made in the last few years, concerning the possibilities to develop a peripheral tissue based α-synuclein biomarker. By analyzing α-synuclein in peripheral nerves from the submandibular gland, the ventricular/colon mucosa and the skin, investigators have found that also solid tissue-based tissues may offer an opportunity to detect increased α-synuclein among patients with Parkinson's disease and other disorders with Lewy body pathology. Also here we will have to await further studies until we know if such biomarkers in the future will have the potential to guide the clinician in their diagnostic workup.

References

1. Irizarry MC, Growdon W, Gomez-Isla T et al (1998) Nigral and cortical Lewy bodies and dystrophic nigral neurites in Parkinson's disease and cortical Lewy body disease contain alpha-synuclein immunoreactivity. J Neuropathol Exp Neurol 57(4):334–337

2. Gómez-Tortosa E, Newell K, Irizarry M et al (1999) Clinical and quantitative pathologic correlates of dementia with Lewy bodies. Neurology 53:1284–1291

3. Jellinger KA (2014) Neuropathology of multiple system atrophy: new thoughts about pathogenesis. Mov Disord 29(14):1720–1741

4. McKeith IG (2000) Clinical Lewy body syndromes. Ann N Y Acad Sci 920:1–8

5. Pereira JB, Svenningsson P, Weintraub D et al (2014) Initial cognitive decline is associated with cortical thinning in early Parkinson disease. Neurology 82(22):2017–2025

6. Donaghy PC, McKeith IG (2014) The clinical characteristics of dementia with Lewy bodies and a consideration of prodromal diagnosis. Alzheimers Res Ther 6(4):46

7. Fanciulli A, Wenning GK (2015) Multiple-system atrophy. N Engl J Med 372(3):249–263

8. Ba F, Martin WR (2015) Dopamine transporter imaging as a diagnostic tool for parkinsonism and related disorders in clinical practice. Parkinsonism Relat Disord 21(2):87–94

9. Kasuga K, Nishizawa M, Ikeuchi T (2012) alpha-Synuclein as CSF and Blood Biomarker of Dementia with Lewy Bodies. Int. J Alzheimers Dis 2012:437025

10. Braak H, Del Tredici K, Rub U et al (2003) Staging of brain pathology related to sporadic Parkinson's disease. Neurobiol Aging 24(2):197–211

11. Braak H, de Vos RA, Bohl J et al (2006) Gastric alpha-synuclein immunoreactive inclusions in Meissner's and Auerbach's plexuses in cases staged for Parkinson's disease-related brain pathology. Neurosci Lett 396(1):67–72

12. Holmqvist S, Chutna O, Bousset L et al (2014) Direct evidence of Parkinson pathology spread from the gastrointestinal tract to the brain in rats. Acta Neuropathol 128(6):805–820

13. Tokuda T, Salem SA, Allsop D et al (2006) Decreased alpha-synuclein in cerebrospinal fluid of aged individuals and subjects with Parkinson's disease. Biochem Biophys Res Commun 349(1):162–166

14. Mollenhauer B, Cullen V, Kahn I et al (2008) Direct quantification of CSF alpha-synuclein by ELISA and first cross-sectional study in

patients with neurodegeneration. Exp Neurol 213(2):315–325

15. Mollenhauer B, Locascio JJ, Schulz-Schaeffer W et al (2011) alpha-Synuclein and tau concentrations in cerebrospinal fluid of patients presenting with parkinsonism: a cohort study. Lancet Neurol 10(3):230–240

16. Wang Y, Shi M, Chung KA et al (2012) Phosphorylated alpha-synuclein in Parkinson's disease. Sci Transl Med 4(121):121ra20

17. Tateno F, Sakakibara R, Kawai T et al (2012) Alpha-synuclein in the cerebrospinal fluid differentiates synucleinopathies (Parkinson Disease, dementia with Lewy bodies, multiple system atrophy) from Alzheimer disease. Alzheimer Dis Assoc Disord 26(3):213–216

18. Parnetti L, Chiasserini D, Bellomo G et al (2011) Cerebrospinal fluid Tau/alpha-synuclein ratio in Parkinson's disease and degenerative dementias. Mov Disord 26(8):1428–1435

19. Mollenhauer B, Trautmann E, Taylor P et al (2013) Total CSF alpha-synuclein is lower in de novo Parkinson patients than in healthy subjects. Neurosci Lett 532:44–48

20. Hong Z, Shi M, Chung KA et al (2010) DJ-1 and alpha-synuclein in human cerebrospinal fluid as biomarkers of Parkinson's disease. Brain 133(Pt 3):713–726

21. van Dijk KD, Bidinosti M, Weiss A et al (2014) Reduced alpha-synuclein levels in cerebrospinal fluid in Parkinson's disease are unrelated to clinical and imaging measures of disease severity. Eur J Neurol 21(3):388–394

22. Shi M, Zhang J (2011) CSF alpha-synuclein, tau, and amyloid beta in Parkinson's disease. Lancet Neurol 10(8):681, author's reply 681-3

23. van Geel WJ, Abdo WF, Melis R et al (2008) A more efficient enzyme-linked immunosorbent assay for measurement of alpha-synuclein in cerebrospinal fluid. J Neurosci Methods 168(1):182–185

24. Bidinosti M, Shimshek DR, Mollenhauer B et al (2012) Novel one-step immunoassays to quantify alpha-synuclein: applications for biomarker development and high-throughput screening. J Biol Chem 287(40):33691–33705

25. Li T, Holmes C, Sham PC, Vallada H, Birkett J, Kirov G, Lesch KP, Powell J, Lovestone S, Collier D (1997) Allelic functional variation of serotonin transporter expression is a susceptibility factor for late onset AD. Neuroreport 8:683–686

26. Hall S, Ohrfelt A, Constantinescu R et al (2012) Accuracy of a panel of 5 cerebrospinal fluid biomarkers in the differential diagnosis of patients with dementia and/or parkinsonian disorders. Arch Neurol 69(11):1445–1452

27. Kang JH, Irwin DJ, Chen-Plotkin AS et al (2013) Association of cerebrospinal fluid beta-amyloid 1-42, T-tau, P-tau181, and alpha-synuclein levels with clinical features of drug-naive patients with early Parkinson disease. JAMA Neurol 70(10):1277–1287

28. Mondello S, Constantinescu R, Zetterberg H et al (2014) CSF alpha-synuclein and UCH-L1 levels in Parkinson's disease and atypical parkinsonian disorders. Parkinsonism Relat Disord 20(4):382–387

29. Parnetti L, Chiasserini D, Persichetti E et al (2014) Cerebrospinal fluid lysosomal enzymes and alpha-synuclein in Parkinson's disease. Mov Disord 29(8):1019–1027

30. Unterberger U, Lachmann I, Voigtlander T et al (2014) Detection of disease-associated alpha-synuclein in the cerebrospinal fluid: a feasibility study. Clin Neuropathol 33(5):329–334

31. Buddhala C, Campbell MC, Perlmutter JS et al (2015) Correlation between decreased CSF alpha-synuclein and Abeta(1)(-)(4)(2) in Parkinson disease. Neurobiol Aging 36(1):476–484

32. Aerts MB, Esselink RA, Abdo WF et al (2012) CSF alpha-synuclein does not differentiate between parkinsonian disorders. Neurobiol Aging 33(2):430, e1-3

33. Park MJ, Cheon SM, Bae HR et al (2011) Elevated levels of alpha-synuclein oligomer in the cerebrospinal fluid of drug-naive patients with Parkinson's disease. J Clin Neurol 7(4):215–222

34. Ohrfelt A, Grognet P, Andreasen N et al (2009) Cerebrospinal fluid alpha-synuclein in neurodegenerative disorders-a marker of synapse loss? Neurosci Lett 450(3):332–335

35. Noguchi-Shinohara M, Tokuda T, Yoshita M et al (2009) CSF alpha-synuclein levels in dementia with Lewy bodies and Alzheimer's disease. Brain Res 1251:1–6

36. Spies PE, Melis RJ, Sjogren MJ et al (2009) Cerebrospinal fluid alpha-synuclein does not discriminate between dementia disorders. J Alzheimers Dis 16(2):363–369

37. Kasuga K, Tokutake T, Ishikawa A et al (2010) Differential levels of alpha-synuclein, beta-amyloid42 and tau in CSF between patients with dementia with Lewy bodies and Alzheimer's disease. J Neurol Neurosurg Psychiatry 81(6):608–610

38. Reesink FE, Lemstra AW, van Dijk KD et al (2010) CSF alpha-synuclein does not discriminate dementia with Lewy bodies from Alzheimer's disease. J Alzheimers Dis 22(1):87–95

39. Wennstrom M, Londos E, Minthon L et al (2012) Altered CSF orexin and alpha-synuclein

levels in dementia patients. J Alzheimers Dis 29(1):125–132

40. Borghi R, Marchese R, Negro A et al (2000) Full length alpha-synuclein is present in cerebrospinal fluid from Parkinson's disease and normal subjects. Neurosci Lett 287(1):65–67

41. Slaets S, Vanmechelen E, Le Bastard N et al (2014) Increased CSF alpha-synuclein levels in Alzheimer's disease: correlation with tau levels. Alzheimers Dement 10(5 Suppl):S290–S298

42. Compta Y, Valente T, Saura J et al (2015) Correlates of cerebrospinal fluid levels of oligomeric- and total-alpha-synuclein in premotor, motor and dementia stages of Parkinson's disease. J Neurol 262(2):294–306

43. Magdalinou NK, Paterson RW, Schott JM et al (2015) A panel of nine cerebrospinal fluid biomarkers may identify patients with atypical parkinsonian syndromes. J Neurol Neurosurg Psychiatry 86(11):1240–1247

44. Kapaki E, Paraskevas GP, Emmanouilidou E et al (2013) The diagnostic value of CSF alpha-synuclein in the differential diagnosis of dementia with Lewy bodies vs. normal subjects and patients with Alzheimer's disease. PLoS One 8(11):e81654

45. Tokuda T, Qureshi MM, Ardah MT et al (2010) Detection of elevated levels of alpha-synuclein oligomers in CSF from patients with Parkinson disease. Neurology 75(20):1766–1772

46. Aasly JO, Johansen KK, Bronstad G et al (2014) Elevated levels of cerebrospinal fluid alpha-synuclein oligomers in healthy asymptomatic LRRK2 mutation carriers. Front Aging Neurosci 6:248

47. Hansson O, Hall S, Ohrfelt A et al (2014) Levels of cerebrospinal fluid alpha-synuclein oligomers are increased in Parkinson's disease with dementia and dementia with Lewy bodies compared to Alzheimer's disease. Alzheimers Res Ther 6(3):25

48. Jakowec MW, Petzinger GM, Sastry S et al (1998) The native form of alpha-synuclein is not found in the cerebrospinal fluid of patients with Parkinson's disease or normal controls. Neurosci Lett 253(1):13–16

49. Giasson BI, Jakes R, Goedert M et al (2000) A panel of epitope-specific antibodies detects protein domains distributed throughout human alpha-synuclein in Lewy bodies of Parkinson's disease. J Neurosci Res 59(4):528–533

50. Barbour R, Kling K, Anderson JP et al (2008) Red blood cells are the major source of alpha-synuclein in blood. Neurodegener Dis 5(2):55–59

51. Kruse N, Persson S, Alcolea D et al (2015) Validation of a quantitative cerebrospinal fluid alpha-synuclein assay in a European-wide inter-laboratory study. Neurobiol Aging 36(9): 2587–2596

52. Foulds PG, Mitchell JD, Parker A et al (2011) Phosphorylated alpha-synuclein can be detected in blood plasma and is potentially a useful biomarker for Parkinson's disease. FASEB J 25(12):4127–4137

53. Gao L, Tang H, Nie K et al (2015) Cerebrospinal fluid alpha-synuclein as a biomarker for Parkinson's disease diagnosis: a systematic review and meta-analysis. Int J Neurosci 125(9):645–654

54. Sako W, Murakami N, Izumi Y et al (2014) Reduced alpha-synuclein in cerebrospinal fluid in synucleinopathies: evidence from a meta-analysis. Mov Disord 29(13):1599–1605

55. Zetterberg H, Petzold M, Magdalinou N (2014) Cerebrospinal fluid alpha-synuclein levels in Parkinson's disease--changed or unchanged? Eur J Neurol 21(3):365–367

56. Winner B, Jappelli R, Maji SK et al (2011) In vivo demonstration that alpha-synuclein oligomers are toxic. Proc Natl Acad Sci U S A 108(10):4194–4199

57. Rockenstein E, Nuber S, Overk CR et al (2014) Accumulation of oligomer-prone alpha-synuclein exacerbates synaptic and neuronal degeneration in vivo. Brain 137(Pt 5):1496–1513

58. Sierks MR, Chatterjee G, McGraw C et al (2011) CSF levels of oligomeric alpha-synuclein and beta-amyloid as biomarkers for neurodegenerative disease. Integr Biol (Camb) 3(12):1188–1196

59. Brannstrom K, Lindhagen-Persson M, Gharibyan AL et al (2014) A generic method for design of oligomer-specific antibodies. PLoS One 9(3), e90857

60. Lesage S, Brice A (2009) Parkinson's disease: from monogenic forms to genetic susceptibility factors. Hum Mol Genet 18(R1):R48–R59

61. Schmid AW, Fauvet B, Moniatte M et al (2013) Alpha-synuclein post-translational modifications as potential biomarkers for Parkinson disease and other synucleinopathies. Mol Cell Proteomics 12(12):3543–3558

62. Fujiwara H, Hasegawa M, Dohmae N et al (2002) alpha-Synuclein is phosphorylated in synucleinopathy lesions. Nat Cell Biol 4(2): 160–164

63. Stewart T, Sossi V, Aasly JO et al (2015) Phosphorylated alpha-synuclein in Parkinson's disease: correlation depends on disease severity. Acta Neuropathol Commun 3:7

64. Wennstrom M, Surova Y, Hall S et al (2013) Low CSF levels of both alpha-synuclein and the alpha-synuclein cleaving enzyme neurosin in patients with synucleinopathy. PLoS One 8(1), e53250

65. El-Agnaf OM, Salem SA, Paleologou KE et al (2003) Alpha-synuclein implicated in Parkinson's disease is present in extracellular biological fluids, including human plasma. FASEB J 17(13):1945–1947

66. El-Agnaf OM, Salem SA, Paleologou KE et al (2006) Detection of oligomeric forms of alpha-synuclein protein in human plasma as a potential biomarker for Parkinson's disease. FASEB J 20(3):419–425

67. Lee PH, Lee G, Park HJ et al (2006) The plasma alpha-synuclein levels in patients with Parkinson's disease and multiple system atrophy. J Neural Transm 113(10):1435–1439

68. Duran R, Barrero FJ, Morales B et al (2010) Plasma alpha-synuclein in patients with Parkinson's disease with and without treatment. Mov Disord 25(4):489–493

69. Foulds PG, Diggle P, Mitchell JD et al (2013) A longitudinal study on alpha-synuclein in blood plasma as a biomarker for Parkinson's disease. Sci Rep 3:2540

70. Li QX, Mok SS, Laughton KM et al (2007) Plasma alpha-synuclein is decreased in subjects with Parkinson's disease. Exp Neurol 204(2):583–588

71. Laske C, Fallgatter AJ, Stransky E et al (2011) Decreased alpha-synuclein serum levels in patients with Lewy body dementia compared to Alzheimer's disease patients and control subjects. Dement Geriatr Cogn Disord 31(6):413–416

72. Gorostidi A, Bergareche A, Ruiz-Martinez J et al (2012) Alphalpha-synuclein levels in blood plasma from LRRK2 mutation carriers. PLoS One 7(12), e52312

73. Shi M, Zabetian CP, Hancock AM et al (2010) Significance and confounders of peripheral DJ-1 and alpha-synuclein in Parkinson's disease. Neurosci Lett 480(1):78–82

74. Mata IF, Shi M, Agarwal P et al (2010) SNCA variant associated with Parkinson disease and plasma alpha-synuclein level. Arch Neurol 67(11):1350–1356

75. Besong-Agbo D, Wolf E, Jessen F et al (2013) Naturally occurring alpha-synuclein autoantibody levels are lower in patients with Parkinson disease. Neurology 80(2):169–175

76. Smith LM, Schiess MC, Coffey MP et al (2012) Alpha-Synuclein and anti-alpha-synuclein antibodies in Parkinson's disease, atypical Parkinson syndromes, REM sleep behavior disorder, and healthy controls. PLoS One 7(12):e52285

77. Malek N, Swallow D, Grosset KA et al (2014) Alpha-synuclein in peripheral tissues and body fluids as a biomarker for Parkinson's disease—a systematic review. Acta Neurol Scand 130(2):59–72

78. Shi M, Liu C, Cook TJ et al (2014) Plasma exosomal alpha-synuclein is likely CNS-derived and increased in Parkinson's disease. Acta Neuropathol 128(5):639–650

79. Devic I, Hwang H, Edgar JS et al (2011) Salivary alpha-synuclein and DJ-1: potential biomarkers for Parkinson's disease. Brain 134(Pt 7), e178

80. Beach TG, Adler CH, Sue LI et al (2010) Multi-organ distribution of phosphorylated alpha-synuclein histopathology in subjects with Lewy body disorders. Acta Neuropathol 119(6):689–702

81. Lebouvier T, Chaumette T, Damier P et al (2008) Pathological lesions in colonic biopsies during Parkinson's disease. Gut 57(12):1741–1743

82. Lebouvier T, Neunlist M, Bruley S (2010) des Varannes, et al., Colonic biopsies to assess the neuropathology of Parkinson's disease and its relationship with symptoms. PLoS One 5(9), e12728

83. Shannon KM, Keshavarzian A, Mutlu E et al (2012) Alpha-synuclein in colonic submucosa in early untreated Parkinson's disease. Mov Disord 27(6):709–715

84. Pouclet H, Lebouvier T, Coron E et al (2012) A comparison between rectal and colonic biopsies to detect Lewy pathology in Parkinson's disease. Neurobiol Dis 45(1):305–309

85. Pouclet H, Lebouvier T, Coron E et al (2012) A comparison between colonic submucosa and mucosa to detect Lewy pathology in Parkinson's disease. Neurogastroenterol Motil 24(4): e202–e205

86. Pouclet H, Lebouvier T, Coron E et al (2012) Lewy pathology in gastric and duodenal biopsies in Parkinson's Disease. Mov Disord 27(6):708

87. Sanchez-Ferro A, Rabano A, Catalan MJ et al (2015) In vivo gastric detection of alpha-synuclein inclusions in Parkinson's disease. Mov Disord 30(4):517–524

88. Beach TG, Adler CH, Dugger BN et al (2013) Submandibular gland biopsy for the diagnosis of Parkinson disease. J Neuropathol Exp Neurol 72(2):130–136

89. Del Tredici K, Hawkes CH, Ghebremedhin E et al (2010) Lewy pathology in the submandibular gland of individuals with incidental Lewy body disease and sporadic Parkinson's disease. Acta Neuropathol 119(6):703–713

90. Donadio V, Incensi A, Leta V et al (2014) Skin nerve alpha-synuclein deposits: a biomarker for idiopathic Parkinson disease. Neurology 82(15):1362–1369

91. Mu L, Sobotka S, Chen J et al (2013) Alpha-synuclein pathology and axonal degeneration of the peripheral motor nerves innervating pharyngeal muscles in Parkinson disease. J Neuropathol Exp Neurol 72(2):119–129

Chapter 15

Imaging as a Diagnostic Tool in Parkinson's Disease

Johan Wikström and Torsten Danfors

Abstract

Magnetic resonance imaging (MRI) and nuclear imaging techniques are complementary methods to visualize biological changes on a morphological as well as a molecular level. Together they are useful tools to establish an early diagnosis of Parkinson's disease (PD) and to differentiate between PD and other neurodegenerative disorders. Magnetic resonance imaging has the advantage of having a superior spatial resolution and being more widely available. The method could support the diagnosis of PD by detecting volume loss in specific regions, e.g., substantia nigra (SN), but also by unraveling functional changes associated with PD, such as decreased activation of motor regions by motor activating tasks, decreased white matter integrity, and metabolic changes in certain brain regions. Nuclear medicine imaging techniques, such as positron emission tomography (PET) and single photon emitted tomography (SPECT), can be used to detect dopamine deficiency, functional metabolic neuronal impairments and pathological accumulation of certain proteins in the nervous system. Similar to MRI, both PET and SPECT may also be used to aid in the differential diagnosis between Parkinson's disease and other parkinsonian syndromes.

Key words Magnetic resonance imaging, MRI, Parkinson's disease, Magnetic resonance spectroscopy, Functional MRI, Resting state functional MRI, Diffusion weighted imaging, Diffusion tensor imaging, Magnetic transfer imaging, PET, SPECT, Dopamine transporter, PE2I, FDG, Amyloid, Tau, Alpha-synuclein

Abbreviations

FDG	Fluorodeoxyglucose
PET	Positron emission tomography
DAT	Dopamine transporter
SPECT	Single photon emitted computed tomography
NPH	Normal pressure hydrocephalus
VASC	Vascular parkinsonism
MSA	Multiple system atrophy
PD	Parkinson's disease
CBD	Corticobasal degeneration

Martin Ingelsson and Lars Lannfelt (eds.), *Immunotherapy and Biomarkers in Neurodegenerative Disorders*, Methods in Pharmacology and Toxicology, DOI 10.1007/978-1-4939-3560-4_15, © Springer Science+Business Media New York 2016

1 MRI of Parkinson's Disease

1.1 Introduction

Magnetic resonance imaging (MRI) is a technique without the use of ionizing radiation, producing images with high soft tissue contrast in arbitrary imaging planes. The technique has proven especially useful for investigations of the central nervous system, with marked improvement of gray–white matter differentiation compared to computed tomography. In addition to morphological images, MRI permits functional evaluation of nervous tissue by several different complementary methods, by which information can be obtained on location of activated areas (functional MRI), white matter tract integrity (diffusion tensor imaging), white matter tract connections (tractography), and metabolite concentrations (MR spectroscopy).

1.2 Methods

1.2.1 Morphological Techniques

Morphological images are routinely obtained with T1- and T2-weighted and FLAIR sequences, and reflect above all differences in tissue water content, but also other factors, such as iron content, can influence the signal. Iron causes local magnetic field perturbations, which cause signal intensity loss, most notably on T2-weighted sequences. A way of quantifying this effect is to measure the tissue specific parameter T2, or R2 (R2=1/T2). Besides these sequences, diffusion weighted imaging (DWI) has been proposed as a method for improved delineation of subcortical gray matter, e.g., substantia nigra (SN) [1]. In DWI, the contrast is mostly dependent on differences in local water diffusion rate, which can be restricted by for example cell membranes, causing increased signal intensity in areas with diffusion restriction on diffusion weighted images. Another method for improving delineation of pathology is magnetic transfer (MT) imaging, which exploits differences in magnetization between free protons and protons bound to macromolecules to enhance contrast between healthy and pathological neural tissue [2].

1.2.2 Functional MRI Techniques

Functional MRI methods include diffusion tensor imaging (DTI), functional MRI (f-MRI), and MR spectroscopy (MRS). DTI is a method that extracts information about the degree of directionality of water diffusion in a tissue. In free water, diffusion is equal in all directions (isotropic), whereas in brain tissue, the diffusion is higher along the direction of the axons (anisotropic). DTI permits quantification of the diffusion in different directions and calculation of the so-called fractional anisotropy (FA), which is a scalar ranging from zero to one. An FA of zero corresponds to isotropic diffusion and an FA of one corresponds to maximally anisotropic diffusion (diffusion in only one direction). Apart from quantification of degree of diffusion anisotropy, the FA permits 3D visualization of nerve fiber tracts (tractography). This is accomplished by calculation of the direction with highest diffusion in each voxel and then drawing paths between neighboring voxels along these directions.

With f-MRI the nerve cell activation in different brain areas during a task is indirectly visualized through the resultant local paradoxical increase in blood oxygen content which increases the MR signal. Images acquired during task performance are compared with images at rest and the difference is calculated. From this difference, parametric images showing activated areas are produced. Besides task related f-MRI there is also resting state f-MRI; in which the variation in brain activity at rest is studied and areas with synchronous activation are identified. DTI and resting state f-MRI are thus different, but complementary, methods for investigation of brain connectivity.

MRS exploits small differences in rotation frequency of the protons' magnetic moment between different chemical compounds for estimation of concentration of different metabolites. MRS may be performed for different nuclei. Most often hydrogen containing compounds are studied (H-MRS). Common metabolites studied with H-MRS include N-acetylaspartate (NAA), choline (Cho), creatine (Cr) and lactate (La). NAA decreases in conditions with nerve cell loss or dysfunction, choline is related to cell membrane synthesis and degradation, creatine is a more or less stable metabolite which is often used for normalization purposes, and lactate is a marker of ischemia. The second most studied nucleus is phosphor (P-MRS), which is especially interesting for the study of energy metabolism. Metabolites studied with P-MRS include phosphocreatine (PCr) and adenosine triphosphate (ATP).

1.3 MRI Findings in Parkinson's Disease

Many MRI studies have focused on possible changes in the nigrostriatal complex. Some studies have found volume reductions of the substantia nigra, especially the pars compacta [3] but other studies have not been able to reproduce this [1, 4]. A decrease in putamen volume was found in early PD compared to controls, and a significantly more pronounced decrease was seen in advanced PD [5]. Furthermore, findings suggesting increased iron content in the substantia nigra (SN) have been observed [6–8]. A voxel based magnetization transfer imaging study showed reduced tissue integrity (neuronal loss and/or myelin reduction) within the SN in patients with Parkinson's disease (PD) compared to age-matched controls [9]. Significant morphological changes have thus been found in several studies, but it remains to be established if these measures can be used for reliable identification of PD.

Different functional MRI techniques have also been explored in PD patients. Using DTI, FA reductions in the SN consistent with histopathological findings of axonal loss have been described, but results are somewhat inconsistent between studies [10–18]. A promising finding from Vaillancourt et al. [14] was a pronounced FA reduction in the posterior part of SN in 14 early PD patients compared with 14 age matched controls, with 100 % sensitivity and specificity. Reductions in FA in PD patients have also been found in motor, premotor, and supplementary motor cortex [15, 19] as well as in premotor white matter tracts [15]. Reduced connectivity between SN and ipsilateral thalamus and putamen was also shown using DTI technique [10].

Metabolite changes have been observed in PD patients using mainly hydrogen [20–24] but also phosphorous MRS [21]. Regions with metabolite changes include SN, and basal ganglia but also cortical structures. Reduction in NAA/Cr ratio, suggesting reduction of normally functioning neurons, have been described in both SN [25] and putamen [23]. On the other hand, conflicting results were observed in other studies, reporting increase in NAA/Cr ratio in the SN [20] and no change in NAA concentration in the basal ganglia in PD compared to controls [26]. Hattingen et al. reported reduced levels of high-energy phosphates (ATP and PCr) in striatum and midbrain in both early and advanced PD [21], while Weiduschat et al. found no significant metabolite changes in early PD either with H- or P-MRS [27]. Reasons for conflicting results include differences in ROI placement and different methods for defining the investigated anatomical structures. Comparisons between different studies are especially difficult for the SN, where the small size makes partial volume effects a significant problem.

F-MRI studies have shown changes in motor network connectivity in PD patients [28–30]. Reduced activation during a motor task in PD patients was also reported in the anterior part of SMA and in the right dorsal prefrontal cortex but increased activation in primary motor cortex, posterior SMA, and anterior cingulate cortex, possibly reflecting compensatory changes [31]. However, it remains to be shown if these techniques can aid in the diagnosis of PD.

1.3.1 Differential Diagnosis

Morphological MR sequences have an important role for excluding atypical Parkinson syndromes. In multiple system atrophy (MSA), typical findings are volume loss in the pons and cerebellar vermis and signal intensity changes in the pons producing the so-called "hot cross bun sign" (Fig. 1) [32]. In progressive supranuclear palsy (PSP), there is marked volume reduction of the mesencephalon causing the so-called "hummingbird sign" (Fig. 2) [33]. Different area measurements have been proposed for differentiation between PD, MSA, and PSP [34, 35] and a Parkinsonism Index has been described which could identify patients with PSP [35]. Du et al. studied the SN in PD and controls, using R2 measurements to assess differences in brain iron accumulation and FA measurements to assess differences in nerve cell integrity [16]. PD patients had lower FA and higher R2 than controls, and ROC analysis showed best diagnostic performance for the combination of R2 and FA, followed by R2 alone. Further, with H-MRS, differences in NAA concentrations in the lentiform nucleus in MSA and PSP compared with PD patients have been reported [26], which

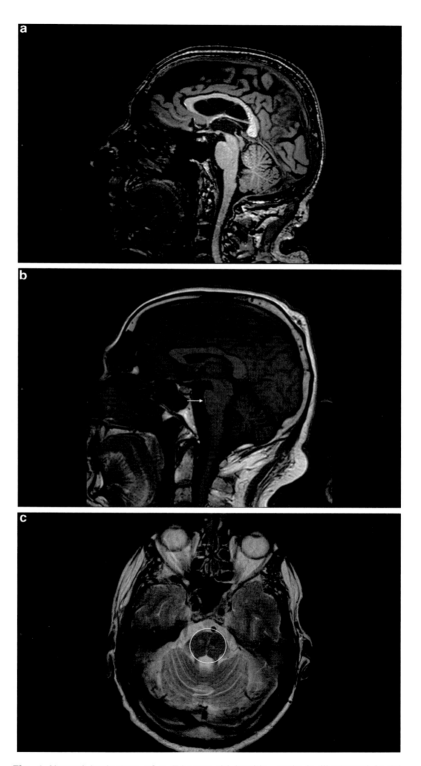

Fig. 1 Normal brainstem of a 74-year-old healthy male is illustrated in (**a**). Compare this to findings of a 63-year-old male with multiple system atrophy (MSA), where a marked volume reduction of pons is observed (*arrow* in **b**), and typical signal intensity changes are observed in the pons, producing the characteristic "hot cross bun sign" (**c**)

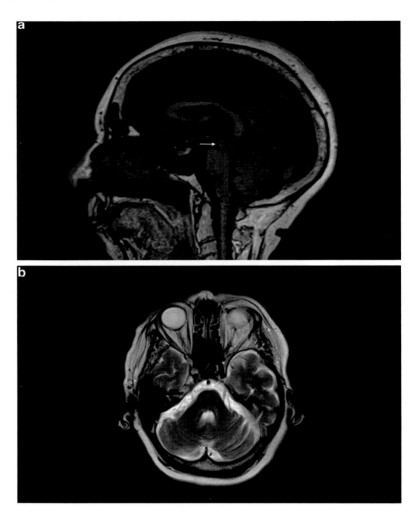

Fig. 2 Images of a 73-year-old woman with progressive supranuclear palsy, with volume reduction of mesencephalon producing the so-called hummingbird sign (*arrow* in **a**), but normal volume and signal intensity in the pons (**a**, **b**)

might be used for differentiation between the disorders. Differences in rostral to caudal NAA/Cr ratios have also been detected between PD and atypical Parkinsonian syndromes [36]. In corticobasal degeneration, there is typically asymmetrical parietal and paracentral cortical volume loss, sometimes associated with adjacent subcortical signal intensity changes and ipsilateral cerebral peduncle atrophy [37]. Infarcts in strategic locations can also cause symptoms mimicking idiopathic PD. Such infarcts are typically found within basal ganglia and frontal white matter [38].

1.3.2 Treatment Monitoring

The degree of FA reduction in the SN in PD has been shown to correlate with disease severity [13], making this a possible biomarker for treatment monitoring. In a H-MRS study of PD patients without treatment, reductions in NAA/Cr and Cho/Cr ratios compared with controls were observed [22], which could be interpreted as evidence of nerve cell loss/dysfunction and disturbance of cell membrane metabolism, respectively. After 6 months treatment with the dopamine agonist Pergolide, these ratios were partly normalized, with a significant change in Cho/Cr ration compared with baseline, making this another potential treatment monitoring biomarker.

2 Nuclear Medicine and Molecular Imaging in Parkinson's Disease

2.1 Introduction

The dopamine deficiency, the functional metabolic neuronal impairments and the specific proteins accumulating in the nervous system in Parkinson's disease can be assessed with nuclear medicine and molecular imaging techniques. This chapter focuses on how PET and SPECT may be used to aid in the differential diagnostic procedure for Parkinson's disease and other parkinsonian syndromes.

Parkinson's disease (PD) is recognized as the second most common neurodegenerative disorder after Alzheimer's disease (AD) and affects about 1 % of the population. The definite diagnosis of idiopathic PD requires a histopathologic analysis with the finding of intraneuronal inclusions of Lewy bodies in the substantia nigra pars compacta. A clinical diagnosis of PD poses a great challenge but studies suggest that there is a 90 % concordance between the clinical diagnosis from a movement disorder expert and the histologic conformation [39, 40].

Parkinsonism is a neurological condition with a symptom complex characterized by tremor, hypokinesia, rigidity, and postural instability. The most common and typical cause for parkinsonism is PD. Atypical parkinsonian syndromes (APS) (also known as Parkinson-plus syndromes) include multiple system atrophy, progressive supranuclear palsy, and corticobasal degeneration. These disorders are clinically difficult to separate from each other and from PD. Other common and important differential diagnoses of parkinsonism are essential tremor, drug induced parkinsonism, dopa-responsive and cervical dystonia, normal pressure hydrocephalus, and vascular parkinsonism. Dementia with Lewy bodies (DLB) is the second most common type of dementia after AD and shares symptoms of cognitive and motor disabilities with both AD and PD. DLB is typically also accompanied by visual hallucinations and fluctuations in alertness and attention. Dementia can be a feature also of late stage Parkinson's disease (PDD) and is then considered to be a separate entity of dementia.

Therapy options for patients with parkinsonism include both medication and surgical interventions. Only patients with PD will benefit from high doses of dopaminergic drugs while others will mostly experience side effects, which sometimes may be severe. For patients with essential tremor treatment is primarily pharmacological but less benign cases can be helped by deep brain stimulation, an invasive procedure that is also used for PD. However, the target stimulation area differs in these conditions, further highlighting the demand for accurate diagnosis. Another important differential diagnosis is drug-induced parkinsonism, where dopaminergic imaging can help to exclude PD. Any drug that blocks the action of dopamine, i.e., dopamine antagonists, may cause parkinsonism. Not only neuroleptics (typically haloperidol) but also cardiac anti-arrhythmic substances (cordarone) and antidepressive drugs (lithium) may cause parkinsonism. Typically, such adverse effects can be seen in a patient with psychiatric symptoms and parkinsonism where removal of the drug is unwanted. Vascular parkinsonism is another important differential diagnosis, where the symptoms may mimic PD or APD [41].

Dementia is often a late stage symptom of PD, but can also be an early disease manifestation of DLB. The symptoms of DLB may overlap not only with PD but also with AD and is therefore often misdiagnosed early in disease. For clinicians it is important to know that patients with DLB often have a marked sensitivity to neuroleptic drugs and acetylcholinesterase inhibitors should then be the drug of choice [42]. Normally it is not difficult to clinically differentiate between DLB and PDD. They share the same cortical pathology but the pattern and timescale of evolution are different. Treatment of patients with PDD is mainly focused on reducing dopaminergic and anticholinergic drugs. PDD patients may not react in the same way as patients with DLB on treatment with neuroleptics. Instead they will experience increasing extrapyramidal symptoms making them unsuitable for this treatment. If antipsychotic treatment is necessary atypical neuroleptics should be used.

2.2 Presynaptic Dopaminergic Imaging

The dopaminergic system can be visualized in different ways. The nigrostriatal pathway terminates in the striatum and dopamine is released into the synapses. The function of dopamine terminals can be examined by estimating the availability of dopamine transporters (DAT). This has been done with a number of different SPECT and PET tracers, such as ^{123}I Iometopan (beta-CIT), ^{123}I Ioflupane (FP-CIT), ^{11}C- or ^{18}F-WIN 34,428 (^{11}C-CFT, ^{18}F-CFT) and ^{11}C- or ^{18}F-PE2I. Also, the dopadecarboxylase activity and dopamine turnover can be measured with ^{18}F-3,4-dihydroxyphenylalanine (^{18}F-DOPA) and the vesicle monoamine transporter availability with ^{18}F- or ^{11}C-dihydrotetrabenazine (DHTB).

Many of the SPECT ligands are commercially available and widely used. The uptake reflects the number of functionally intact dopamine producing neurons in the substantia nigra. In early and even in the preclinical stage of the disease loss of DAT may be identified [43, 44]. This reduction is bilaterally reduced with the most severe changes in the dorsal part of the putamen contralateral to the affected limb [45]. Symptoms of clinical parkinsonism occur when PD patients have lost 40–50 % of posterior dopamine function in the putamen [46]. As a compensatory mechanism the remaining functioning neurons increase their dopamine production to preserve function of the striatal motor circuit.

With DAT imaging it is also possible to distinguish between essential tremor that is not due to dopamine deficiency and tremor due to idiopathic parkinsonian diseases [47, 48] with a high specificity and sensitivity. This becomes particularly important when evaluating different possible treatments including deep brain stimulation. It is also possible to distinguish AD from PD and DLB with DAT imaging [49].

2.3 Postsynaptic Dopaminergic Imaging

When dopamine (DA) is released into the synaptic cleft, it binds to specific G-protein coupled DA receptors on the postsynaptic neuron. There are two major groups of DA receptors; D1- (D1 and D5) and D2- like (D2-4) groups. D2/D3 receptors may be visualized with ^{123}I-IBZM SPECT [50] or ^{11}C-Raclopride PET [51, 52]. The visualization of postsynaptic D2/D3 receptors in parts of the brain outside the striatum is challenging because of their relatively low concentrations [53–55]. In the striatum, studies of the postsynaptic dopamine receptors have mainly been used in psychiatric research [56, 57] or psychological studies related to stress [58, 59]. Moreover, the technique has been used to study obesity [60–64], drug abuse [65] and pathological gambling [66]. The latter can sometimes be associated either with Parkinson's disease or treatment with dopamine agonists [67].

In PD and APS postsynaptic SPECT has shown a decrease of D2 receptor binding [68]. The possibility to differentiate between PD and APS with the aid of IBZM SPECT has been tested [69] also in combination with FP-CIT. A combination of FP-CIT and IBZM rendered a sensitivity of 89 % but a specificity of only 50 % [70].

2.4 Extracerebral Imaging

In Parkinson's disease the sympathetic myocardial innervation may be altered. This can be measured with ^{123}I metaiodobenzylguanidine (MIBG), a norepinephrine (noradrenaline, NA) analogue that competes with the same cellular transporter mechanisms of postganglionic adrenergic neurons. It accumulates in organs with high sympathetic activation such as the liver, adrenal and salivary glands, the spleen, and the heart. Low uptake of MIBG was found in patients with autonomic symptoms [71] and in PD where it correlates with disease severity [72]. Many studies have found variances in the sympathetic innervation of the heart with impaired function in PD and preserved function in APS [73–75]. Lately, low MIBG uptake has also been associated with affection of the postganglionic presynaptic cardiac sympathetic nerve endings with accumulation of Lewy bodies in both PD and APS [76]. The parasympathetic function may also be impaired in patients with Parkinson's disease. 5-[(11)C]-methoxy-donepezil is a high-affinity ligand for acetylcholinesterase and can be used to visualize cholinergic neurons [77]. In patients with Parkinson's disease uptake is decreased in the small intestine and pancreas suggesting a parasympathetic denervation of internal organs [78].

2.5 Brain Metabolism: Regional Fluorodeoxyglucose Metabolism

The human brain depends on glucose as its primary source of energy and glucose utilization can be measured with ^{18}F-fluorodeoxyglucose (^{18}F-FDG), a glucose analogue that is phosphorylated and trapped inside the cell after passing through the cell membrane.

Multiple studies have investigated the pattern of regional cerebral glucose metabolism in PD. It has proven to be useful in the differentiation between PD and APS [79]. In early stage of PD the uptake in the lentiform nucleus is normal or increased [80, 81] and disease progression is associated with increased glucose metabolism in the internal globus pallidus, the dorsal part of the pons, primary motor cortex, and the subthalamic nucleus [82]. Patients with PDD also have an impaired cortical glucose metabolism similar to that seen in AD but with no beta-amyloid deposition suggesting that the dementia in PD is a unique biological process [83].

2.6 The Combination of Dopaminergic and Metabolic or Perfusion Imaging

DAT imaging does not have the possibility to sensitively discriminate between PD and APS syndromes alone. In typical clinical cases FDG PET may be valuable but the uptake is often unspecific and vascular or degenerative alterations other than the primary neurodegenerative changes may be coexisting, which can distort the specific uptake patterns. However, a combination of these two imaging modalities has been found useful. The FDG patterns of patients with parkinsonism and normal DAT imaging were examined and in this group no typical findings of either PD or APD were found [84]. For this reason DAT imaging may help to exclude patients with vascular or other forms of parkinsonism and improve the sensitivity of FDG PET.

Recently a new imaging tracer for human use, the high affinity DAT compound N-(3-iodoprop-2 E-enyl)-2beta-carbomethoxy-3beta-(4-methylphenyl)nortropane (PE2I) has been developed and labelled with ^{11}C [85] and ^{18}F [86]. The main advantage to previous ligands is the more specific binding with high selectivity for DAT over the serotonin- and norepinephrine transporters. The high contrast also allows for quantification of DAT receptor availability in the midbrain (substantia nigra) [85, 87]

Dynamic collection of ^{11}C-PE2I image data allows for calculation of both cerebral perfusion (regional perfusion relative to cerebellum) and binding potential (BP) [88] (Fig. 3). Since both cerebral perfusion and glucose metabolism reflect neuronal activity we performed a study where dual information of DAT availability and cerebral perfusion from PET PE2I was compared to FP-CIT SPECT and FDG PET on a group of patients with PD and APS

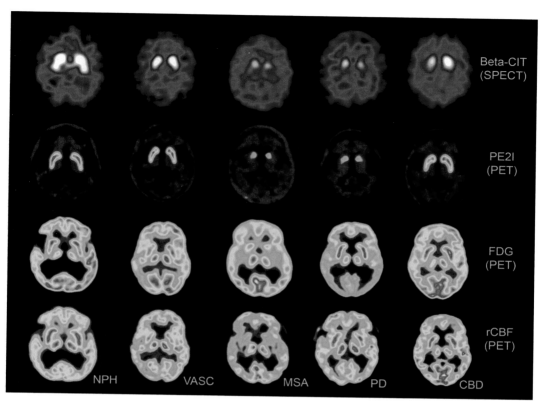

Fig. 3 Representative images using four different tracers with either SPECT or PET. Illustrations from the *top* to *bottom* row: The presynaptic dopamine transporter protein ^{123}I beta-Cit (DAT SPECT), ^{11}C PE2I (DAT PET), ^{18}F fluorodeoxyglucose (FDG PET), and the relative cerebral perfusion (rCBF) calculated from the dynamic ^{11}C PE2I scan. The DAT SPECT color scale was adjusted so that the signal from the occipital lobe was similar between subjects. DAT PET is measured in absolute values, i.e., binding potential (BP), and the color scale varies between BP 0 and 10. The color scale in the FDG images represents standard uptake values (SUV) and in the rCBF cerebral blood flow relative to the pons. In these images the color scale was adjusted so that the maximum intensity was often reached in the basal ganglia or in the occipital lobe

[89]. In this study a high correlation between PE2I BP and FP-CIT SPECT was found, with a somewhat weaker correlation between FDG PET and relative cerebral perfusion.

2.7 Beta-Amyloid-, Tau- and Alpha-Synuclein Imaging in PD

Imaging of the specific proteins that are accumulating in the nervous system in neurodegenerative diseases has the potential to improve diagnostic accuracy. The Pittsburg compound B (PIB), an amyloid binding tracer developed by William Klunk, was evaluated on AD patients in a collaboration with the Uppsala University PET Centre and Karolinska institute [90, 91]. [11]C PIB has primarily been used for research studies in AD and a number of amyloid binding tracers labelled with ^{18}F have now emerged. In April 2012, ^{18}F florbetapir (Amyvid; Eli Lilly) was the first amyloid tracer to be approved by the US Food and Drug Administration (FDA) to identify Aβ plaque accumulation. The initial conclusion was that a positive scan does not establish the diagnosis of AD because high binding may also be present in adults with normal cognition, although a negative scan indicates that the cognitive impairment is less likely due to AD. However, post mortem studies of amyloid deposition with correlations to amyloid imaging later showed that not all patients with AD pathology have a positive scan and that amyloid imaging only accurately reflects the dense, neuritic, plaques [92]. These results in combination with low effectiveness of the current available treatments has led to a decrease in the clinical impact of an amyloid scan [93] and a statement from the Centers for Medicare and Medicare Services (CMS) that amyloid imaging may be covered by the Social Security Act only in two scenarios. Firstly, to exclude AD in "narrowly defined and clinically difficult differential diagnoses, such as AD vs frontotemporal dementia (FTD)"; and secondly to ensure that only amyloid positive subjects are being enrolled in clinical studies of novel treatment and prevention strategies (CAG-00431 N). Amyloid binding tracers have also been tested for the diagnostic procedure of Parkinson's disease (PD), Parkinson's disease with dementia (PDD), and dementia with Lewy bodies (DLB) [94]. The studies have shown that the tested ligands could not detect any amyloid deposition in PD and that they only infrequently (2/12) or nonsignificantly could reveal amyloid presence in PDD whereas a significant deposition (11/13) could be found in DLB [95]. These results correspond well to the neuropathological findings [96]. Thus, this type of imaging can be useful in discriminating between cognitive dysfunction due to amyloid deposition, as in AD or DLB, and other pathological backgrounds, as in PD.

^{18}F FDDNP is a PET tracer by which tau fibrillary aggregates can be visualized in vivo. This tracer was first evaluated on tauopathies like AD [18, 97, 98] and Down's syndrome [99] but has now also been explored for the use on parkinsonian disorders. In a study on 15 subjects with progressive supranuclear palsy the uptake was compared with early stage PD and with healthy controls (HC). High uptake was then found in subcortical areas in all progressive supranuclear palsy patients regardless of disease severity and with increasing levels of uptake as the disease progressed [100].

Alpha synuclein aggregates in Lewy bodies (LB) and Lewy neurites (LN) are the predominant protein in the typical pathology of PD, DLB, and multiple system atrophy. Lately, LBs and LNs have also been reported to be present in the enteric nervous system [101–103] and in the skin [104] of patients with PD suggesting that loss of dopaminergic neurons occur late in PD and that there might be a cell-to-cell transmission of alpha-synuclein. These findings highlight the need for noninvasive methods to measure the presence and distribution of LB and LN in whole body measurements. Ongoing efforts to develop tracers for alpha-synuclein pathology [105] may provide a method to visualize and measure the level of protein accumulation in clinical studies and identify patients similar to amyloid imaging in AD.

2.8 Neuro-inflammation and Parkinson's Disease

Microglia are immune cells that reside inside of the blood–brain barrier and are part of the first immune defense in the central nervous system (CNS). These cells become activated in response to injury, infectious agents, or other pathological changes in the CNS. The mitochondria of activated microglia express a translocator protein (TSPO, previously called peripheral benzodiazepine receptor). A number of different PET ligands against this protein have been developed, of which the most commonly used is ^{11}C PK11195 [106]. This tracer has been proven useful to detect neuroinflammation in PD [107] and there is evidence that the neuroinflammation precedes the other pathological processes in PD and PDD [108].

3   Conclusions

Deciding on the cause of parkinsonism is crucial in the management of Parkinson's disease. DAT SPECT imaging has the possibility to exclude Parkinson's disease, multiple system atrophy, corticobasal degeneration, and progressive supranuclear palsy. Further differentiation of the disorders within this group is difficult but can be done with FDG PET. With newer DAT PET tracers it is possible to measure binding in absolute terms (binding potential), which can potentially improve the diagnostic procedure and also provide a biomarker for disease progression.

Another important and clinically difficult situation is to differentiate between AD and dementia with Lewy bodies. Also here a pathological DAT imaging can help to exclude AD. With imaging it is more difficult to separate patients with Parkinson's disease dementia and dementia with Lewy bodies but the medical history with motor symptoms preceding dementia is normally diagnostic.

Finally, imaging of specific accumulating proteins such as amyloid-beta, tau and alpha-synuclein is important not only for clinical diagnostics but also to provide a tool in the search and monitoring of new potentially disease modifying therapies.

References

1. Adachi M, Hosoya T, Haku T et al (1999) Evaluation of the substantia nigra in patients with Parkinsonian syndrome accomplished using multishot diffusion-weighted MR imaging. AJNR Am J Neuroradiol 20(8):1500–1506

2. Wolff SD, Balaban RS (1989) Magnetization transfer contrast (MTC) and tissue water proton relaxation in vivo. Magn Reson Med 10(1):135–144

3. Pujol J, Junque C, Vendrell P et al (1992) Reduction of the substantia nigra width and motor decline in aging and Parkinson's disease. Arch Neurol 49(11):1119–1122

4. Oikawa H, Sasaki M, Tamakawa Y et al (2002) The substantia nigra in Parkinson disease: proton density-weighted spin-echo and fast short inversion time inversion-recovery MR findings. AJNR Am J Neuroradiol 23(10):1747–1756

5. Geng DY, Li YX, Zee CS (2006) Magnetic resonance imaging-based volumetric analysis of basal ganglia nuclei and substantia nigra in patients with Parkinson's disease. Neurosurgery 58(2):256–262. doi:10.1227/01.NEU.0000 194845.19462.7B, discussion 256-262

6. Gorell JM, Ordidge RJ, Brown GG et al (1995) Increased iron-related MRI contrast in the substantia nigra in Parkinson's disease. Neurology 45(6):1138–1143

7. Graham JM, Paley MN, Grunewald RA et al (2000) Brain iron deposition in Parkinson's disease imaged using the PRIME magnetic resonance sequence. Brain 123(Pt 12): 2423–2431

8. Martin WR (2009) Quantitative estimation of regional brain iron with magnetic resonance imaging. Parkinsonism Relat Disord 15(Suppl 3):S215–S218. doi:10.1016/ S1353-8020(09)70818-1

9. Morgen K, Sammer G, Weber L et al (2011) Structural brain abnormalities in patients with Parkinson disease: a comparative voxel-based analysis using T1-weighted MR imaging and magnetization transfer imaging. AJNR Am J Neuroradiol 32(11):2080–2086. doi:10.3174/ajnr.A2837

10. Menke RA, Scholz J, Miller KL et al (2009) MRI characteristics of the substantia nigra in Parkinson's disease: a combined quantitative T1 and DTI study. Neuroimage 47(2):435–441. doi:10.1016/j.neuroimage.2009.05.017

11. Peran P, Cherubini A, Assogna F et al (2010) Magnetic resonance imaging markers of Parkinson's disease nigrostriatal signature. Brain 133(11):3423–3433. doi:10.1093/ brain/awq212

12. Rolheiser TM, Fulton HG, Good KP et al (2011) Diffusion tensor imaging and olfactory identification testing in early-stage Parkinson's disease. J Neurol 258(7):1254–1260. doi:10.1007/s00415-011-5915-2

13. Chan LL, Rumpel H, Yap K et al (2007) Case control study of diffusion tensor imaging in Parkinson's disease. J Neurol Neurosurg Psychiatry 78(12):1383–1386. doi:10.1136/ jnnp.2007.121525

14. Vaillancourt DE, Spraker MB, Prodoehl J et al (2009) High-resolution diffusion tensor imaging in the substantia nigra of de novo Parkinson disease. Neurology 72(16):1378–1384. doi:10.1212/01.wnl.0000340982.01727.6e

15. Yoshikawa K, Nakata Y, Yamada K et al (2004) Early pathological changes in the parkinsonian brain demonstrated by diffusion tensor MRI. J Neurol Neurosurg Psychiatry 75(3): 481–484

16. Du G, Lewis MM, Styner M et al (2011) Combined R2* and diffusion tensor imaging changes in the substantia nigra in Parkinson's disease. Mov Disord 26(9):1627–1632. doi:10.1002/mds.23643

17. Focke NK, Helms G, Pantel PM et al (2011) Differentiation of typical and atypical Parkinson syndromes by quantitative MR imaging. AJNR Am J Neuroradiol 32(11):2087–2092. doi:10.3174/ajnr. A2865

18. Xia CF, Arteaga J, Chen G et al (2013) [(18) F]T807, a novel tau positron emission tomography imaging agent for Alzheimer's disease. Alzheimers Dement 9(6):666–676. doi:10.1016/j.jalz.2012.11.008

19. Zhan W, Kang GA, Glass GA et al (2012) Regional alterations of brain microstructure in Parkinson's disease using diffusion tensor imaging. Mov Disord 27(1):90–97. doi:10.1002/mds.23917

20. Choe BY, Park JW, Lee KS et al (1998) Neuronal laterality in Parkinson's disease with unilateral symptom by in vivo 1H magnetic resonance spectroscopy. Invest Radiol 33(8):450–455

21. Hattingen E, Magerkurth J, Pilatus U et al (2009) Phosphorus and proton magnetic resonance spectroscopy demonstrates mitochondrial dysfunction in early and advanced Parkinson's disease. Brain 132(Pt 12):3285–3297. doi:10.1093/brain/awp293

22. Lucetti C, Del Dotto P, Gambaccini G et al (2007) Influences of dopaminergic treatment on motor cortex in Parkinson disease: a MRI/ MRS study. Mov Disord 22(15):2170–2175. doi:10.1002/mds.21576

23. Abe K, Terakawa H, Takanashi M et al (2000) Proton magnetic resonance spectroscopy of patients with parkinsonism. Brain Res Bull 52(6):589–595

24. Griffith HR, Okonkwo OC, O'Brien T et al (2008) Reduced brain glutamate in patients with Parkinson's disease. NMR Biomed 21(4):381–387. doi:10.1002/nbm.1203

25. Heerschap AZ, J.; de Koster, A.; Thijssen,H; Horstink, M Metabolite levels at three brain locations in parkinsonism as viewed by proton MRS. In: SMRM, 12th Annual Meeting, New York, 1993. p 234

26. Guevara CA, Blain CR, Stahl D et al (2010) Quantitative magnetic resonance spectroscopic imaging in Parkinson's disease, progressive supranuclear palsy and multiple system atrophy. Eur J Neurol 17(9):1193–1202. doi:10.1111/j.1468-1331.2010.03010.x

27. Weiduschat N, Mao X, Beal MF et al (2013) Usefulness of proton and phosphorus MR spectroscopic imaging for early diagnosis of Parkinson's disease. J Neuroimaging. doi:10.1111/jon.12074

28. Helmich RC, Derikx LC, Bakker M et al (2010) Spatial remapping of cortico-striatal

connectivity in Parkinson's disease. Cereb Cortex 20(5):1175–1186. doi:10.1093/cercor/bhp178

29. Palmer SJ, Li J, Wang ZJ et al (2010) Joint amplitude and connectivity compensatory mechanisms in Parkinson's disease. Neuroscience 166(4):1110–1118. doi:10.1016/j.neuroscience.2010.01.012

30. Wu T, Wang L, Chen Y et al (2009) Changes of functional connectivity of the motor network in the resting state in Parkinson's disease. Neurosci Lett 460(1):6–10. doi:10.1016/j.neulet.2009.05.046

31. Sabatini U, Boulanouar K, Fabre N et al (2000) Cortical motor reorganization in akinetic patients with Parkinson's disease: a functional MRI study. Brain 123(Pt 2):394–403

32. Watanabe H, Saito Y, Terao S et al (2002) Progression and prognosis in multiple system atrophy: an analysis of 230 Japanese patients. Brain 125(Pt 5):1070–1083

33. Kato N, Arai K, Hattori T (2003) Study of the rostral midbrain atrophy in progressive supranuclear palsy. J Neurol Sci 210(1-2):57–60

34. Gama RL, Tavora DF, Bomfim RC et al (2010) Morphometry MRI in the differential diagnosis of parkinsonian syndromes. Arq Neuropsiquiatr 68(3):333–338

35. Quattrone A, Nicoletti G, Messina D et al (2008) MR imaging index for differentiation of progressive supranuclear palsy from Parkinson disease and the Parkinson variant of multiple system atrophy. Radiology 246(1):214–221. doi:10.1148/radiol.2453061703

36. Groger A, Bender B, Wurster I et al (2013) Differentiation between idiopathic and atypical parkinsonian syndromes using three-dimensional magnetic resonance spectroscopic imaging. J Neurol Neurosurg Psychiatry 84(6):644–649. doi:10.1136/jnnp-2012-302699

37. Koyama M, Yagishita A, Nakata Y et al (2007) Imaging of corticobasal degeneration syndrome. Neuroradiology 49(11):905–912. doi:10.1007/s00234-007-0265-6

38. Zijlmans JC (2010) The role of imaging in the diagnosis of vascular parkinsonism. Neuroimaging Clin N Am 20(1):69–76. doi:10.1016/j.nic.2009.08.006

39. Hughes AJ, Daniel SE, Ben-Shlomo Y et al (2002) The accuracy of diagnosis of parkinsonian syndromes in a specialist movement disorder service. Brain 125(Pt 4):861–870

40. Hughes AJ, Daniel SE, Lees AJ (2001) Improved accuracy of clinical diagnosis of Lewy body Parkinson's disease. Neurology 57(8):1497–1499

41. Benitez-Rivero S, Marin-Oyaga VA, Garcia-Solis D et al (2013) Clinical features and 123I-FP-CIT SPECT imaging in vascular parkinsonism and Parkinson's disease. J Neurol Neurosurg Psychiatry 84(2):122–129. doi:10.1136/jnnp-2012-302618

42. Fernandez HH, Wu CK, Ott BR (2003) Pharmacotherapy of dementia with Lewy bodies. Expert Opin Pharmacother 4(11):2027–2037. doi:10.1517/14656566.4.11.2027

43. Filippi L, Manni C, Pierantozzi M et al (2005) 123I-FP-CIT semi-quantitative SPECT detects preclinical bilateral dopaminergic deficit in early Parkinson's disease with unilateral symptoms. Nucl Med Commun 26(5):421–426

44. Booij J, Knol RJ (2007) SPECT imaging of the dopaminergic system in (premotor) Parkinson's disease. Parkinsonism Relat Disord 13(Suppl 3):S425–S428. doi:10.1016/S1353-8020(08)70042-7

45. Marek KL, Seibyl JP, Zoghbi SS et al (1996) [123I] beta-CIT/SPECT imaging demonstrates bilateral loss of dopamine transporters in hemi-Parkinson's disease. Neurology 46(1):231–237

46. Marek K, Innis R, van Dyck C et al (2001) [123I]beta-CIT SPECT imaging assessment of the rate of Parkinson's disease progression. Neurology 57(11):2089–2094

47. Benamer TS, Patterson J, Grosset DG et al (2000) Accurate differentiation of parkinsonism and essential tremor using visual assessment of [123I]-FP-CIT SPECT imaging: the [123I]-FP-CIT study group. Mov Disord 15(3):503–510

48. Hamilton D, List A, Butler T et al (2006) Discrimination between parkinsonian syndrome and essential tremor using artificial neural network classification of quantified DaTSCAN data. Nucl Med Commun 27(12):939–944. doi:10.1097/01.mnm.0000243369.80765.24

49. Kemp PM, Hoffmann SA, Holmes C et al (2005) The contribution of statistical parametric mapping in the assessment of precuneal and medial temporal lobe perfusion by 99mTc-HMPAO SPECT in mild Alzheimer's and Lewy body dementia. Nucl Med Commun 26(12):1099–1106

50. Kung HF, Alavi A, Chang W et al (1990) In vivo SPECT imaging of CNS D-2 dopamine receptors: initial studies with iodine-123-IBZM in humans. J Nucl Med 31(5):573–579

51. Ehrin E, Farde L, de Paulis T et al (1985) Preparation of 11C-labelled Raclopride, a new potent dopamine receptor antagonist: preliminary PET studies of cerebral dopamine receptors in the monkey. Int J Appl Radiat Isot 36(4):269–273

52. Farde L, Halldin C, Stone-Elander S et al (1987) PET analysis of human dopamine receptor subtypes using 11C-SCH 23390 and 11C-raclopride. Psychopharmacology (Berl) 92(3):278–284

53. Suhara T, Sudo Y, Okauchi T et al (1999) Extrastriatal dopamine D2 receptor density and affinity in the human brain measured by 3D PET. Int J Neuropsychopharmacol 2(2):73–82. doi:10.1017/S1461145799001431

54. Okubo Y, Olsson H, Ito H et al (1999) PET mapping of extrastriatal D2-like dopamine receptors in the human brain using an anatomic standardization technique and [11C] FLB 457. Neuroimage 10(6):666–674. doi:10.1006/nimg.1999.0502

55. Olsson H, Halldin C, Swahn CG et al (1999) Quantification of [11C]FLB 457 binding to extrastriatal dopamine receptors in the human brain. J Cereb Blood Flow Metab 19(10):1164–1173. doi:10.1097/00004647-199910000-00013

56. Tateno A, Arakawa R, Okumura M et al (2013) Striatal and extrastriatal dopamine D2 receptor occupancy by a novel antipsychotic, blonanserin: a PET study with [11C]raclopride and [11C]FLB 457 in schizophrenia. J Clin Psychopharmacol 33(2):162–169. doi:10.1097/JCP.0b013e3182825bce

57. Talvik M, Nordstrom AL, Okubo Y et al (2006) Dopamine D2 receptor binding in drug-naive patients with schizophrenia examined with raclopride-C11 and positron emission tomography. Psychiatry Res 148(2-3):165–173. doi:10.1016/j.pscychresns.2006.05.009

58. Montgomery AJ, Mehta MA, Grasby PM (2006) Is psychological stress in man associated with increased striatal dopamine levels?: A [11C]raclopride PET study. Synapse 60(2):124–131. doi:10.1002/syn.20282

59. Pruessner JC, Champagne F, Meaney MJ et al (2004) Dopamine release in response to a psychological stress in humans and its relationship to early life maternal care: a positron emission tomography study using [11C] raclopride. J Neurosci 24(11):2825–2831. doi:10.1523/JNEUROSCI.3422-03.2004

60. Kessler RM, Zald DH, Ansari MS et al (2014) Changes in dopamine release and dopamine D2/3 receptor levels with the development of mild obesity. Synapse 68(7):317–320. doi:10.1002/syn.21738

61. Eisenstein SA, Antenor-Dorsey JA, Gredysa DM et al (2013) A comparison of D2 receptor specific binding in obese and normal-weight individuals using PET with (N-[(11)C]methyl)benperidol. Synapse 67(11):748–756. doi:10.1002/syn.21680

62. Wang GJ, Volkow ND, Thanos PK et al (2004) Similarity between obesity and drug addiction as assessed by neurofunctional imaging: a concept review. J Addict Dis 23(3):39–53. doi:10.1300/J069v23n03_04

63. Wang GJ, Volkow ND, Logan J et al (2001) Brain dopamine and obesity. Lancet 357(9253):354–357

64. Steele KE, Prokopowicz GP, Schweitzer MA et al (2010) Alterations of central dopamine receptors before and after gastric bypass surgery. Obes Surg 20(3):369–374. doi:10.1007/s11695-009-0015-4

65. Nader MA, Czoty PW (2005) PET imaging of dopamine D2 receptors in monkey models of cocaine abuse: genetic predisposition versus environmental modulation. Am J Psychiatry 162(8):1473–1482. doi:10.1176/appi.ajp.162.8.1473

66. Boileau I, Payer D, Chugani B et al (2013) The D2/3 dopamine receptor in pathological gambling: a positron emission tomography study with [11C]-(+)-propyl-hexahydro-naphthoxazin and [11C]raclopride. Addiction 108(5):953–963. doi:10.1111/add.12066

67. Steeves TD, Miyasaki J, Zurowski M et al (2009) Increased striatal dopamine release in Parkinsonian patients with pathological gambling: a [11C] raclopride PET study. Brain 132(Pt 5):1376–1385. doi:10.1093/brain/awp054

68. Hierholzer J, Cordes M, Venz S et al (1998) Loss of dopamine-D2 receptor binding sites in Parkinsonian plus syndromes. J Nucl Med 39(6):954–960

69. Kim YJ, Ichise M, Ballinger JR et al (2002) Combination of dopamine transporter and D2 receptor SPECT in the diagnostic evaluation of PD, MSA, and PSP. Mov Disord 17(2):303–312

70. Mo SJ, Linder J, Forsgren L et al (2010) Pre- and postsynaptic dopamine SPECT in the early phase of idiopathic parkinsonism: a population-based study. Eur J Nucl Med Mol Imaging 37(11):2154–2164. doi:10.1007/s00259-010-1520-3

71. Hirayama M, Hakusui S, Koike Y et al (1995) A scintigraphical qualitative analysis of peripheral vascular sympathetic function with meta-[123I]iodobenzylguanidine in neurological patients with autonomic failure. J Auton Nerv Syst 53(2-3):230–234

72. Satoh A, Serita T, Tsujihata M (1997) Total defect of metaiodobenzylguanidine (MIBG) imaging on heart in Parkinson's disease: assessment of cardiac sympathetic denervation. Nihon Rinsho 55(1):202–206

73. Goldstein DS, Holmes C, Li ST et al (2000) Cardiac sympathetic denervation in Parkinson disease. Ann Intern Med 133(5):338–347

74. Spiegel J, Mollers MO, Jost WH et al (2005) FP-CIT and MIBG scintigraphy in early Parkinson's disease. Mov Disord 20(5):552–561. doi:10.1002/mds.20369

75. Takatsu H, Nagashima K, Murase M et al (2000) Differentiating Parkinson disease from multiple-system atrophy by measuring cardiac iodine-123 metaiodobenzylguanidine accumulation. JAMA 284(1):44–45

76. Orimo S (2012) The clinical significance of MIBG myocardial scintigraphy in Parkinson disease. Brain Nerve 64(4):403–412

77. Gjerloff T, Jakobsen S, Nahimi A et al (2014) In vivo imaging of human acetylcholinesterase density in peripheral organs using 11C-donepezil: dosimetry, biodistribution, and kinetic analyses. J Nucl Med 55(11):1818–1824. doi:10.2967/jnumed.114.143859

78. Gjerloff T, Fedorova T, Knudsen K et al (2015) Imaging acetylcholinesterase density in peripheral organs in Parkinson's disease with 11C-donepezil PET. Brain 138(Pt 3):653–663. doi:10.1093/brain/awu369

79. Eckert T, Barnes A, Dhawan V et al (2005) FDG PET in the differential diagnosis of parkinsonian disorders. Neuroimage 26(3):912–921. doi:10.1016/j.neuroimage.2005.03.012

80. Eidelberg D, Moeller JR, Ishikawa T et al (1995) Early differential diagnosis of Parkinson's disease with 18F-fluorodeoxyglucose and positron emission tomography. Neurology 45(11):1995–2004

81. Eggers C, Hilker R, Burghaus L et al (2009) High resolution positron emission tomography demonstrates basal ganglia dysfunction in early Parkinson's disease. J Neurol Sci 276(1-2):27–30. doi:10.1016/j.jns.2008.08.029

82. Huang C, Tang C, Feigin A et al (2007) Changes in network activity with the progression of Parkinson's disease. Brain 130(Pt 7):1834–1846. doi:10.1093/brain/awm086

83. Jokinen P, Scheinin N, Aalto S et al (2010) [(11)C]PIB-, [(18)F]FDG-PET and MRI imaging in patients with Parkinson's disease with and without dementia. Parkinsonism Relat Disord 16(10):666–670. doi:10.1016/j.parkreldis.2010.08.021

84. Eckert T, Feigin A, Lewis DE et al (2007) Regional metabolic changes in parkinsonian patients with normal dopaminergic imaging. Mov Disord 22(2):167–173. doi:10.1002/mds.21185

85. Jucaite A, Odano I, Olsson H et al (2006) Quantitative analyses of regional [11C]PE2I binding to the dopamine transporter in the human brain: a PET study. Eur J Nucl Med Mol Imaging 33(6):657–668. doi:10.1007/s00259-005-0027-9

86. Schou M, Steiger C, Varrone A et al (2009) Synthesis, radiolabeling and preliminary in vivo evaluation of [18F]FE-PE2I, a new probe for the dopamine transporter. Bioorg Med Chem Lett 19(16):4843–4845. doi:10.1016/j.bmcl.2009.06.032

87. Hirvonen J, Johansson J, Teras M et al (2008) Measurement of striatal and extrastriatal dopamine transporter binding with high-resolution PET and [11C]PE2I: quantitative modeling and test-retest reproducibility. J Cereb Blood Flow Metab 28(5):1059–1069. doi:10.1038/sj.jcbfm.9600607

88. Jonasson M, Appel L, Engman J et al (2013) Validation of parametric methods for [(1)(1)C]PE2I positron emission tomography. Neuroimage 74:172–178. doi:10.1016/j.neuroimage.2013.02.022

89. Appel L, Jonasson M, Danfors T et al (2015) Use of 11C-PE2I Positron Emission Tomography in Differential Diagnosis of Parkinsonian Disorders. J Nucl Med. doi:10.2967/jnumed.114.148619

90. Klunk WE, Engler H, Nordberg A et al (2003) Imaging the pathology of Alzheimer's disease: amyloid-imaging with positron emission tomography. Neuroimaging Clin N Am 13(4):781–789, ix

91. Klunk WE, Engler H, Nordberg A et al (2004) Imaging brain amyloid in Alzheimer's disease with Pittsburgh Compound-B. Ann Neurol 55(3):306–319. doi:10.1002/ana.20009

92. Cairns NJ, Ikonomovic MD, Benzinger T et al (2009) Absence of Pittsburgh compound B detection of cerebral amyloid beta in a patient with clinical, cognitive, and cerebrospinal fluid markers of Alzheimer disease: a case report. Arch Neurol 66(12):1557–1562. doi:10.1001/archneurol.2009.279

93. Pearson SD, Ollendorf DA, Colby JA (2014) Amyloid-beta positron emission tomography in the diagnostic evaluation of alzheimer disease: summary of primary findings and conclusions. JAMA Intern Med 174(1):133–134. doi:10.1001/jamainternmed.2013.11711

94. Brooks DJ (2009) Imaging amyloid in Parkinson's disease dementia and dementia with Lewy bodies with positron emission tomography. Mov Disord 24(Suppl 2):S742–S747. doi:10.1002/mds.22581

95. Edison P, Rowe CC, Rinne JO et al (2008) Amyloid load in Parkinson's disease dementia and Lewy body dementia measured with [11C]PIB positron emission tomography. J Neurol Neurosurg Psychiatry 79(12):1331–1338. doi:10.1136/jnnp.2007.127878

96. Aarsland D, Perry R, Brown A et al (2005) Neuropathology of dementia in Parkinson's

disease: a prospective, community-based study. Ann Neurol 58(5):773–776. doi:10.1002/ana.20635

97. Tolboom N, Yaqub M, van der Flier WM et al (2009) Detection of Alzheimer pathology in vivo using both 11C-PIB and 18F-FDDNP PET. J Nucl Med 50(2):191–197. doi:10.2967/jnumed.108.056499

98. Ossenkoppele R, Tolboom N, Foster-Dingley JC et al (2012) Longitudinal imaging of Alzheimer pathology using [11C]PIB, [18F]FDDNP and [18F]FDG PET. Eur J Nucl Med Mol Imaging 39(6):990–1000. doi:10.1007/s00259-012-2102-3

99. Nelson LD, Siddarth P, Kepe V et al (2011) Positron emission tomography of brain beta-amyloid and tau levels in adults with Down syndrome. Arch Neurol 68(6):768–774. doi:10.1001/archneurol.2011.104

100. Kepe V, Bordelon Y, Boxer A et al (2013) PET imaging of neuropathology in tauopathies: progressive supranuclear palsy. J Alzheimers Dis 36(1):145–153. doi:10.3233/JAD-130032

101. Lebouvier T, Chaumette T, Damier P et al (2008) Pathological lesions in colonic biopsies during Parkinson's disease. Gut 57(12):1741–1743. doi:10.1136/gut.2008.162503

102. Lebouvier T, Neunlist M, Bruley des Varannes S et al (2010) Colonic biopsies to assess the neuropathology of Parkinson's disease and its relationship with symptoms. PLoS One 5(9), e12728. doi:10.1371/journal.pone.0012728

103. Hilton D, Stephens M, Kirk L et al (2014) Accumulation of alpha-synuclein in the bowel of patients in the pre-clinical phase of Parkinson's disease. Acta Neuropathol 127(2):235–241. doi:10.1007/s00401-013-1214-6

104. Donadio V, Incensi A, Leta V et al (2014) Skin nerve alpha-synuclein deposits: a biomarker for idiopathic Parkinson disease. Neurology 82(15):1362–1369. doi:10.1212/WNL.0000000000000316

105. Neal KL, Shakerdge NB, Hou SS et al (2013) Development and screening of contrast agents for in vivo imaging of Parkinson's disease. Mol Imaging Biol 15(5):585–595. doi:10.1007/s11307-013-0634-y

106. McGeer PL, Itagaki S, Boyes BE et al (1988) Reactive microglia are positive for HLA-DR in the substantia nigra of Parkinson's and Alzheimer's disease brains. Neurology 38(8):|1285–1291

107. Gerhard A, Pavese N, Hotton G et al (2006) In vivo imaging of microglial activation with [11C](R)-PK11195 PET in idiopathic Parkinson's disease. Neurobiol Dis 21(2):404–412

108. Edison P, Ahmed I, Fan Z et al (2013) Microglia, amyloid, and glucose metabolism in Parkinson's disease with and without dementia. Neuropsychopharmacology 38(6):938–949. doi:10.1038/npp.2012.255

Chapter 16

Mass Spectrometry-Based Proteomics in Biomarker Discovery for Neurodegenerative Diseases

Sravani Musunuri, Ganna Shevchenko, and Jonas Bergquist

Abstract

Several neurodegenerative disorders such as Alzheimer's disease (AD), Parkinson's disease (PD), Huntington's disease (HD), Machado–Joseph disease (MJD), and amyotrophic lateral sclerosis (ALS) lead to disease-specific changes in the neuronal proteins. The usage of rapidly evolving proteomic technologies, such as mass spectrometry (MS), has opened new avenues to detect the changes in the protein expression in disease vs. control samples for understanding biochemical pathogenesis in neurodegenerative disorders. Efficient sample preparation is an integral part of a successful MS-based proteomics. Apart from the identification, quantification of the proteins is needed to investigate the alterations between proteome profiles from different sample sets. This chapter provides an overview of the sample collection, preparation, identification, and quantification of proteins using MS in the biomarker discovery for the neurodegenerative diseases.

Key words Alzheimer's disease, Biological samples, Mass spectrometry, Neuroproteomics, Parkinson's disease, Protein purification, Sample preparation, Separation techniques, Qualitative analysis, Quantitative analysis

1 Introduction

The word "proteome" was coined for the first time by Marc R. Wilkins in 1994 and derived from PROTEins expressed by a genOME [1]. The proteome refers to all the proteins produced by an organism, much like the genome is the entire set of genes. The genome is a static blueprint but the proteome is dynamic in nature, changing constantly in response to thousands of intra- and extracellular factors such as disease conditions, drugs, stress, developmental cue, and environmental factors [2]. Proteomics is the study of an organism's complete complement of proteins expressed by the generic material of an organism. Neuroproteomics is the branch of proteomics that focuses on the qualitative and quantitative aspects of tissue/organelle proteomes of the nervous system. More than 1000 disorders are associated with abnormalities in the

Martin Ingelsson and Lars Lannfelt (eds.), *Immunotherapy and Biomarkers in Neurodegenerative Disorders*, Methods in Pharmacology and Toxicology, DOI 10.1007/978-1-4939-3560-4_16, © Springer Science+Business Media New York 2016

neuronal activity and cellular dysfunctions, ranging from rare to common illnesses [3, 4]. A database search in ISI web of knowledge for the terms neurodegenerative diseases AND proteomics between years 2000 and 2014 revealed a total number of 868 published articles (Fig. 1).

There has been a growing interest in applying proteomics for the clinical diagnostic procedure of neurodegenerative diseases. The aims of clinical proteomics are to identify the absolute or relative changes in the protein levels that are likely to reflect the effects of the disease, to improve the accuracy of clinical diagnosis by identifying the biomarkers that are associated with pathophysiological mechanism, and to improve the drug therapy by discovering novel proteins which can act as drug targets [5]. Identification and characterization of complex neuronal proteome are essential to understand the neuronal functions. Therefore, comprehensive proteome profiling is beneficial to identify and discover new prognostic and diagnostic biomarkers, and also to develop therapeutic agents for neurological disorders. Although there are several approaches to achieve proteome profiling, many of them share common features. Typical proteomic workflow includes sample collection, preparation, protein/peptide separation, identification, quantification, and subsequent confirmation and validation (Fig. 2).

The fast development of proteomic research has led to many new experimental methods which can be distinguished either by gel-based or gel-free analysis. In both methodological approaches, mass spectrometry has increasingly become the method of choice

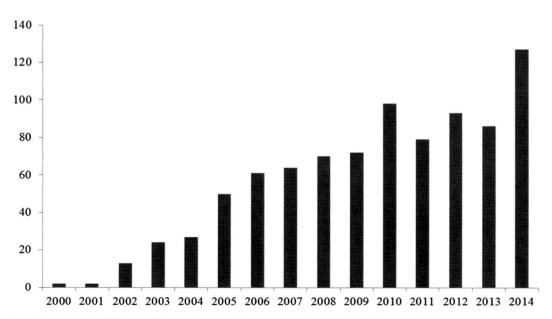

Fig. 1 Number of published articles with search terms neurodegenerative diseases AND proteomics from year 2000 until 2014 (*source*: ISI web of knowledge)

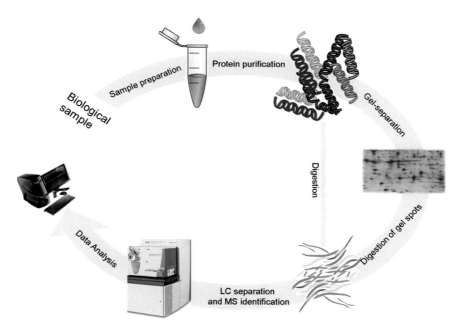

Fig. 2 General proteomics workflow: Sample collection from different sources (disease and healthy), sample preparation, protein or peptide separation, identification using mass spectrometry, quantification and validation of the biomarker candidates

for in-depth profiling of complex protein/peptide mixtures derived from biological samples. Two types of approaches, namely "bottom-up" and "top-down", are used in proteomics (Fig. 3). In the most commonly employed bottom-up approach, proteins are converted into peptides by enzymatic or chemical digestion and analysis is done by using MS or tandem MS, whereas the top-down approach is used to study intact proteins or large protein fragments by direct analysis with MS and MS/MS [6].

2 Challenges in MS-Based Neuroproteomics

Proteomic studies of several neurological disorders have led to the identification of a large number of protein alterations and modifications between healthy and disease groups. However, in order to translate the current proteomic technologies from bench to bedside there is a need to overcome some of the limitations in the pre-analytical phase and analytical methods. Starting from sample collection, storage, preparation, analysis until the final outcome, each step should be monitored with outmost vigilance to produce the proteomics data with minimum errors.

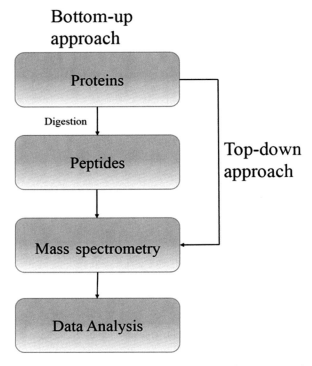

Fig. 3 Schematic representation of bottom-up and top-down approaches in proteomics workflow

2.1 Pre-analytical Phase

In studies involving biological samples, the variations and errors in in vitro diagnostics arise during the pre-analytical phase. The pre-analytical processes such as study design, sample collection, transport, processing, and storage can have dramatic impact on the proteomic results. Many of the neurological disorders are age related and more common with elderly patients. Therefore, inter- and intra- assay variability due to various physiological factors such as age, sex, possibility of other disease, and drug treatment complicates the data analysis. Several technical, disease-unrelated factors such as *postmortem* time interval for tissue samples, long-term storage at room temperature, and repeated freeze-thaw cycles may also influence the stability of proteins.

After establishing the clinical question and selecting the biological source based on the question, it is pivotal to collect and store the samples under appropriate conditions to prevent protein degradation. Samples should preferably be collected in cryogenic vials or tubes and frozen immediately by using liquid nitrogen or dry ice and stored at −80 °C until further usage. Anticoagulants such as ethylenediaminetetraacetic acid tetrasodium salt dihydrate (EDTA) can be added to plasma/blood samples and centrifuged for 10 min at 400 g prior to aliquoting the samples [7]. Cerebrospinal fluid (CSF) samples are collected on ice in a chilled plastic tube, by lumbar puncture in the lateral decubitus position in the L4–L5 vertebral interspace. Samples are mixed gently and centrifuged for 10 min at 2000 g. The supernatant is collected to eliminate cell and other insoluble material and aliquoted into small sample volumes prior to freezing at –80 °C [7]. Microdialysis (MD) is another sampling technique useful to collect the small hydrophilic molecules, cytokines, and proteins to monitor neuro-intensive care patients [8]. All steps should be handled by wearing gloves and clean environment to e.g., minimize, the keratin contamination in the samples.

2.2 Biological Samples

Choosing the right biological sample for the proteomic studies is of utmost importance in order to arrive at correct conclusions. Proteomic studies in neurodegenerative disorders such as Alzheimer's disease, Parkinson's disease, or amyotrophic lateral sclerosis employ various central nervous system (CNS) tissues (brain biopsy, spinal cord, etc.), body fluids (blood, plasma, serum, CSF, urine, saliva), or cell cultures (Table 1).

In many neurodegenerative disorders the treatment will be more effective if started in early stages of disease. But current clinical diagnosis of such disorders cannot be made until the disease has progressed to the point that dementia or motoric

Table 1
Different biological sources, their advantages, and limitation in the neuroproteomic research

Biological source	Advantages	Limitations
CNS tissue samples (brain, spinal cord)	• To monitor changes in the disease-specific area • Used for screening biomarkers in discovery phase	• Invasive for patient • Limited availability of effected tissue • Different *postmortem* times can give variable results
CSF	• Reflect the changes in CNS as it is in close proximity to brain and spinal cord • Good for large-scale screening in validation phase of biomarkers	• Need depletion in order to remove highly abundant proteins • Moderately invasive due to lumbar puncture
Plasma	• Most preferred clinical diagnostic sample • Low invasive and easier sampling	• Blood is one of the most complex human proteomes which has very large dynamic range • Might not reflect a linear relationship between changes of proteins in diseased CNS tissue and in blood • Less sensitive and specific for neurological disorder diagnosis • Results from plasma are poorly reproducible in CNS diseases due to effect of inflammatory or metabolic influences

dysfunctions arise. Thus, there is a demand to have biomarkers which support diagnosis of the disease in early stages in order to improve the therapeutic prospects. Additionally, it is extremely important to find reliable biomarkers that can distinguish different neurodegenerative disorders to initiate an early treatment [9]. Several transgenic animal models such as mouse, zebrafish, *Caenorhabditis elegans*, and *Drosophila melanogaster* have been used to model human neurodegenerative conditions [10]. These models are invaluable in the study of changes in the proteome during the preclinical stages, understanding the disease progression, and testing therapeutic strategies. Genetically engineered mice are the most popular animal models used to mimic the diverse range of human neurodegenerative disorders. So far, several mouse models have been established for neurological disorders, of which the list can be seen at http://www.alzforum.org/res/com/tra/default. asp. However, these models serve only as the approximate representation of the clinical scenarios of patients and neurological disorders. Also their use as translational models of human-specific neurodegenerative diseases is limited due to the phylogenetic distance of these species from humans.

2.3 Low-Abundant Proteins

Global proteomics is a highly complex and challenging task due to large heterogeneity of proteins. Hence, the analysis of low-abundant proteins, which usually serve as biomarker candidates, has become a very difficult and demanding task. Membrane proteins (MPs) are distributed throughout the different compartments of the nervous system and they occupy center stage in developmental processes and neurotransmission. In the nervous system MPs participate in axonal guidance, synaptic release, and reuptake [5]. A majority of the current drug targets (~70–80 %) are represented by MPs, which also act as epitopes for vaccine design [11, 12]. Comprehensive analysis of brain MPs remains a challenge because of their highly hydrophobic nature and low abundance. Despite their biological and biomedical importance, MPs are still comprised in the underrepresented subset of the CNS studies. In order to overcome the challenges pertaining to MPs, various pre-fractionation techniques can be employed for the enrichment. One such example of pre-fractionation technique is the use of cloud point extraction using nonionic detergents. By increasing temperature above a certain temperature, called cloud point temperature, nonionic polyoxyethylene detergents become cloudy and upon centrifugation separate into two phases: aqueous phase and surfactant-rich phase. The nonionic detergent solution exhibits liquid-liquid-phase separation at the cloud point temperature and can be applied to enrich the MPs from brain tissue [13, 14].

3 Sample Preparation

Sample preparation is the crucial and foremost step that dictates the final outcome of the analysis. There is no universal sample preparation technique that could be applied to all possible biological samples, and it is practical to optimize the procedure for a particular sample. The saying that goes "Garbage in, garbage out" holds true for proteomics as much as for other scientific fields. The selection of sample preparation and separation techniques plays a major role in determining the end result. The workflow employed during sample preparation steps typically involves extraction, protein purification, enrichment, and tryptic digestion of proteins into peptides. Analysis of tryptic peptides is achieved by using high-resolution MS.

3.1 Extraction

Extraction conditions should be optimized depending on the characteristics of the biological tissue, the nature of protein to be studied, the subsequent assay or analytical steps used, and the desired outcome [14]. Efficient cell disruption is a prerequisite for comprehensive proteome analysis. Cell lysis can be achieved by mechanical disruption of biological tissue/cells using a blender, an ultrasonication device (bath/probe), a french press, a mortar and pestle, and a glass bead agitator or by applying a detergent-based lysis. A combination of two or more of these techniques might prove more efficient in extraction of proteins from organelles. Cell disruption causes the release of endogenous enzymes, such as proteases and phosphatases, which will degrade the proteins in the extracts resulting in reduction of the protein yield during isolation and purification. Protease inhibitor cocktail and ethylenediaminetetraacetic acid (EDTA) were added to the tissue homogenates for inhibition of serine, cysteine, acid proteases, aminopeptidases, and metalloproteases. Along with the protease inhibitors and detergents, other additives like organic acids, organic solvents, and chaotropes can also be used in the lysis buffer in order to improve extraction and solubilization [13]. Ionic detergents are extremely efficient in solubilizing and denaturing the proteins [7, 15] but are incompatible with isoelectric focusing (IEF) of the two-dimensional gel electrophoresis (2-DE) and interfere with the MS analysis by suppressing ionization by electrospray ionization (ESI). Nonionic detergents are considered as mild compared to the ionic detergents and the glycosidic detergents at low concentrations (0.01–0.1 %) are fairly compatible with ESI [15]. Zwitterionic detergents have intermediate properties and act as better solubilizing agents compared to nonionic detergents but not as strong as ionic detergents [16]. Additionally they are generally compatible with trypsin digestion as well as ESI-MS [15].

3.2 Protein Purification

Addition of salts, buffers, and detergents is necessary in order to maintain pH and ionic strength of the buffer as well for the solubilization of MPs. The presence of salts, detergents, nucleic acids, and lipid polysaccharides in the extracts hampers the tryptic digestion and also interferes during the gel electrophoresis and analysis steps, thus reducing the efficiency of the analytical technique. Currently, there are several sample cleanup techniques available, of which dialysis [17], ultrafiltration [18], gel filtration [19], precipitation [20, 21], and solid-phase extraction [22] are used in proteomic sample preparation to remove interfering contaminants. The choice of the protein purification techniques depends on the tissue characteristics, e.g., lipids are abundant in brain, so selective precipitation using organic solvents is the common protein purification technique employed to efficiently remove lipids together with nucleic acids while retaining maximum protein recoveries [23, 24].

3.3 Immunodepletion of Highly Abundant Proteins

The major analytical challenge of the proteome analysis of complex body fluids such as CSF and plasma is the broad dynamic range of protein concentrations present in the mixture, spanning over 10–15 orders of magnitude [25]. Therefore, depletion of highly abundant proteins, such as albumin, IgG, and transferrin, by immunoaffinity chromatography is often desired prior to the proteome analysis of plasma and CSF [26–29]. The advantage of fractionation is reduced complexity and higher sample loading capabilities for the low-abundant proteins, which in turn can lead to almost a tenfold increase in the number of proteins identified [30]. Studies by Schutzer et al. showed an increase in 70 % protein identification yield using immunoaffinity-depleted CSF samples [31, 32]. Hexapeptide ligand libraries can also be employed to enrich the low-abundant proteins from CSF samples [33].

3.4 Denaturation, Reduction, Alkylation, and Protein Digestion

Prior to the digestion, denaturation, reduction, and alkylation of proteins are performed by adding various reagents. Proteins are subjected to simultaneous denaturation and reduction by a combination of heat and chemical reagents in order to reduce the native disulfide bonds in proteins. Alkylating agents help to retain thiol groups in solution by preventing inter- and intramolecular disulfide formation between cysteines in the protein by covalent addition of carbamidomethyl groups.

Another crucial sample preparation step that needs consideration in the bottom-up approach is the digestion of proteins into peptides. The classical approaches for protein digestion involve enzymatic or nonenzymatic chemical cleavage of proteins to generate peptide fragments for the identification, characterization, and quantification by MS. Enzymatic digestion by trypsin is the common choice in a proteomics workflow due to the generation of peptides of practical length and favorable charge suited for tandem

MS sequencing by collision-induced dissociation (CID). Apart from commonly used tryptic digestion, a plethora of other enzymes or chemicals (Table 2) can be considered depending on the desired outcome. Enzymes such as Glu-C, Lys-C, and Asp-N generate large peptide fragments (15–50 amino acids) which can be used for middle-down proteomics. However, single-protease digestion might not be enough to generate the required number of peptides for successful identification of a protein. Therefore, a combination of several enzymes can be applied to improve the sequence coverage and the number of identified peptides and proteins. Employing a multiple enzyme digestion strategy for CNS samples [34] helps to obtain maximal proteome coverage which might be beneficial when fishing for novel biomarker candidates. The conventional heating method employed with most of the proteases (37 °C with overnight digestion) is often time consuming. Several techniques were employed to increase the rate of digestion, and thereby achieve a more accelerated throughput. Such strategies include the use of microwave-assisted digestion, solvents, ultrasonic bath, ultrasonic probes, infrared irradiation, high pressure, on-chip immobilized enzymes, immobilized enzyme reactors, and magnetic particle-immobilized enzymes [35–39].

4 Separation Techniques

Separation of a huge number of proteins or peptides derived from a complex biological sample is a prerequisite step prior to the MS detection. A number of separation techniques are available for proteome analysis of which gel-based and gel-free approaches are commonly employed for protein/peptide separation (Fig. 2).

4.1 Gel Electrophoresis

Gel electrophoresis is the most common approach that provides simultaneous separation and visualization of complex protein mixtures to detect the differential protein expression. The traditional gel-based separation techniques involve sodium dodecyl sulfate-polyacrylamide gels (SDS-PAGE) and 2-DE to separate intact proteins or protein complexes followed by in-gel digestion of proteins into peptides. SDS-PAGE separates denatured proteins depending on the charge and molecular weight. SDS denatures proteins and imparts negative charge to the proteins in proportion to the mass enabling them to move towards the positive end of the gel.

2-DE works by separating proteins based on the two physical properties. In the first dimension proteins are separated based on their isoelectric point (pI) and in the second dimension on their molecular weight using SDS-PAGE. Visualization of proteins is achieved by staining, which can be processed prior to in-gel digestion before MS identification or by antibody-based techniques,

Table 2
Commonly used enzymes and chemicals for protein digestion

Name	Specificity	Optimal pH	Pros	Cons
Trypsin	C-terminal side of Arg, Lys	7–9	Conventional digestion technique in proteomics Highly specific Generates peptides with favorable length and charge for tandem MS sequencing by CID Useful for both in-solution and in-gel digestion	Protease efficiency is affected if the posttranslational modification site is in proximity of the proteolytic site Usage of trypsin alone might not provide complete proteome coverage Might sometimes produce peptides which are too small or too large to provide sequence information
Chymotrypsin	C-terminal side of Tyr, Phe, Trp, and Leu	7–9	Useful for hydrophobic protein digestion [98] Improves sequence coverage if used in combination with trypsin	Less specific compared to trypsin Cleaves too frequently resulting in small peptides that lack an adequate sequence context
Glu-C	C-terminus side of Asp and Glu	4–9	Improves sequence coverage if used in combination with trypsin Useful for middle-down proteomics	Not recommended for in-gel digestion
rLys-C	C-terminus side of Lys	8–9	Highly specific Retains activity under 8 M urea denaturing conditions Less expensive compared to native Lys-C	Not suitable to use alone for bottom-up approach Can be used in combination with trypsin to increase the sequence coverage
Lys-N	N-terminal side Lys	7–9	Retains activity at 0.1 % SDS, 6 M urea, and temperatures up to 70 °C Requires less time for digestion at higher temperature	Not suitable for bottom-up approach

(continued)

Table 2
(continued)

Name	Specificity	Optimal pH	Pros	Cons
Proteinase K	Peptide bond adjacent to the carboxyl group of aliphatic and aromatic amino acids with blocked α-amino groups	7.5–9.0	Retains activity at 0.1–0.5 % SDS, urea, and temperatures up to 50 °C Exposes the antigen-binding sites of paraffin-embedded tissue for antibody labeling [99] Useful for digestion of prions from brain tissue during transmissible spongiform encephalopathy research [100]	Nonspecific cleavage
Cyanogen bromide	C-terminus side of Met	Acidic	Specific and efficient compared to other chemical cleavage	The yield may drop near to zero if the bond to be cleaved is formed by a Met-Ser or Met-Thr sequence CNBr is toxic and sensitive to oxidation [101]
N-bromo-succinimide [102]	C-terminus side of Trp, Tyr, His		Useful to determine structure of smaller peptides [101]	Might give low yield due to partial cleavage Attacks the sulfur-containing amino acids leading to unspecific cleavage [101]

e.g., by western blotting. 2-DE, although the most commonly used conventional separation technique in combination with MS, has inherent limitations. 2-DE does not give a true representation of the entire proteome due to its inability to detect low-abundant proteins because of limited sample capacity and limited detection sensitivity. Also 2-DE has several challenges, such as separation of transmembrane proteins and limited throughput due to time-consuming analysis of each single spot to identify protein/s. Some of the issues with 2-DE can be addressed by its advanced version, two-dimensional difference gel electrophoresis (2D-DIGE) which was introduced in 1997. 2D-DIGE provides multiplexing of up to three different protein samples, by labeling them with different fluorescent dyes and separating them on a single gel. 2D-DIGE has increased reproducibility in terms of quantitation when compared to classical 2-DE and has higher sensitivity compared to normal staining methods [40].

4.2 Liquid Chromatography Separation

Shotgun methods, where proteins are digested into peptides and then separated by liquid chromatography (LC), provide alternatives to gel-based proteomics. Ion-exchange, affinity, size-exclusion, and reverse-phase (RP) LC are common techniques used in the gel-free proteomics. LC techniques work with both bottom-up and top-down approach, i.e., for the separation of proteolytic peptides or intact proteins. The sample is carried with the mobile phase and separates based on its interaction with stationary phase. Polypeptides/analyte mixture can be eluted sequentially from the stationary phase using gradient elution by increasing the concentration of organic solvent in the mobile phase during separation. The column used in RP-LC is usually packed with silica particles attached with alkyl chains of varying lengths from C_4 to C_{18}, of which C_{18} was commonly used for separation of peptides. RP-LC has become a standard method in shotgun proteomics due to its high resolving power, good detection sensitivity, and compatibility with ESI-MS. Capillary electrophoresis (CE) can also be used in combination with MS either as an off-line or an online separation technique [41, 42].

5 Mass Spectrometry

Mass spectrometry has emerged as an indispensable tool for the identification of proteins/peptides, providing accurate mass measurements for peptides as well as amino acid sequence information. The basic components of mass spectrometer are an ion source to convert molecules into gas-phase ions, a mass analyzer to separate the ionized analytes based on their mass-to-charge ratio (m/z), a detector to record the number of ions at specific m/z value, and vacuum pumps to prevent the collision of ions with residual gas and assist the ions' uninhibited movements within the instrument. The introduction of two soft ionization techniques, electrospray ionization [43] and matrix-assisted laser desorption/ionization (MALDI) [44], for the analysis of proteins and peptides has greatly increased the MS application in the proteomics field. The heart of the MS instrumentation is the mass analyzer. Five different types of mass analyzers, quadrupole (Q), ion trap (quadrupole ion trap, QIT; linear ion trap, LTQ), time-of-flight (TOF), fourier-transform ion cyclotron resonance (FTICR), and Orbitrap, are commonly used [45, 46]. These mass analyzers can be used either alone or in combination with each other.

5.1 Electrospray Ionization

ESI is a technique which facilitates a soft ionization of large biomolecules such as proteins and peptides without in-source fragmentation [43]. ESI employs high electric field (3–5 kV/cm) to produce a mist of droplets carrying excess charge at the surface.

The droplet size is reduced in the ion source region due to the solvent evaporation by counterflow of heated drying gas. As the droplets evaporate, the ions move close and due to Coulombic repulsive forces between ions, the explosion of droplet occurs, resulting in smaller droplets. This process is repeated until solvent-free ions are formed that can pass through the mass analyzer. In positive-ion mode, the droplets will carry positive charge forming $[M+H]^+$ and $[M+Na]^+$ adducts. Nanoelectrospray with lower flow rates in the range of 1–1000 nl/min is an important development of this ionization method. Low injection flow rate has the advantage of producing long-lasting signals with less sample consumption.

5.2 Matrix-Assisted Laser Desorption/ Ionization

Matrix-assisted laser desorption/ionization, introduced in 1988 by Hillenkamp and Karas, is a soft ionization technique [44]. MALDI process utilizes two different substances: analyte and matrix. The analyte is a biological sample of interest, whereas the matrix usually is a UV-absorbing weak organic acid that surrounds the analyte and assists in the ionization process. The analyte is co-crystallized with large excess molars of matrix, followed by the laser irradiation of the analyte-matrix mixture. This results in the absorption of laser radiation by matrix resulting in the indirect vaporization of the analyte. Unlike ESI, the samples are analyzed directly on MALDI without prior separation by chromatographic techniques. MALDI provides sensitive and significant analysis of complex peptide mixture by combining with off-line separation techniques, LC [47] or CE [42, 48] techniques. MALDI imaging mass spectrometry (IMS) has been applied to thin tissue sections (5–20 μm thick) to investigate the distribution of neuropeptides in the biological systems such as brain and spinal cord [49]. MALDI-IMS offers the advantage of determining the molecular changes associated with disease progression on discrete tissue locations.

6 Protein Identification

Protein identification in a bottom-up approach is based on the analysis of peptides generated by tryptic digestion. The peptide ions are subjected to precursor ion scan, which provides information on the m/z ion. A single-peptide precursor ion is isolated and fragmented further by colliding with inert gas molecules. This process is called collision-induced dissociation and it generates MS/MS spectra for the identification of the amino acid sequence of the peptide fragments. The experimental MS and MS/MS spectra can be matched against hypothetical peptide fragments generated from an in silico protein database to identify the proteins in the sample.

7 Mass Spectrometry-Based Quantitative Proteomics

Detecting changes in the protein or peptide abundance in response to a disease compared to a non-diseased state in biological samples is the major goal of quantitative clinical proteomics [50]. Recent developments in instrumentation have greatly improved the accuracy and sensitivity of the detection for MS-based quantitative proteomics [9].

7.1 Absolute vs. Relative Quantitation

Absolute quantitation involves spiking of known concentration of synthetic, isotope-labeled reference peptide into the experimental sample, and performing LC-MS/MS analysis. Quantification is achieved by comparing the signal intensities of the target peptide in the experimental sample to the reference peptide [51]. Relative quantitation involves comparing the alterations in the individual proteins/peptides between different experimental samples by employing either label-free or labeling strategies (Fig. 4). Differential proteomic methods based on labeling strategies include in vivo metabolic labeling and in vitro enzymatic or chemical labeling.

7.2 Label-Free Approach

Label-free methods can be used for both absolute and relative quantitation, for clinical screening of large sample sets and biomarker discovery experiments without using isotope-labeled components. A label-free quantitative approach is based on the observation that intensity in ESI-MS is linearly proportional to the concentration of the ions being detected [52]. Label-free methods involve either spectral counting or measurement of the ion peak intensity. Therefore, the relative peptide levels between samples can be determined by measuring peak intensities from LC-MS

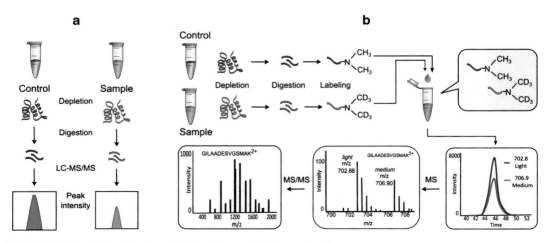

Fig. 4 Label-free (**a**) and isotope labeling (**b**) quantitative approaches

[52]. Spectral counting methods involve comparing the sum of MS/MS spectra from a peptide across multiple samples, which is shown to correlate with protein abundance [52]. Label-free quantitation is straightforward and inexpensive but the experiments need to be carefully controlled to account for any variations, since each sample is prepared and analyzed by LC-MS or LC-MS/MS separately.

7.3 Stable Isotope Labeling Quantitative Approaches

Different labeling approaches involve labeling of proteins/peptides with stable heavy isotopes (^{15}N, ^{18}O, ^{2}H, ^{13}C) either metabolically in cells or post-metabolically by enzymatic or chemical reactions. The light- and heavy-labeled peptide ions are chemically identical (except for ^{2}H). They exhibit identical LC elution profiles but distinctively different MS spectra and are separated by the difference in their mass. The peak intensities of differentially labeled peptides are compared to determine the change in the abundance between different sample sets.

Two of the most popular metabolic labeling approaches are ^{15}N labeling and stable isotope labeling with amino acids in cell culture (SILAC) [53]. ^{15}N labeling technique replaces all nitrogen atoms throughout the proteome, whereas SILAC method involves labeling of one or several amino acids (typically arginine or lysine) with heavy isotopes and adding them to the growth medium to incorporate the labels into proteins. SILAC is used to quantify in vivo changes and the level of quantitation bias from processing errors is low because samples can be combined in the beginning of the sample preparation step. Previously, SILAC has been limited to cell cultures; however in past few years its applicability has been expanded by labeling entire organisms [54–57]. SILAC has also been used for quantification of mouse brain by using culture-derived isotope tags as internal standards [58].

For samples that are not suited for metabolic labeling, such as human body fluids or tissues [59], and when the experimental time is limited, enzymatic or chemical labeling can be applied for quantitative proteomic analyses. The enzymatic labeling approach involves the use of trypsin- or Glu-C-catalyzed incorporation of ^{18}O atoms into C-terminus of the proteolytic peptides during or after protein digestion [60, 61]. Enzymatic labeling has disadvantages, such as incomplete labeling due to the slow back exchange of ^{18}O and ^{16}O, and difference in the rate of incorporation of label for each peptide which complicates the data analysis [62, 63]. Another commonly used stable isotope labeling strategy entails the incorporation of stable isotope-containing tags into proteins or peptides through a chemical reaction. Chemical labeling strategy involves the usage of isotopic and isobaric tags for labeling, e.g., isotope-coded protein labeling (ICPL), isotope-coded affinity tag (ICAT), isotope tags for relative and absolute quantification (iTRAQ), tandem mass tags (TMT), and dimethyl labeling (DML).

The ICPL approach employs the usage of deuterium-free (light) or deuterium-containing (heavy) form, to derivatize the free amino groups in the protein mixtures. Protein samples are reduced and alkylated prior to labeling. Light- and heavy-labeled protein samples are mixed, digested, and analyzed by MS. The labelled proteins differ by 4 Da mass in the acquired MS spectra. The drawback of ICPL is an isotopic effect of deuterated tags that interferes with the LC elution of the peptides leading to retention time shifts.

The iTRAQ technique employs the amine-reactive isobaric tags to label peptides at the N-terminus and the lysine side chains. iTRAQ can be applied to a wide range of tissue samples including CSF [64, 65]. Eight isobaric labels are available in iTRAQ making it possible to label and compare up to eight samples simultaneously. Each of the labels consists of three groups: reporter (114, 115, 116, 117 Da for 4-plex and 113, 114, 115, 116, 117, 118, 119, 121 Da for 8-plex), balancer, and reactive groups that are attached to N-terminus and lysine residues of the peptide. The peptides labeled with isotopic tags appear as a single unresolved precursor at the same m/z in MS spectrum. Upon fragmentation in MS/MS, the reporter group split from the peptide and form small fragments at low m/z (114–121 Da). A relative quantification of peptide is enabled by measuring the reporter ion fragment intensities. However, the data generated with iTRAQ has is disadvantageous due to the variance heterogeneity and underestimation of the ratio due to the compression of ratios towards one [66].

Stable isotope dimethylation is a rapid and inexpensive chemical labeling strategy, which employs formaldehyde for methylation of primary amines of N-terminus and lysine residues of tryptic peptides via Schiff base formation and subsequent reduction by cyanoborohydride [67, 68]. Three isotopomeric labels—light, medium, and heavy containing formaldehyde (CH_2O), deuterated formaldehyde (CD_2O), and ^{13}C-labeled deuterated formaldehyde ($^{13}CD_2O$)—can be employed for DML. Sodium cyanoborohydride is added to light and medium labels, whereas deuterated sodium cyanoborohydride is added to the heavy-labeled mixtures for reduction. DML can be applied to neurological samples such as brain [69] and spinal cord [70] and including other biological tissues.

In MS-based quantitative proteomics, many options are available with their own set of advantages and disadvantages. The choice of method depends on the type and number of samples to be compared, the biological source and complexity of samples, analytical needs (e.g., precision, accuracy, and absolute or relative quantification is needed), and the cost and time required for the analysis [71].

8 Mass Spectrometry-Based Proteomics Discoveries in Alzheimer's Disease and Parkinson's Disease

The neurodegenerative diseases (e.g., Alzheimer's disease, Parkinson's disease, multiple sclerosis, amyotrophic lateral sclerosis) are a large group of disorders characterized by irreversible loss of neurons of brain and spinal cord tissue. The progressive neurodegeneration in turn leads to shared disease symptoms, e.g., impaired memory and learning functions, communication difficulties, as well as changes in personality. The neuropathology of these diseases is linked to the aggregation and accumulation of misfolded proteins that leads to the formation of intra- and extracellular aggregates, such as amyloid-β plaques in AD and Lewy bodies in PD.

Typically, the clinical diagnosis of such diseases cannot be made until the disease has progressed to the point that cognitive or motoric dysfunctions arise. Although significant improvement in clinical diagnosis and care for patients with these diseases has been made, there is still no curative treatment for any of these disorders. However, along with the development of such drugs, there is an increasing need for identification, development, and validation of biomarkers for diagnosing different forms of dementia that meet the criteria of precision, specificity, and repeatability.

In the following section, we focus on biomarker discovery for the two most common CNS disorders, Alzheimer's disease (AD) and Parkinson's disease (PD), using MS-based proteomic methods and summarize the recent advances in this field. The overview of recently published neuroproteomic studies differentiating between AD, PD, and control samples, including the source of CNS samples, applied MS-based techniques and the biomarker candidates discovered are listed in Table 3.

8.1 Alzheimer's Disease

Alzheimer's disease is the most common form of neurodegenerative disease, accounting for 50–60 % of all diagnosed cases [72]. Although the exact etiology of AD remains to be defined, the disease is histopathologically characterized by deposition of the aggregated β-amyloid (Aβ) peptide in the form of extracellular senile plaques and hyperphosphorylated tau protein in the form of intracellular neurofibrillary tangles along with massive neuronal and synaptic degeneration. Analysis of the 42-amino acid-form of Aβ (Aβ42), total tau (tTau), and hyperphosphorylated tau (pTau) in CSF are validated AD biomarkers and AD patients show decreased values of Aβ42 and increased values of tTau or pTau.

During the last years MS-based proteomic technologies have been applied quite intensively to study AD-related changes in protein levels of CSF and plasma samples as well as of *postmortem* brain tissues. Classic proteomics platforms, such as 2-DE in combination

Table 3
An overview of recently published neuroproteomic studies differentiating between AD, PD, and control samples, including the source of CNS samples, separation technologies, applied mass spectrometry-based techniques, main results, and validated differential abundant proteins between diseased cases and controls by independent technology

Source	Quantitative method	Proteins/peptides identified, quantified/altered proteins	Validation by independent technique	Year	Reference
Alzheimer's disease					
Brain tissue (neocortex)	DML, LC MS/MS, WB	62 differentially regulated proteins	Sarcoplasmic/endoplasmic reticulum calcium ATPase2, lysosome-associated membrane glycoprotein 1, 14-3-3 protein gamma and alpha-enolase	2014	[78]
Brain tissue (neocortex)	DML, LC MS/MS	69 differentially regulated proteins	–	2014	[69]
Serum	SRM MS	Significant decrease of serum ApoE levels in AD patients (45) versus control (43)	Apolipoprotein E	2014	[83]
Brain tissue (cortex)	MALDI-TOF MS	36 differentially regulated synaptic proteins	–	2013	[103]
CSF	Immunoaffinity enrichment, LC-MS/MS	Twofold increase of tau	Tau	2014	[104]
CSF	MRM, ELISA	12 differentially regulated proteins	Aβ1–40, Aβ1–42, retinol-binding protein, and cystatin C	2013	[84]
CSF	Immunoprecipitation, LC MS/MS	Significant increases in soluble amyloid precursor protein α and β levels	–	2013	[85]
CSF	SRM MS	Significant decrease in level of Aβ42, Aβ42 Aβ40, and Aβ38.		2013	[82]
Brain tissue (cortex)	1-DE, LC MS/MS, WB	25 differentially regulated proteins	IRSp53 and internexin	2013	[105]
Plasma	2-DE, LC MS/MS	20 differentially regulated proteins	–	2012	[73]

Sample	Method	Findings	Protein	Year	Ref
Brain tissue (cortex)	LC MS/MS, WB	197 differentially regulated proteins	PKC-gamma and NUMBL	2012	[79]
Brain tissue (substantia nigra)	Nano-UPLC MS/MS, WB	19 differentially regulated proteins	Heat-shock 70 kDa protein 2	2012	[81]
Brain tissue (cortex)	LC MS/MS, WB	13 differentially regulated proteins	Ubiquitin carboxy-terminal hydrolase 1 and syntaxin-binding protein 1	2012	[80]
Brain tissue (cortex, hippocampus, and cerebellum)	Immunoprecipitation, MALDI-TOF MS	Decrease in level of aβ4−42, aβ1−40, − and aβ1−42 isoforms in AD brains		2011	[86]
CSF	2-DE, LC MS/MS, ELISA	47 novel candidate protein biomarkers	Neuronal cell adhesion molecule, YKL-40, chromogranin A, carnosinase I	2011	[74]
CSF	Immunoprecipitation, LC MS/MS	Elevated neurogranin levels in AD and MCI patients	Neurogranin	2010	[87]
Plasma	2-DE, LC MS/MS	Significant increases in clusterin/ apolipoprotein J level in AD patients versus controls	Clusterin	2010	[76]
Plasma	2-DE, LC MS/MS	18 differentially regulated proteins	−	2009	[77]
CSF	2-DE, LC MS/MS, WB	Significant changes in levels of contactin-1, contactin-2, carnosine dipeptidase 1, 120 kDa isoform precursor of neural cell adhesion molecule 1, α-dystroglycan, secreted protein acidic and rich in cysteine-like protein 1 precursor, isoform 2 of calsyntenin 1, neuronal pentraxin receptor	Neural cell adhesion molecule 1, alpha-dystroglycan, and neuronal pentraxin receptor	2009	[75]

(continued)

Table 3
(continued)

Parkinson's disease

Source	Quantitative method	Proteins/peptides identified, quantified/altered proteins	Validation by independent technique	Year	Reference
Plasma	2-DE, LC MS/MS	Nine different proteins (haptoglobin,– transthyretin, apolipoprotein A-1, serum amyloid P component, apolipoprotein E, complement factor H, fibrinogen γ, thrombin, complement C3) were identified as a potential diagnostic pattern		2013	[89]
CSF	2-DE, MALDI-TOF MS, WB	21 differentially regulated proteins	Superoxide dismutase and tetranectin	2013	[106]
CSF	iTRAQ, MRM	16 differentially regulated proteins in PD	Tyrosine-kinase non-receptor-type 13 and netrin G	2012	[96]
CSF	2-DE, LC-MS	Six proteins, fibrinogen, transthyretin, apolipoprotein E, clusterin, apolipoprotein A-1, and glutathione-S-transferase-Pi, were found to be different	–	2012	[90]
Serum	2-DE, LC MS/MS, iTRAQ, WB	26 proteins were differentially expressed. Significant increases of sero-transferrin and clusterin levels and decrease of complement component 4B, apolipoprotein A-I, α-2-antiplasmin, and coagulation factor V levels in PD patients versus controls	Apolipoprotein A–I, sero-transferrin, and a-2-antiplasmin	2012	[93]

Sample	Method	Finding	Key proteins	Year	Ref
Brain tissues (superior parietal gyrus)	Immunoprecipitation, LC MS/MS, WB	Novel isoforms of alpha-synuclein	N-terminally acetylated full-length α-syn and two N-terminally acetylated truncated forms of α-syn	2012	[95]
Plasma	2-DE MS, ELISA	Two proteins: IgG kappa L and human serum amyloid P component were found differentially expressed	Serum amyloid P component	2011	[107]
Serum	MALDI-TOF-MS combined with magnetic bead-based weak cation exchange	Five differentially regulated proteins	–	2011	[108]
CSF	2D DIGE, MALDI-TOF MS, WB	Eight differentially regulated proteins by MS analysis	Tetranectin and apolipoprotein A	2011	[109]
CSF	2-DE, MALDI-TOF MS, WB	Significant increases in transthyretin and haptoglobin levels in PD patents	Transthyretin and haptoglobin	2010	[92]
Serum	2-DE, LC MS/MS, WB	15 differentially regulated proteins by MS analysis	KIAA0325 protein, myosin heavy-chain IIx/d, and transthyretin	2010	[91]
CSF	2-DE, LC MS/MS, WB	Eight differentially regulated proteins	Tetranectin and apolipoprotein A-I	2010	[110]
CSF	LC MS/MS, WB, ELISA	Two differentially regulated proteins: DJ-1 and alpha-synuclein	DJ-1 and alpha-synuclein	2010	[97]
CSF	2-DE, LC MS/MS	14 differentially regulated proteins	–	2009	[94]
CSF	2-DE, MALDI-TOF MS, WB	Six differentially regulated proteins (serum albumin precursor, serum albumin chain-A, mutant globin, proline-rich repeat 14, hemoglobin β fragment, and serum transferrin N-terminal lobe)	Hemoglobin β fragment was attenuated and serum transferrin N-terminal lobe	2009	[111]

with MS or MS/MS techniques, have been widely used in many of the studies in biomarker discovery for AD. Recently, Henkel et al. [73] reported the analysis of plasma samples of AD patients using 2-DE and LC MS/MS approach. They identified 20 potential plasma biomarkers, ten of which are involved in either the pathophysiology of AD or the Aβ-peptide processing pathway. The 2-DE study [74] revealed altered levels of 47 novel candidate protein biomarkers in AD as compared to control CSF samples. Decreased levels of three novel proteins (neuronal cell adhesion molecule (NCAM), chromogranin A, carnosinase I) and increased levels of novel YKL-40 were further confirmed by ELISA measurements. The same approach was applied by Yin et al. [75], when they identified a large number of significantly regulated proteins in AD CSF samples. Additionally, they showed that the increased level of neural cell adhesion molecule 1 in the CSF of AD patients compared with normal controls is higher than that of PD patients, indicating that NCAM1 is a possible marker for distinguishing AD from PD. Moreover, Thambisetty et al. [76] have found increased levels of clusterin and apolipoprotein J proteins in plasma of the AD patient samples compared to controls using a combination of 2-DE and LC MS/MS. In another 2-DE study, Song et al. [77] detected a panel of 18 signal proteins as markers of AD and mild cognitive impairment.

Gel-free shotgun approach combined with different quantitative proteomic techniques is also widely used for identification and quantification of possible AD protein biomarkers. Musunuri et al. [69] employed a stable isotope DML MS approach to find differentially expressed proteins in AD brain tissue, detecting 69 proteins that were altered between AD and non-neurological control cases. A quantitative proteomic strategy based on the cloud-point extraction method for the separation and enrichment of hydrophobic MPs in combination with DML labeling followed by nanoLC-MS/MS analysis was also employed by Musunuri et al. [78] to quantitatively identify protein expression changes in AD temporal neocortex samples. 62 proteins were found to be differentially expressed including three novel highly hydrophobic transmembrane proteins: downregulated sarcoplasmic/endoplasmic reticulum calcium ATPase2 and up-regulated orphan sodium- and chloride-dependent neurotransmitter transporter NTT4 and C9orf5. Label-free quantitative proteomics was used to investigate the protein expression in the brain cortex [79, 80] and substantia nigra [81] of AD patients, leading to the identification of 197, 13, and 19 differentially expressed proteins, respectively.

Several target MS-based proteomic studies for the determination and quantification of aβ peptides in CSF and brain tissue have been published recently. Pannee et al. [82] have applied multiple reaction monitoring (MRM) MS technique to quantify Aβ42, Aβ40, and Aβ38 in human CSF. Apolipoprotein E has also been measured in serum using this approach, showing a significant decrease of its level in serum of AD patients [83]. A nanoLC-MRM/MS approach was applied by Choi et al. [84] for the measurements of the Aβ1–40, Aβ1–42, retinol-binding protein, and cystatin C in human CSF.

Immunoaffinity enrichment technique, e.g., immunoprecipitation followed by high-resolution MS, was used to analyze the levels of two species of the amyloid precursor protein (APP), sAPPα and sAPPβ, in CSF from AD and non-demented controls [85]. However, this study led to the conclusion that sAPPα and sAPPβ levels are unaltered in AD and none of the sAPP variants could be used to distinguish between the patient groups studied.

Immunoprecipitation in combination with MALDI-TOF/MS or LC-MS/MS was used by Portelius et al. [86] for the determination of the Aβ isoform pattern in the cerebellum, cortex, and hippocampus of AD subjects. The Authors showed that the dominating Aβ isoforms in all three different brain regions are Aβ4–42, Aβ1–40, and Aβ1–42. Thorsell et al. [87] have also applied immunoprecipitation and LC-MS/MS analysis to determine neurogranin in AD CSF samples. The results revealed a significant increase in the neurogranin levels in the CSF from AD patients and a trend towards increasing levels in the MCI group.

8.2 Parkinson's Disease

Parkinson's disease is the second most common progressive degenerative CNS disorder after AD. It is characterized by motor function impairment caused by loss of the dopamine (DA)-containing neurons in the brainstem and the presence of intracellular protein inclusions in the substantia nigra, known as Lewy bodies. It is suggested that the abnormal accumulation of proteins, particularly heavily ubiquitinated alpha-synuclein (α-syn), may play role in the pathogenesis of PD [88].

MS-based proteomic approaches, particularly a combination of 2-DE and LC-MS/MS, have been widely applied to study protein expression changes in CSF, plasma, and brain tissue samples from patients diagnosed with PD. Recently, Alberio et al. [89] reported a list of potential PD biomarkers, proposed by different authors and visible in 2-DE plasma maps of 90 subjects, and developed a panel of nine PD-related plasma proteins (haptoglobin, transthyretin, apolipoprotein A-1, serum amyloid P component, apolipoprotein E, complement factor H, fibrinogen γ, thrombin, complement C3) using 2-DE MS/MS approach. Increased levels of transthyretin and haptoglobin were also identified in serum and CSF samples from PD patients using 2-DE in combination with LC-MS/MS [90, 91] or MALDI-TOF MS [92]. 2-DE MS/MS coupled with iTRAQ labeling was employed by Zhang et al. [93] to quantitatively identify protein expression changes in PD serum samples. 26 proteins were found to be differentially expressed including up-regulated sero-transferrin and clusterin and downregulated complement component 4B, apolipoprotein A-I, alpha -2-antiplasmin, and coagulation factor V. Guo et al. [94] applied 2-DE-LC-MS/MS approach for the identification of 14 differentially expressed proteins in the CSF of PD patients and demonstrated for the first time that the levels of autotoxin and SOD1 are up-regulated in CSF samples from PD patients.

Targeted proteomics has also been used to elucidate PD-related proteome signatures. Recently Öhrfelt et al. [95] employed a combination of immunoprecipitation method and LC-MS/MS to detect and identify known and novel isoforms of alpha-synuclein in PD brain tissue homogenates, including N-terminally acetylated full-length α-syn and two N-terminally acetylated truncated forms of α-syn. Lehnert et al. [96] detected 16 differentially expressed proteins in CSF of PD patients using iTRAQ labeling method. Validation of these candidates was carried out by MRM method, confirming however that only tyrosine-kinase non-receptor-type 13 and netrin G1 were significantly changed in PD and control subjects. Hong et al. [97] have recently performed the largest proteomic study on CSF levels of alpha-synuclein and observed reduced levels of α-syn in more than 100 PD patients compared to both 50 AD patients and 132 non-neurological control cases. Additionally, DJ-1 was found to be significantly decreased in PD cases versus controls or AD patients with further confirmation by Western blot and ELISA.

9   Conclusion

The instrument and methodological development in the field of mass spectrometry and proteomics have dramatically increased the number of applications in neurodegenerative disease research. By carefully controlling the pre-analytical phase and sample preparation steps, the bias in the results can be minimized leading to successful identification and quantification of protein biomarker candidates. At present a large number of promising findings are validated within different laboratories around the world and the outcome has a very high likelihood of rendering in-depth molecular understanding of the physiological changes found in patients with neurodegeneration. Combining the current knowledge with the rapidly evolving technological developments will significantly contribute to the screening and discovery of new biomarkers specific for neurodegenerative diseases in the near future.

Acknowledgments

This research was supported by Uppsala Berzelii Technology Centre for Neurodiagnostics, with financing from the Swedish Governmental Agency for Innovation Systems and The Swedish

Research Council 621-2011-4423. We acknowledge Dr. Denys Shevchenko for technical assistance with Fig. 4.

References

1. Wilkins MR, Pasquali C, Appel RD, Ou K, Golaz O, Sanchez JC, Yan JX, Gooley AA, Hughes G, Humphery-Smith I, Williams KL, Hochstrasser DF (1996) From proteins to proteomes: large scale protein identification by two-dimensional electrophoresis and amino acid analysis. Bio/Technology 14(1): 61–65

2. Wu CC, MacCoss MJ (2002) Shotgun proteomics: tools for the analysis of complex biological systems. Curr Opin Mol Ther 4(3): 242–250

3. Li K (2011) Neuroproteomics: Deciphering Brain Function and Disorders. In: Li KW (ed) Neuroproteomics, vol 57, Neuromethods. Humana Press, New York, pp 3–9. doi:10.1007/978-1-61779-111-6_1

4. neuroscience Tsf (2002) Brain facts: The society for neuroscience. The Society for Neuroscience, Washington, pp 4–5

5. Davidsson P, Sjogren M (2005) The use of proteomics in biomarker discovery in neurodegenerative diseases. Dis Markers 21(2): 81–92

6. Speers AE, Wu CC (2007) Proteomics of integral membrane proteins--theory and application. Chem Rev 107(8):3687–3714

7. Bergquist J, Palmblad M, Wetterhall M, Hakansson P, Markides KE (2002) Peptide mapping of proteins in human body fluids using electrospray ionization Fourier transform ion cyclotron resonance mass spectrometry. Mass Spectrom Rev 21(1):2–15. doi:10.1002/mas.10016

8. Dahlin AP, Wetterhall M, Caldwell KD, Larsson A, Bergquist J, Hillered L, Hjort K (2010) Methodological aspects on microdialysis protein sampling and quantification in biological fluids: an in vitro study on human ventricular CSF. Anal Chem 82(11):4376–4385. doi:10.1021/ac1007706

9. Ekegren T, Hanrieder J, Bergquist J (2008) Clinical perspectives of high-resolution mass spectrometry-based proteomics in neuroscience: exemplified in amyotrophic lateral sclerosis biomarker discovery research. J Mass Spectrom 43(5):559–571. doi:10.1002/jms.1409

10. Raslan AA, Kee Y (2013) Tackling neurodegenerative diseases: animal models of Alzheimer's disease and Parkinson's disease. Genes Genom 35(4):425–440

11. Bunger S, Roblick UJ, Habermann JK (2009) Comparison of five commercial extraction kits for subsequent membrane protein profiling. Cytotechnology 61(3):153–159. doi:10.1007/s10616-009-9249-1

12. Qoronfleh MW, Benton B, Ignacio R, Kaboord B (2003) Selective Enrichment of Membrane Proteins by Partition Phase Separation for Proteomic Studies. J Biomed Biotechnol 2003(4):249–255. doi:10.1155/S1110724303209244

13. Shevchenko G, Musunuri S, Wetterhall M, Bergquist J (2012) Comparison of extraction methods for the comprehensive analysis of mouse brain proteome using shotgun-based mass spectrometry. J Proteome Res 11(4):2441–2451. doi:10.1021/pr201169q

14. Wetterhall M, Shevchenko G, Artemenko K, Sjodin MO, Bergquist J (2011) Analysis of membrane and hydrophilic proteins simultaneously derived from the mouse brain using cloud-point extraction. Anal Bioanal Chem 400(9):2827–2836

15. Loo RR, Dales N, Andrews PC (1994) Surfactant effects on protein structure examined by electrospray ionization mass spectrometry. Protein Sci 3(11):1975–1983

16. Seddon AM, Curnow P, Booth PJ (2004) Membrane proteins, lipids and detergents: not just a soap opera. Biochim Biophys Acta 1666(1-2):105–117

17. Manabe T, Miyamoto H, Inoue K, Nakatsu M, Arai M (1999) Separation of human cerebrospinal fluid proteins by capillary isoelectric focusing in the absence of denaturing agents. Electrophoresis 20(18): 3677–3683

18. Lai CC, Her GR (2000) Analysis of phospholipase A2 glycosylation patterns from venom of individual bees by capillary electrophoresis/electrospray ionization mass spectrometry using an ion trap mass spectrometer. Rapid Commun Mass Spectrom 14(21):2012–2018

19. Ouyang J, Wang J, Deng R, Long Q, Wang X (2003) High-level expression, purification, and characterization of porcine somatotropin in Pichia pastoris. Protein Expr Purif 32(1):28–34

20. Jiang L, He L, Fountoulakis M (2004) Comparison of protein precipitation methods for sample preparation prior to proteomic analysis. J Chromatogr 1023(2):317–320

21. Shevchenko G, Sjodin MO, Malmstrom D, Wetterhall M, Bergquist J (2010) Cloud-point extraction and delipidation of porcine brain proteins in combination with bottom-up mass spectrometry approaches for proteome analysis. J Proteome Res 9(8): 3903–3911

22. Rappsilber J, Ishihama Y, Mann M (2003) Stop and go extraction tips for matrix-assisted laser desorption/ionization, nanoelectrospray, and LC/MS sample pretreatment in proteomics. Anal Chem 75(3):663–670

23. Freeman WM, Hemby SE (2004) Proteomics for protein expression profiling in neuroscience. Neurochem Res 29(6):1065–1081

24. Bodzon-Kulakowska A, Bierczynska-Krzysik A, Dylag T, Drabik A, Suder P, Noga M, Jarzebinska J, Silberring J (2007) Methods for samples preparation in proteomic research. J Chromatogr B Anal Technol Biomed Life Sci 849(1-2):1–31

25. Anderson NL, Anderson NG (1998) Proteome and proteomics: New technologies, new concepts, and new words. Electrophoresis 19(11):1853–1861

26. Schutzer SE, Angel TE, Liu T, Schepmoes AA, Xie F, Bergquist J, Vecsei L, Zadori D, Camp DG 2nd, Holland BK, Smith RD, Coyle PK (2013) Gray matter is targeted in first-attack multiple sclerosis. PLoS One 8(9), e66117. doi:10.1371/journal.pone.0066117

27. Wetterhall M, Zuberovic A, Hanrieder J, Bergquist J (2010) Assessment of the partitioning capacity of high abundant proteins in human cerebrospinal fluid using affinity and immunoaffinity subtraction spin columns. J Chromatogr B Anal Technol Biomed Life Sci 878(19):1519–1530. doi:10.1016/j.jchromb.2010.04.003

28. Ramstrom M, Zuberovic A, Gronwall C, Hanrieder J, Bergquist J, Hober S (2009) Development of affinity columns for the removal of high-abundance proteins in cerebrospinal fluid. Biotechnol Appl Biochem 52(Pt 2):159–166. doi:10.1042/BA20080015

29. Ramstrom M, Hagman C, Mitchell JK, Derrick PJ, Hakansson P, Bergquist J (2005) Depletion of high-abundant proteins in body fluids prior to liquid chromatography fourier transform ion cyclotron resonance mass spectrometry. J Proteome Res 4(2):410–416. doi:10.1021/pr049812a

30. Zhang J, Goodlett DR, Peskind ER, Quinn JF, Zhou Y, Wang Q, Pan C, Yi E, Eng J, Aebersold RH, Montine TJ (2005) Quantitative proteomic analysis of age-related changes in human cerebrospinal fluid. Neurobiol Aging 26(2):207–227

31. Schutzer SE, Angel TE, Liu T, Schepmoes AA, Clauss TR, Adkins JN, Camp DG, Holland BK, Bergquist J, Coyle PK, Smith RD, Fallon BA, Natelson BH (2011) Distinct cerebrospinal fluid proteomes differentiate post-treatment Lyme disease from chronic fatigue syndrome. PLoS One 6(2), e17287. doi:10.1371/journal.pone.0017287

32. Schutzer SE, Liu T, Natelson BH, Angel TE, Schepmoes AA, Purvine SO, Hixson KK, Lipton MS, Camp DG, Coyle PK, Smith RD, Bergquist J (2010) Establishing the proteome of normal human cerebrospinal fluid. PLoS One 5(6), e10980. doi:10.1371/journal.pone.0010980

33. Sjodin MO, Bergquist J, Wetterhall M (2010) Mining ventricular cerebrospinal fluid from patients with traumatic brain injury using hexapeptide ligand libraries to search for trauma biomarkers. J Chromatogr B Anal Technol Biomed Life Sci 878(22):2003–2012. doi:10.1016/j.jchromb.2010.05.036

34. Biringer RG, Amato H, Harrington MG, Fonteh AN, Riggins JN, Huhmer AF (2006) Enhanced sequence coverage of proteins in human cerebrospinal fluid using multiple enzymatic digestion and linear ion trap LC-MS/MS. Brief Funct Genomic Proteomic 5(2):144–153. doi:10.1093/bfgp/ell026

35. Capelo JL, Carreira R, Diniz M, Fernandes L, Galesio M, Lodeiro C, Santos HM, Vale G (2009) Overview on modern approaches to speed up protein identification workflows relying on enzymatic cleavage and mass spectrometry-based techniques. Anal Chim Acta 650(2):151–159. doi:10.1016/j.aca.2009.07.034

36. Hustoft HK, Reubsaet L, Greibrokk T, Lundanes E, Malerod H (2011) Critical assessment of accelerating trypsination methods. J Pharm Biomed Anal 56(5):1069–1078. doi:10.1016/j.jpba.2011.08.013

37. Bao H, Liu T, Chen X, Chen G (2008) Efficient in-gel proteolysis accelerated by infrared radiation for protein identification. J Proteome Res 7(12):5339–5344. doi:10.1021/pr800572e

38. Pramanik BN, Mirza UA, Ing YH, Liu YH, Bartner PL, Weber PC, Bose AK (2002) Microwave-enhanced enzyme reaction for protein mapping by mass spectrometry: a new approach to protein digestion in minutes. Protein Sci 11(11):2676–2687. doi:10.1110/ps.0213702

39. Yamaguchi H, Miyazaki M, Honda T, Briones-Nagata MP, Arima K, Maeda H (2009) Rapid and efficient proteolysis for proteomic analysis by protease-immobilized microreactor. Electrophoresis 30(18):3257–3264. doi:10.1002/elps.200900134

40. May C, Brosseron F, Chartowski P, Meyer HE, Marcus K (2012) Differential proteome analysis using 2D-DIGE. Methods Mol Biol 893:75–82. doi:10.1007/978-1-61779-885-6_6

41. Wetterhall M, Palmblad M, Hakansson P, Markides KE, Bergquist J (2002) Rapid analysis of tryptically digested cerebrospinal fluid using capillary electrophoresis-electrospray ionization-Fourier transform ion cyclotron resonance-mass spectrometry. J Proteome Res 1(4):361–366

42. Zuberovic A, Wetterhall M, Hanrieder J, Bergquist J (2009) CE MALDI-TOF/TOF MS for multiplexed quantification of proteins in human ventricular cerebrospinal fluid. Electrophoresis 30(10):1836–1843. doi:10.1002/elps.200800714

43. Fenn JB, Mann M, Meng CK, Wong SF, Whitehouse CM (1989) Electrospray ionization for mass spectrometry of large biomolecules. Science 246(4926):64–71

44. Karas M, Hillenkamp F (1988) Laser desorption ionization of proteins with molecular masses exceeding 10,000 daltons. Anal Chem 60(20):2299–2301

45. Han X, Aslanian A, Yates JR 3rd (2008) Mass spectrometry for proteomics. Curr Opin Chem Biol 12(5):483–490. doi:10.1016/j.cbpa.2008.07.024

46. Bergquist J (2003) FTICR mass spectrometry in proteomics. Curr Opin Mol Ther 5(3):310–314

47. Ekegren T, Hanrieder J, Aquilonius SM, Bergquist J (2006) Focused proteomics in post-mortem human spinal cord. J Proteome Res 5(9):2364–2371. doi:10.1021/pr060237f

48. Zuberovic A, Hanrieder J, Hellman U, Bergquist J, Wetterhall M (2008) Proteome profiling of human cerebrospinal fluid: exploring the potential of capillary electrophoresis with surface modified capillaries for analysis of complex biological samples. Eur J Mass Spectrom 14(4):249–260. doi:10.1255/ejms.929

49. Hanrieder J, Ekegren T, Andersson M, Bergquist J (2013) MALDI imaging of post-mortem human spinal cord in amyotrophic lateral sclerosis. J Neurochem 124(5):695–707. doi:10.1111/jnc.12019

50. Ong SE, Mann M (2005) Mass spectrometry-based proteomics turns quantitative. Nat Chem Biol 1(5):252–262

51. Bronstrup M (2004) Absolute quantification strategies in proteomics based on mass spectrometry. Expert Rev Proteomics 1(4):503–512

52. Liu H, Sadygov RG, Yates JR 3rd (2004) A model for random sampling and estimation of relative protein abundance in shotgun proteomics. Anal Chem 76(14):4193–4201

53. Oda Y, Huang K, Cross FR, Cowburn D, Chait BT (1999) Accurate quantitation of protein expression and site-specific phosphorylation. Proc Natl Acad Sci U S A 96(12):6591–6596

54. Gouw JW, Krijgsveld J, Heck AJ (2010) Quantitative proteomics by metabolic labeling of model organisms. Mol Cell Proteomics 9(1):11–24. doi:10.1074/mcp.R900001-MCP200

55. Westman-Brinkmalm A, Abramsson A, Pannee J, Gang C, Gustavsson MK, von Otter M, Blennow K, Brinkmalm G, Heumann H, Zetterberg H (2011) SILAC zebrafish for quantitative analysis of protein turnover and tissue regeneration. J Proteome 75(2):425–434. doi:10.1016/j.jprot.2011.08.008

56. Doherty MK, Whitehead C, McCormack H, Gaskell SJ, Beynon RJ (2005) Proteome dynamics in complex organisms: using stable isotopes to monitor individual protein turnover rates. Proteomics 5(2):522–533. doi:10.1002/pmic.200400959

57. Kruger M, Moser M, Ussar S, Thievessen I, Luber CA, Forner F, Schmidt S, Zanivan S, Fassler R, Mann M (2008) SILAC mouse for quantitative proteomics uncovers kindlin-3 as an essential factor for red blood cell function. Cell 134(2):353–364. doi:10.1016/j.cell.2008.05.033

58. Ishihama Y, Sato T, Tabata T, Miyamoto N, Sagane K, Nagasu T, Oda Y (2005) Quantitative mouse brain proteomics using culture-derived isotope tags as internal standards. Nat Biotechnol 23(5):617–621. doi:10.1038/nbt1086

59. Xie F, Liu T, Qian WJ, Petyuk VA, Smith RD (2011) Liquid Chromatography-Mass Spectrometry-based Quantitative Proteomics. J Biol Chem 286(29):25443–25449

60. Yao X, Freas A, Ramirez J, Demirev PA, Fenselau C (2001) Proteolytic 18O labeling for comparative proteomics: model studies with two serotypes of adenovirus. Anal Chem 73(13):2836–2842

61. Reynolds KJ, Yao X, Fenselau C (2002) Proteolytic 18O labeling for comparative proteomics: evaluation of endoprotease Glu-C as the catalytic agent. J Proteome Res 1(1):27–33

62. Johnson KL, Muddiman DC (2004) A method for calculating 16O/18O peptide ion ratios for the relative quantification of proteomes. J Am Soc Mass Spectrom 15(4):437–445

63. Ramos-Fernandez A, Lopez-Ferrer D, Vazquez J (2007) Improved method for differential expression proteomics using trypsin-catalyzed 18O labeling with a correction for labeling efficiency. Mol Cell Proteomics 6(7):1274–1286

64. Fuvesi J, Hanrieder J, Bencsik K, Rajda C, Kovacs SK, Kaizer L, Beniczky S, Vecsei L, Bergquist J (2012) Proteomic analysis of cerebrospinal fluid in a fulminant case of multiple sclerosis. Int J Mol Sci 13(6):7676–7693. doi:10.3390/ijms13067676

65. Hanrieder J, Wetterhall M, Enblad P, Hillered L, Bergquist J (2009) Temporally resolved differential proteomic analysis of human ventricular CSF for monitoring traumatic brain injury biomarker candidates. J Neurosci Methods 177(2):469–478

66. Karp NA, Huber W, Sadowski PG, Charles PD, Hester SV, Lilley KS (2010) Addressing accuracy and precision issues in iTRAQ quantitation. Mol Cell Proteomics 9(9):1885–1897. doi:10.1074/mcp.M900628-MCP200

67. Hsu JL, Huang SY, Chow NH, Chen SH (2003) Stable-isotope dimethyl labeling for quantitative proteomics. Anal Chem 75(24):6843–6852

68. Ji C, Guo N, Li L (2005) Differential dimethyl labeling of N-termini of peptides after guanidination for proteome analysis. J Proteome Res 4(6):2099–2108

69. Musunuri S, Wetterhall M, Ingelsson M, Lannfelt L, Artemenko K, Bergquist J, Kultima K, Shevchenko G (2014) Quantification of the brain proteome in Alzheimer's disease using multiplexed mass spectrometry. J Proteome Res 13(4):2056–2068. doi:10.1021/pr401202d

70. Sui P, Watanabe H, Ossipov MH, Porreca F, Bakalkin G, Bergquist J, Artemenko K (2013) Dimethyl-labeling-based protein quantification and pathway search: a novel method of spinal cord analysis applicable for neurological studies. J Proteome Res 12(5):2245–2252. doi:10.1021/pr4001064

71. Elliott MH, Smith DS, Parker CE, Borchers C (2009) Current trends in quantitative proteomics. J Mass Spectrom 44(12):1637–1660

72. Blennow K, de Leon MJ, Zetterberg H (2006) Alzheimer's disease. Lancet 368(9533):387–403

73. Henkel AW, Muller K, Lewczuk P, Muller T, Marcus K, Kornhuber J, Wiltfang J (2012) Multidimensional plasma protein separation technique for identification of potential Alzheimer's disease plasma biomarkers: a pilot study. J Neural Transm 119(7):779–788

74. Perrin RJ, Craig-Schapiro R, Malone JP, Shah AR, Gilmore P, Davis AE, Roe CM, Peskind ER, Li G, Galasko DR, Clark CM, Quinn JF, Kaye JA, Morris JC, Holtzman DM, Townsend RR, Fagan AM (2011) Identification and Validation of Novel Cerebrospinal Fluid Biomarkers for Staging Early Alzheimer's Disease. PLoS One 6(1)

75. Yin GN, Lee HW, Cho JY, Suk K (2009) Neuronal pentraxin receptor in cerebrospinal fluid as a potential biomarker for neurodegenerative diseases. Brain Res 1265:158–170

76. Thambisetty M, Simmons A, Velayudhan L, Hye A, Campbell J, Zhang Y, Wahlund LO, Westman E, Kinsey A, Guntert A, Proitsi P, Powell J, Causevic M, Killick R, Lunnon K, Lynham S, Broadstock M, Choudhry F, Howlett DR, Williams RJ, Sharp SI, Mitchelmore C, Tunnard C, Leung R, Foy C, O'Brien D, Breen G, Furney SJ, Ward M, Kloszewska I, Mecocci P, Soininen H, Tsolaki M, Vellas B, Hodges A, Murphy DGM, Parkins S, Richardson JC, Resnick SM, Ferrucci L, Wong DF, Zhou Y, Muehlboeck S, Evans A, Francis PT, Spenger C, Lovestone S (2010) Association of Plasma Clusterin Concentration With Severity, Pathology, and Progression in Alzheimer Disease. Arch Gen Psychiatry 67(7):739–748

77. Song F, Poljak A, Smythe GA, Sachdev P (2009) Plasma biomarkers for mild cognitive impairment and Alzheimer's disease. Brain Res Rev 61(2):69–80

78. Musunuri S, Kultima K, Richard BC, Ingelsson M, Lannfelt L, Bergquist J, Shevchenko G (2014) Micellar extraction possesses a new advantage for the analysis of Alzheimer's disease brain proteome. Anal Bioanal Chem. doi:10.1007/s00216-014-8320-8

79. Andreev VP, Petyuk VA, Brewer HM, Karpievitch YV, Xie F, Clarke J, Camp D, Smith RD, Lieberman AP, Albin RL, Nawaz Z, El Hokayem J, Myers AJ (2012) Label-Free Quantitative LC-MS Proteomics of Alzheimer's Disease and Normally Aged Human Brains. J Proteome Res 11(6):3053–3067

80. Donovan LE, Higginbotham L, Dammer EB, Gearing M, Rees HD, Xia QW, Duong DM, Seyfried NT, Lah JJ, Levey AI (2012) Analysis of a membrane-enriched proteome from postmortem human brain tissue in Alzheimer's disease. Proteom Clin Appl 6(3-4):201–211

81. Chen S, Lu FF, Seeman P, Liu F (2012) Quantitative Proteomic Analysis of Human Substantia Nigra in Alzheimer's Disease, Huntington's Disease and Multiple Sclerosis. Neurochem Res 37(12):2805–2813

82. Pannee J, Portelius E, Oppermann M, Atkins A, Hornshaw M, Zegers I, Hojrup P, Minthon L, Hansson O, Zetterberg H, Blennow K, Gobom J (2013) A Selected Reaction Monitoring (SRM)-Based Method for Absolute Quantification of A beta(38), A beta(40), and A beta(42) in Cerebrospinal Fluid of Alzheimer's Disease Patients and Healthy Controls. J Alzheimers Dis 33(4):1021–1032

83. Han SH, Kim JS, Lee Y, Choi H, Kim JW, Na DL, Yang EG, Yu MH, Hwang D, Lee C, Mook-Jung I (2014) Both Targeted Mass Spectrometry and Flow Sorting Analysis Methods Detected the Decreased Serum Apolipoprotein E Level in Alzheimer's Disease Patients. Mol Cell Proteomics 13(2):407–419

84. Choi YS, Hou SY, Choe LH, Lee KH (2013) Targeted human cerebrospinal fluid proteomics for the validation of multiple Alzheimer's disease biomarker candidates. J Chromatogr B 930:129–135

85. Brinkmalm G, Brinkmalm A, Bourgeois P, Persson R, Hansson O, Portelius E, Mercken M, Andreasson U, Parent S, Lipari F, Ohrfelt A, Bjerke M, Minthon L, Zetterberg H, Blennow K, Nutu M (2013) Soluble amyloid precursor protein alpha and beta in CSF in Alzheimer's disease. Brain Res 1513:117–126

86. Portelius E, Bogdanovic N, Gustavsson MK, Volkmann I, Brinkmalm G, Zetterberg H, Winblad B, Blennow K (2011) Mass spectrometric characterization of brain amyloid beta isoform signatures in familial and sporadic Alzheimer's disease. Acta Neuropathol 120(2):185–193

87. Thorsell A, Bjerke M, Gobom J, Brunhage E, Vanmechelen E, Andreasen N, Hansson O, Minthon L, Zetterberg H, Blennow K (2010) Neurogranin in cerebrospinal fluid as a marker of synaptic degeneration in Alzheimer's disease. Brain Res 1362:13–22

88. Olanow CW, Prusiner SB (2009) Is Parkinson's disease a prion disorder? Proc Natl Acad Sci U S A 106(31):12571–12572

89. Alberio T, Bucci EM, Natale M, Bonino D, Di Giovanni M, Bottacchi E, Fasano M (2013) Parkinson's disease plasma biomarkers: An automated literature analysis followed by experimental validation. J Proteome 90:107–114

90. Maarouf CL, Beach TG, Adler CH, Shill HA, Sabbagh MN, Wu T, Walker DG, Kokjohn TA, Roher AE (2012) Cerebrospinal fluid biomarkers of neuropathologically diagnosed Parkinson's disease subjects. Neurol Res 34(7):669–676

91. Zhao X, Xiao WZ, Pu XP, Zhong LJ (2010) Proteome analysis of the sera from Chinese Parkinson's disease patients. Neurosci Lett 479(2):175–179

92. Arguelles S, Venero JL, Garcia-Rodriguez S, Tomas-Camardiel M, Ayala A, Cano J, Machado A (2010) Use of haptoglobin and transthyretin as potential biomarkers for the preclinical diagnosis of Parkinson's disease. Neurochem Int 57(3):227–234

93. Zhang XP, Yin XF, Yu HH, Liu XH, Yang FY, Yao J, Jin H, Yang PY (2012) Quantitative proteomic analysis of serum proteins in patients with Parkinson's disease using an isobaric tag for relative and absolute quantification labeling, two-dimensional liquid chromatography, and tandem mass spectrometry. Analyst 137(2):490–495

94. Guo JG, Sun ZW, Xiao SF, Liu DP, Jin GH, Wang ES, Zhou JN, Zhou JW (2009) Proteomic analysis of the cerebrospinal fluid of Parkinson's disease patients. Cell Res 19(12):1401–1403

95. Ohrfelt A, Zetterberg H, Andersson K, Persson R, Secic D, Brinkmalm G, Wallin A, Mulugeta E, Francis PT, Vanmechelen E, Aarsland D, Ballard C, Blennow K, Westman-Brinkmalm A (2012) Identification of Novel alpha-Synuclein Isoforms in Human Brain Tissue by using an Online NanoLC-ESI-FTICR-MS Method. Neurochem Res 36(11):2029–2042

96. Lehnert S, Jesse S, Rist W, Steinacker P, Soininen H, Herukka SK, Tumani H, Lenter M, Oeckl P, Ferger B, Hengerer B, Otto M (2012) iTRAQ and multiple reaction monitoring as proteomic tools for biomarker search in cerebrospinal fluid of patients with Parkinson's disease dementia. Exp Neurol 234(2):499–505

97. Hong Z, Shi M, Chung KA, Quinn JF, Peskind ER, Galasko D, Jankovic J, Zabetian CP, Leverenz JB, Baird G, Montine TJ, Hancock AM, Hwang H, Pan C, Bradner J, Kang UJ, Jensen PH, Zhang J (2010) DJ-1 and alpha-synuclein in human cerebrospinal fluid as biomarkers of Parkinson's disease. Brain 133:713–726

98. Vermachova M, Purkrtova Z, Santrucek J, Jolivet P, Chardot T, Kodicek M (2011) New protein isoforms identified within Arabidopsis thaliana seed oil bodies combining chymotrypsin/trypsin digestion and peptide fragmentation analysis. Proteomics 11(16):3430–3434. doi:10.1002/pmic.201000603

99. Mizutani Y, Tsuge S, Shiogama K, Shimomura R, Kamoshida S, Inada K, Tsutsumi Y (2009) Enzyme-labeled antigen method: histochemi-

cal detection of antigen-specific antibody-producing cells in tissue sections of rats immunized with horseradish peroxidase, ovalbumin, or keyhole limpet hemocyanin. J histochem Cytochem 57(2):101–111. doi:10.1369/jhc.2008.952259

100. Langeveld JP, Wang JJ, Van de Wiel DF, Shih GC, Garssen GJ, Bossers A, Shih JC (2003) Enzymatic degradation of prion protein in brain stem from infected cattle and sheep. J Infect Dis 188(11):1782–1789. doi:10.1086/379664

101. Waxdal MJ (1971) Selective cleavage of proteins. J Agric Food Chem 19(4):632–637

102. Witkop B, Ramachandran K (1964) Progress in Non-Enzymatic Selective Modification and Cleavage of Proteins. Metab Clin Exp 13(SUPPL):1016–1025

103. Chang RYK, Nouwens AS, Dodd PR, Etheridge N (2013) The synaptic proteome in Alzheimer's disease. Alzheimers Dement 9(5):499–511

104. McAvoy T, Lassman ME, Spellman DS, Ke Z, Howell BJ, Wong O, Zhu L, Tanen M, Struyk A, Laterza OF (2013) Quantification of tau in cerebrospinal fluid by immunoaffinity enrichment and tandem mass spectrometry. Clin Chem 60(4):683–689

105. Zhou JY, Jones DR, Duong DM, Levey AI, Lah JJ, Peng JM (2013) Proteomic analysis of postsynaptic density in Alzheimer's Disease. Clin Chim Acta 420:62–68

106. Wang ES, Yao HB, Chen YH, Wang G, Gao WW, Sun YR, Guo JG, Hu JW, Jiang CC, Hu J (2013) Proteomic Analysis of the Cerebrospinal Fluid of Parkinson's Disease Patients Pre- and Post-Deep Brain Stimulation. Cell Physiol Biochem 31(4-5): 625–637

107. Chen HM, Lin CY, Wang V (2011) Amyloid P component as a plasma marker for Parkinson's disease identified by a proteomic approach. Clin Biochem 44(5-6):377–385

108. Li YH, Wang JA, Zheng XL, Zhang YL, Li X, Yu S, He X, Chan P (2011) Matrix-Assisted Laser Desorption/Ionization Time-of-Flight Mass Spectrometry Combined with Magnetic Beads for Detecting Serum Protein Biomarkers in Parkinson's Disease. Eur Neurol 65(2):105–111

109. Wang ES, Sun Y, Guo JG, Gao X, Hu JW, Zhou L, Hu J, Jiang CC (2011) Tetranectin and apolipoprotein A-I in cerebrospinal fluid as potential biomarkers for Parkinson's disease. Acta Neurol Scand 122(5): 350–359

110. Chen Y, Yu G, Tu WB, Long HC, Jiang SD, Wan JC, Peng GG (2010) Cerebrospinal fluid diagnostic markers for two-dimensional electrophoresis-mass spectrometry in Parkinson's disease patients. Neural Regen Res 5(12):890–894

111. Sinha A, Srivastava N, Singh S, Singh AK, Bhushan S, Shukla R, Singh MP (2009) Identification of differentially displayed proteins in cerebrospinal fluid of Parkinson's disease patients: A proteomic approach. Clin Chim Acta 400(1-2):14–20

INDEX

A

Abeta 4–42 .... 39, 42–44
Aβ protofibrils
    AD immunotherapy 55, 56
    aducanumab 54
    amyloid hypothesis 52
    Arctic AβPP mutation 52
    arctic mutation 55–56
    BAN2401 antibody development 55
    bapineuzumab 53
    crenezumab 54
    gantenerumab 54
    mAb158, transgenic mice 56
    side effects 57–58
    solanezumab 53–54
    soluble Aβ correlates 55
ACI-24, liposome-based vaccine 27, 28
Active immunization
    AN1792 53
    α-syn 65–66
Active immunotherapy 24
    amino acid copolymers 95
    amyloid-β clearance 21–23
    amyloid-β immunotherapy (see Amyloid-β immunotherapy)
    AN1792 .... 23, 24
    B-cell epitopes 94
    benefits and challenges 30, 31
    CD4 and Foxp3 94
    cellular autoimmunity 91
    immunization 94
    microglia-driven neuroinflammatory 94
    PDGFβ 91
    T cells 94
    vaccination 91
    α-syn 91
Active vaccination
    CAD106 11
    vs. passive vaccination 11
Adenosine triphosphate (ATP) 237
Aducanumab 54
AFFITOPE®.. 65
    C-terminal α-syn 96
    human immune system 95
    peptide candidates 96

    vaccines (see Vaccination)
    α-syn transgenic mouse lines 97
    β-syn 97
Aggregate clearance 133
Alpha-synuclein (α-syn) 166
    accumulation and aggregation 88
    active immunization 65, 66
    AD brains 64
    amyloid deposition 246
    amyloid fibrils 74
    antibodies action 68–69
    anti-α-syn antibodies 69
    astrocytes and microglia
        cytokines and chemokines 76
        glial cells 76
        LBs 76
        neurodegenerative diseases 77
        neuronal cells 76
        neuron-released 77
        oligomeric form(s) 77
    bead-based Luminex assay 220
    biotinylated detection antibody 219
    in CSF 216, 218–219
    cytosolic protein 74
    description 64
    disease-modifying alternatives 64, 65
    ELISA 220
    extracellular proteases 77
    glucocerebrosidase 88
    immunohistochemistry 223
    immunoprecipitation protocol 217
    immunostaining 99
    immunotherapy
        AFFiRiS 103
        AFFiRiS PD vaccine 103
        blood–brain barrier 80
        brain 78
        cell lysates 78
        cell-to-cell transmission 78, 79
        human monoclonal antibody 104
        modeling methods 105
        neurotoxicity and neuroinflammation 80
        phase I study 103
        PRX002 104
    intrabodies and single-chain antibodies 67–68

Martin Ingelsson and Lars Lannfelt (eds.), *Immunotherapy and Biomarkers in Neurodegenerative Disorders*, Methods in Pharmacology and Toxicology, DOI 10.1007/978-1-4939-3560-4, © Springer Science+Business Media New York 2016

Alpha-synuclein (α-syn) (cont.)
  LBs 73
  localization and distribution 87–88
  lysosomal activity 77
  meta-analysis studies 221
  monoclonal antibody 217
  mutations 87
  neuroblastoma cell line 78
  neuronal cells 75
  neuronal toxicity 74, 75
  neuropathological findings 246
  neurosin 77
  nigrostriatal neuronal degeneration 216
  oligomeric α-synuclein 223
  oligomers 222
  passive immunization 66–67
  PD pathogenesis 89
  PD patients 220
  parkinsonism 74
  peripheral tissues 229–230
  phosphorylated/oligomeric forms 217
  in plasma...216, 225
  preanalytical sample..................................221
  presynaptic terminals 87
  PS-129 α-synuclein 224
  sensitive techniques 223
  spatial patterns...74
  subclassification, MSA 216
Alzheimer's disease (AD) 21–24, 86,
      157–161, 199, 241
  A4 protein 154
  active immunotherapy, amyloid-beta 10–12
  amyloid cascade hypothesis 4, 5
  APP..155
  atrophy process 181
  autopsy and biomarker...............................157
  Aβ.. 20, 156
  biological process 155
  brain atrophy 156
  clinical research criteria 208
  CSF (see Cerebrospinal fluid (CSF))
  dementia 154
  description 19
  diagnosis 156, 199
  disease-modifying treatment 4
  and Down's syndrome 154
  exome sequencing 156
  genetic factors 156
  higher Aβ levels 5
  immunotherapy 6–7
  MAPT gene 157
  microglial activation and synapse loss 169
  molecular pathways....................................156
  monoclonal antibodies, passive immunotherapy............7–10

  neurofibrillary tangles 155
  neuropathology...154
  NIA-AA criteria..................................207, 208
  N-truncated Aβ peptides.............................38
  passive immunotherapy 8–9
  pathophysiological process.........................200
  PET (see Positron emission tomography (PET))
  pharmacological treatment 6
  plaques 155
  plasma antichymotrypsin protease.............155
  prevalence 4
  prevention 12–13
  progressive dementia..................................20
  pyroglutamate-Aβ 40–43
  stages 5
  standardisation efforts 168–169
  tau pathology..157
  therapeutic approaches
    amyloid-β clearance 21–23
    AN1792...23–24
  visual rating scales....................................186
Amyloid..244–246
  Aβ and tau 204–206
  PET scan 204, 205
Amyloid β (Aβ)
  immunotherapy
    ACC-001.......................................24–26
    ACI-24 27–28
    active vaccine AN1792 52
    AD04...26–27
    CAD106 28–29
    DNA...30
    Lu AF20513 29
    side effects, clinical trials...................57–58
    UB-311...29
    V950 30
  protofibrils (see Aβ protofibrils)
Amyloid cascade hypothesis 4, 5, 13, 20
Amyloid fibril protein β.................................154
Amyloid-related imaging abnormalities
      (ARIAs)...................................11, 12, 57, 58,
      187–188
Amyloid-related imaging abnormalities with edema
      (ARIA-E)............................... 53, 54, 57, 58
Amyloid-related imaging abnormalities with
      microhemorrhages (ARIA-H).........................53
AN 1792, synthetic beta-amyloid peptide 23, 24
Antibodies
  anti-α-syn 64
  α-syn toxic conformations 66–67
Anti-HD intrabodies
  anti-N1-17 intrabodies...............................145
  C4 scFv 143
  HD Drosophila phenotypes.................143, 144

peptide antigens.................................142
VL12.3 144
Anti-tau oligomeric monoclonal antibody (TOMA)...........127
ARIAs. *See* Amyloid-related imaging abnormalities (ARIAs)
Atypical parkinsonian syndromes (APS)..........................241

B

BAN2401 antibody development 55
Bapineuzumab..53, 167
β-site APP-cleaving enzyme 1 (BACE1)......................162
BioArctic Neuroscience.......................................56
Biomarkers
    Aβ oligomers 163
    blood..166–167
    blood-brain barrier 163
    clinical trials..167–168
    CSF BACE1 162
    CSF sAPPα/sAPPβ............................ 162
    dementia 161
    inflammation, oxidative stress and microglial activation
        AD process 166
        CCL2 165
        chitotriosidase.......................................165
        CSF lipocalin 2 164
        cytokines 164
        F2-isoprostanes.......................................165
        neopterin.......................................165
        TREM2 gene.......................................164
    neurodegeneration 163–164
    synaptic proteins 166
    α-synuclein 166
Blood cells 228
Brain Observer MicroBleed scale (BOMBS)...................186

C

C4 scFv
    fibrillar species 144
    HD *Drosophila* phenotypes.....................143, 144
    mouse models 144
CAD106...28
C-C chemokine ligand 2 (CCL2) 165
Cerebral amyloid angiopathy (CAA)...............................182
Cerebral microbleeds (CMB) 182, 188
Cerebrospinal fluid (CSF).......................................216, 217
    AD biomarkers 161
    Aβ42
        ELISA 158
        isoforms 159
        MCI 158
        neuroinflammatory conditions...........................158
        proteolytic clearance pathways...........................157
        tests...160–161
    biomarkers 157, 158, 167–168
    brain and spinal cord 157

P-tau...160–161
T-tau...159–161
CID. *See* Collision-induced dissociation (CID)
Clinical trial
    AFFITOPE® 90
    PDD...87
    tolerability...104
Collision-induced dissociation (CID) 261
Colonic mucosa 229
Crenezumab 54
Creutzfeldt-Jakob disease (CJD)...........................159

D

Deformation-based morphometry (DBM) 192
Dementia...203
Dementia with Lewy bodies (DLB)................... 87, 202, 215
3D FLAIR sequence 186
Differential diagnosis, NAA/Cr ratios 240
Diffusion tensor imaging (DTI)...........................236
Diffusion weighted imaging (DWI)...........................236
DNA amyloid-β immunotherapy...........................30
Dopamine transporter
    autonomic symptoms 243
    DAT imaging 243
    extracerebral imaging...243–244
    FP-CIT SPECT 244
    G-protein coupled DA 243
    nigrostriatal pathway 242
    PD and APS syndromes 244
    postsynaptic D2/D3 receptors 243
    serotonin- and norepinephrine
        transporters 244
    SPECT...242, 243
Dopamine transporters (DAT)...........................204, 242

E

Endosomal sorting complex required for transport
    (ESCRT)...68
Enzyme-linked immunosorbent assay (ELISA)..............158
    bead-based flow cytometric assays...........................220
    CSF α-synuclein...221
    monoclonal capture antibody...........................220
    α-synuclein levels...217
European Medicines Agency (EMA)...........................167

F

Fazekas scale...186, 187
Fibrillar aggregates 43, 74
Fluorescein isothiocyanate (FITC)...........................91
Fluorodeoxyglucose (FDG)...........................200, 201
^{18}F-fluorodeoxyglucose (^{18}F-FDG) 244
Fluorodeoxyglucose metabolism (FDG)
    cerebral glucose metabolism 244
    PDD...244

Frontotemporal dementia (FTD)....................................246
    hypometabolism 201, 202
Functional MRI...236, 237

G

Gantenerumab...54
GCA. *See* Global cortical atrophy (GCA)
Genome wide association studies (GWAS).......................87
Glial cytoplasmic inclusions (GCIs)...............................87
Global Consortium for Biomarker Standardization
    (GCBS) 169
Global cortical atrophy (GCA) 185

H

Heart 230
Hippocampal volumetry 189, 190
Humoral immunization..64
Huntington's disease (HD)
    active vaccination protocol...147
    causes
        polyQ...139
        trinucleotide CAG repeat 139
    immunotherapy 140
    intrabodies
        EM48 scFv..146
        Happ..145, 146
        mechanisms 141
    targeting signal
        intracellular protein degradation...................146, 147
        protein and systemic delivery...............................147
    testing models 142
Hyperacetylation 121
Hyperphosphorylation 121

I

Immunoglobulins 67
Immunotherapy
    against α-syn (*see* Aβ protofibrils; Alpha-synuclein (α-syn))
    neurodegeneration
        active immunotherapy 10–12
        passive immunotherapy.......................................7–10
        prevention, AD...12–13
    α-syn...64–65
International Federation of Clinical Chemistry and
    Laboratory Medicine (IFCC)........................169
Intracellular antibodies (intrabodies) 67–68
Isoprostanes..165

K

Keyhole limpet hemocyanin (KLH)...........................95, 125

L

Leucine-rich repeat kinase 2 (LRRK2) gene....................222
Lewy bodies (LB)..87, 246

Lewy neurites (LN)...246
Linear discriminant analysis (LDA)................................194
Liposome-based vaccine..27
Lu AF20513, therapeutic vaccine......................................29
Lysosome...77, 79,
    131, 147

M

mAb158
    transgenic mice 56
mAbs. *See* Monoclonal antibodies (mAbs)
Magnetic resonance imaging (MRI) 216
    automated segmentation algorithms...........................191
    hippocampal volumes, measurements........................193
    ionizing radiation...236
    morphological techniques...236
    software packages 190–193
    tractography..236
    visual rating 191
Magnetic transfer (MT) imaging 236
Manual outlining..189
Mass spectrometry
    electrospray ionization (ESI) 264–265
    matrix-assisted laser desorption/ionization.................265
    techniques..264
Mass spectrometry-based quantitative proteomics
    absolute *vs.* relative quantitation..............................266
    enzymatic labeling 267
    isotopic and isobaric tags...267
    label-free approach 266–267
    neurological samples 268
    technique 268
MCI. *See* Mild cognitive impairment (MCI)
Medial temporal lobe atrophy (MTA)......................183, 184
Micro hemorrhages (MH) 182
Microbleed anatomical rating scale (MARS) 186
Microbleeds...195
Mild cognitive impairment (MCI)..............................5, 158
ModuloDEEP technology..95
Monoclonal antibodies (mAbs)
    humanized 7
    passive immunotherapy, AD.....................................7–10
Morris water maze (MWM) 100
MRI. *See* Magnetic resonance imaging (MRI)
MTA. *See* Medial temporal lobe atrophy (MTA)
Multiple system atrophy (MSA) 87, 215, 238
Multivariate analysis
    biomarkers 194
    patterns of atrophy...193
    SVM...193

N

National Institute on Aging—Alzheimer's Association
    (NIA-AA) 207, 208
Neocortex..122

Neurodegenerative diseases
    AD
        Aβ isoforms pattern 275
        brain tissue 270
        levels 270
        neurotransmitter transporter 270
        novel proteins 270
        serum 275
        techniques 275
        tTau/pTau 269
    dementia 269
    drug targets 254
    methodological approaches 254
    nervous system 253
    PD
        brain tissue 276
        novel isoforms 276
        serum samples 275
        transthyretin and haptoglobin 275
    proteomics workflow 255
    qualitative and quantitative 253
    separation techniques
        gel electrophoresis 261, 263
        liquid chromatography separation 264
    symptoms 269
    therapeutic agents 254
Neurofibrillary tangles (NFTs) 122, 154
Neurofilament light protein (NFL) 163
Neuroinflammation 207
Neuron loss 41, 42
Neuroproteomics
    advantages and limitation 257
    biological samples 257–258
    carbamidomethyl groups 260
    extraction 259
    highly abundant proteins 260
    low-abundant proteins 258
    pre-analytical phase 256–257
    protein digestion 262–263
    protein purification 260
    sample preparation 259
    techniques 271–274
Neurotransmitter function 203–204
Neutrophil gelatinase-associated lipocalin 164
NIA-AA. *See* National Institute on Aging—Alzheimer's
    Association (NIA-AA)
N-truncated amyloid-β oligomers
    in vitro studies 43–45
    postmortem human brain, evidence 38–40
    preclinical trials 45–47
    pyroglutamate-Aβ, transgenic mouse models 40–43

O

Oligomers 52, 54, 55
Orthogonal partial least squares to latent structures
    (OPLS) 194

P

PA. *See* Posterior or parietal atrophy (PA)
Parkinson's disease (PD) 203
    dementia 242
    DLB 241
    dopaminergic drugs 241
    drug-induced parkinsonism 242
    immunotherapy 64, 65
    monoamine oxidase inhibitors 86
    MRI (*see* Magnetic resonance imaging (MRI))
    neurodegenerative disorder 86
    neuroinflammation 247
    non-motor symptoms 86
    pathological changes 64
    PET and SPECT 241
    α-syn 63, 86, 88
    treatment 240–241
Passive immunotherapy 102, 103
Pattern recognition receptors (PRR) 89
PD01A immunization 102
Peripheral nervous system 230
PET. *See* Positron emission tomography (PET)
Phosphocreatine (PCr) 237
Phosphorylated tau (P-tau) 160
Pittsburg compound B (PIB) 245
Plaques
    AD 39
    amyloid 38, 40–42, 45
    Aβ$_{pE3}$-positive plaques 46
Plasma
    anti-parkinsonian treatment 226
    ELISA-based study 227
    exosomes 228
    immunoprecipitated α-synuclein 227
    immunoprecipitation 225
    Lewy body disorders 227
    LRRK2 mutation 227
    non-affected individuals 225
    P-129 α-synuclein 227
    phosphorylated α-synuclein 226
    post-translational modification 226
    α-synuclein plasma levels 226
Platelet-derived growth factor-β (PDGFβ) 91
Positron emission tomography (PET) 242
    AD
        pathophysiological process 200
        research criteria 200, 205, 207–209
    amyloid 204–206
    [11C]deuterium-deprenyl [11C]DED 207
    diagnostics 199
    glucose metabolism 200–203
    neuroinflammation 207
    neurotransmitter function 203–204
    Tau 206–207
Posterior/parietal atrophy (PA) 186

Progressive supranuclear palsy (PSP) 238
Proof-of-concept (POC) 97
Protein identification...265
Protofibrils. *See* Aβ protofibrils
Pyroglutamate-Aβ, transgenic mouse models 40–43

S

Saliva 228
Senile plaques 154
SILAC. *See* Stable isotope labeling with amino acids
             in cell culture (SILAC)
Single-chain Fvs (scFvs)..142
Single-photon emission computed tomography
             (SPECT)...216, 242
Skin 230
Solanezumab 53–54, 167
Stable isotope labeling with amino acids in cell culture
             (SILAC) 267
Standardized mean difference (SMD)............................222
Submandibular gland..230
Support vector machines (SVM)...............................193
Synucleinopathy 87
             immunotherapy 89–91

T

Tau 206, 245
Tau immunotherapy
             AD...109
             antibody...114
             clinical trials...115
             efficacy and mechanism
                         brain levels 110
                         cell membrane.......................................112
                         cytosol..112
                         endosomal/lysosomal system 110–112
                         epitope 110, 111
             epitope selection 113
             memory loss...110
             phase III Aβ antibody trials............................109
             potential toxicity...113
Tau protein
             active immunization
                         intraperitoneal injections 125
                         KLH..125
                         mice 125
                         NFTs...122
                         peptides..122, 123
                         THY-Tau22 transgenic mice 125
             cell culture system.......................................129
             Drosophila model..129
             human tauopathy brain................................129
             immunotherapy 129, 130

mechanisms 133, 134
microglia and astrocytes...................................132–133
monomeric tau..128
and neurodegenerative disease 121–122
neurons 131–132
oligomers 128, 129
passive immunization
             antibodies..................................122, 124
             anti-tau antibodies 127
             HJ8.5 ....127, 128
             intraperitoneal injections 126
             MC1 126
             PHF1...126
             TOMA...127
             treated *vs.* control mice 126
peripheral sink and cerebrospinal fluid 133
seeding and spreading...................................129
spread/toxicity 130–131
transgenic mouse models 130
Tensor-based morphometry (TBM)...................192
Therapeutic vaccine
             Lu AF20513 29
Total tau (T-tau)...159
Transgenic mouse models
             APP/PS1KI mice 41
             heterozygous TBA2 mice 42
             Tg4-42 mice 42
             5XFAD mice 43
             5XFAD/QC mice.................................42
Trefoil factor 3 (TFF3)..163
Triggering receptor expressed on myeloid cells-2
             (*TREM2*)...164

U

UB-311 immunotherapeutic vaccine...................29
Unified Parkinson's Disease Rating Scale (UPDRS)........221

V

V950...30
Vaccination
             animal models.................................92–93
             ELISPOT assays 97
             microglial cells 100
             neuroinflammation 99
             PDGF-β promoter..............................97
             physiological function....................100–101
             subcortical regions 97
             wild-type animals 98
             α-syn...98
Vasogenic edema 182
Ventricular mucosa 229
Virus-like particles (VLPs) 95

Visinin-like protein 1 (VLP-1) 163
VL12.3 145
Volumetry
    atrophy in posterior regions, PA 186
    GCA...185
    hippocampal 189, 190

MTA..183
    visual rating scales.....................................183
Voxel-based morphometry (VBM)....................192

W

Weight mean difference (WMD) 221